ATTACHMENT PROCESSES IN COUPLE
AND FAMILY THERAPY

ATTACHMENT PROCESSES IN COUPLE AND FAMILY THERAPY

Edited by

Susan M. Johnson
Valerie E. Whiffen

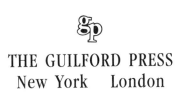

THE GUILFORD PRESS
New York   London

© 2003 The Guilford Press
A Division of Guilford Publications, Inc.
72 Spring Street, New York, NY 10012
www.guilford.com

Paperback edition 2006

Printed in the United States of America

This book is printed on acid-free paper.

Last digit is print number: 9   8   7   6   5   4

Library of Congress Cataloging-in-Publication Data

Attachment processes in couple and family therapy / edited by Susan M.
  Johnson, Valerie E. Whiffen.
      p. cm.
  Includes index.
    ISBN 1-57230-873-7 (hc)   ISBN 1-59385-292-4 (pbk)
    1. Attachment behavior.   2. Marital psychotherapy.   3. Family
  psychotherapy.   I. Johnson, Susan M.   II. Whiffen, Valerie E.
    RC455.4.A84A886 2003
    616.89′156—dc21
                                                        2003000811

About the Editors

Susan M. Johnson, EdD, is Professor of Psychology in the School of Psychology at the University of Ottawa and Director of the Ottawa Couple and Family Institute, Ottawa, Canada. She is the main proponent of emotionally focused couple and family therapy, which she teaches extensively in North America and internationally. In 2005, she received the Distinguished Contribution to Family Systems Research Award from the American Family Therapy Academy. The website for Dr. Johnson's work is *www.eft.ca.* Her most recent publications include *Emotionally Focused Couple Therapy with Trauma Survivors: Strengthening Attachment Bonds* (2002); *The Practice of Emotionally Focused Couple Therapy: Creating Connection, Second Edition* (2004); and *Becoming an Emotionally Focused Couple Therapist: The Workbook* (2005).

Valerie E. Whiffen, PhD, Professor of Psychology in the School of Psychology at the University of Ottawa, has published widely in the area of depression, particularly focusing on women's depression. She approaches the study of depression from an interpersonal perspective, which emphasizes the importance of relationships to emotional well-being. Recently, she has explored the links between depression and factors that seem to place women at greater risk than men for developing depression, specifically childhood sexual abuse and marital distress. In recent publications, she has explored an attachment theory-based understanding of depression that co-occurs with marital distress. Dr. Whiffen teaches graduate courses in adult psychopathology and interpersonal theory. She also supervises the clinical work of practicum students and interns in the American Psychological Association-accredited clinical psychology program at the University of Ottawa. She is a registered clinical psychologist and maintains a private practice specializing in the treatment of depression and marital distress.

Contributors

Pamela C. Alexander, PhD, Office of Research and Technology Development, Albert Einstein Healthcare Network, Philadelphia, Pennsylvania

Thomas N. Bradbury, PhD, Department of Psychology, University of California–Los Angeles, Los Angeles, California

J. Michael Bradley, PhD, Department of Psychiatry, Louisiana State University Health Sciences Center, New Orleans, Louisiana

Vivian J. Carlson, PhD, Department of Child Study/Education/Special Education, Saint Joseph College, West Hartford, Connecticut

Rebecca J. Cobb, PhD, Department of Psychology, University of California–Los Angeles, Los Angeles, California

Nancy J. Cohen, PhD, CPsych, Hincks–Dellcrest Centre, and Department of Psychiatry, University of Toronto, Toronto, Ontario, Canada

Joanne Davila, PhD, Department of Psychology, State University of New York at Stony Brook, Stony Brook, New York

Guy S. Diamond, PhD, Center for Family Intervention Science, Children's Hospital of Philadelphia, Philadelphia, Pennsylvania

Robin L. Harwood, PhD, School of Family Studies, University of Connecticut, Storrs, Connecticut

Cindy Hazan, PhD, Department of Human Development, Cornell University, Ithaca, New York

Roy Holland, MD, FRCP, Maples Adolescent Centre, Burnaby, British Columbia, Canada

Susan M. Johnson, EdD, School of Psychology, University of Ottawa and the Ottawa Couple and Family Institute, Ottawa, Ontario, Canada

Gordon J. Josephson, PhD candidate, School of Psychology, University of Ottawa, Ottawa, Ontario, Canada

Roger Kobak, PhD, Department of Psychology, University of Delaware, Newark, Delaware

Terry M. Levy, PhD, Evergreen Psychotherapy Center, Evergreen, Colorado

Mirek Lojkasek, PhD, CPsych, Hincks–Dellcrest Centre and Department of Psychiatry, University of Toronto, Toronto, Ontario, Canada

Toni Mandelbaum, BA, Department of Psychology, University of Delaware, Newark, Delaware

Samuel F. Mikail, PhD, ABPP, The Southdown Institute, Aurora, Ontario, Canada, and The Institute of Rehabilitation Research and Development, Ottawa, Ontario, Canada

Mario Mikulincer, PhD, Department of Psychology, Bar-Ilan University, Ramat Gan, Israel

Marlene M. Moretti, PhD, Department of Psychology, Simon Fraser University, Burnaby, British Columbia, Canada

Elisabeth Muir, BSc, Hincks–Dellcrest Centre, Toronto, Ontario, Canada

Michael Orlans, MA, Evergreen Psychotherapy Center, Evergreen, Colorado

Gail Palmer, MSW, Ottawa Couple and Family Institute, Ottawa, Ontario, Canada

Dory A. Schachner, PhD candidate, Department of Psychology, University of California–Davis, Davis, California

Elaine Scharfe, PhD, Department of Psychology, Trent University, Peterborough, Ontario, Canada

Phillip R. Shaver, PhD, Department of Psychology, University of California–Davis, Davis, California

Richard S. Stern, PhD, Center for Family Intervention Science, Children's Hospital of Philadelphia, Philadelphia, Pennsylvania

Valerie E. Whiffen, PhD, School of Psychology, University of Ottawa, Ottawa, Ontario, Canada

Preface

This book originated with a research conference sponsored by the American Family Therapy Association (AFTA) in October 2000 in Niagara on the Lake in Ontario, Canada. At this conference, developmental and social psychologists, who had studied and extended Bowlby's attachment theory over the last 30 years, interacted with couple and family therapists. This book is, in a sense, an attempt to continue that dialogue. It also had its roots in the shared dialogues and stories of hundreds of clients who, in the way they describe their realities and relationships, constantly remind us of the tangible significance of attachment theory for people's everyday lives and interactions.

This book reflects that couple and family therapy as a discipline is entering a new era. In the past, couple and family therapy has been thought of as a technique in search of a theory. We believe what has been missing is a coherent, rich, and researchable theory of love and bonding. We suggest that attachment theory, at last, can begin to fill this gap. In this new era, attachment theory, together with research on basic responses and patterns of interaction in distressed as well as satisfying relationships, and research on the impact of specific interventions, offer the therapist a guide to the terrain of primary relationships and how to transform them.

Although John Bowlby, the father of attachment theory, was a reserved Englishman, he was also a rebel who defied his analytic training and insisted that reality is defined not just in the minds and fantasies of individuals but also in compelling interactions with significant others. He learned from such figures as Konrad Lorenz, who studied imprinting; Karl Ludwig von Bertalanffy, the father of systems theory; and Harry Harlow, who studied primates and their need for soothing contact and comfort from significant others. Bowlby believed love was the crowning achievement of human evolution; we believe he has something of profound significance to say to professionals who work with love relationships that can help them to help their clients.

John Bowlby always intended his theory to be a clinical theory that would offer therapists a guide to intervention in troubled relationships. At last, 30 years after the first book in his famous attachment trilogy was published, his theory is beginning to be applied systematically to clinical intervention in distressed couples and families. Until very recently, only developmental and social psychologists have actively used attachment theory, while clinicians have focused elsewhere. This may reflect the tendency in Western societies in general, and in clinical theories in particular, to systematically pathologize dependency.

PLAN OF THE BOOK

This book is divided into four parts. The first part focuses on attachment theory and its relevance for clinical practice. The second part focuses on models of clinical intervention already developed that use the attachment perspective. The third part focuses on ways in which attachment theory can facilitate intervention with particular populations and at particular times in the lifespan. The fourth part focuses on how attachment-oriented interventions can address particular problems.

In the first part, some of the key social psychologists and theorists who have contributed to the recent explosion of research on attachment elaborate on the nature of human attachment. In Chapter 1, Johnson provides an introduction to the main tenets of attachment theory and its relevance to the field of couple and family therapy. In Chapter 2, Shaver, one of the researchers who first insisted on the relevance of attachment theory for adult relationships, and his colleagues Schachner and Mikulincer, elaborate on the clinical applications of attachment research for couple therapy. In Chapter 3, Hazan writes on the nature of the bonds between mates and the issue of mate selection. In Chapter 4, Scharfe, an active attachment researcher, summarizes the research on the development and continuity of attachment across the lifespan. Chapter 5, by Carlson and Harwood, looks at attachment from a cross-cultural perspective and helps the clinician add the factor of cultural differences to his or her view of attachment patterns in family relationships. This section is intended to offer the clinician insight into the cutting edge of attachment theory, research on attachment, and its clinical implications.

In Part II, clinicians who have used attachment theory to design models of intervention set out these models and offer examples of how they work to create change in couples and families. Chapter 6, by Johnson, presents attachment theory as a guide to couple therapy in general and as it is implemented in the emotionally focused model of couple therapy (EFT), now one of the best-documented and validated models of couple interventions. In Chapter 7, Davila, who has completed research on many aspects of attachment theory, including how habitual attachment responses change, summarizes research on attachment processes and how this research can be applied to behavioral approaches to couple therapy. In Chapter 8, Kobak and Mandelbaum discuss the nature of the attachment approach to child problems. Kobak has published extensively on how attachment theory allows us to understand the problems that adolescents face, as well as on adult attachment. Chapters 9 and 10 present the family interventions formulated by Levy and Orlans (Chapter 9) for different kinds of families, including adoptive families, and by Diamond and Stern (Chapter 10) for families struggling with a disturbed or depressed adolescent.

In Part III, the focus is on the use of attachment interventions at particular times in the lifespan and in different kinds of relationships. This part reflects Bowlby's concept that attachment constitutes one of the key elements of human functioning from the cradle to the grave and is the basic building block of many different kinds of close relationships. In Chapter 11, Cohen, Muir, and Lojkasek offer a model of intervention for mothers and infants that can facilitate the growth of secure bonding. In Chapter 12, Moretti and Holland offer attachment as a framework for intervening when adolescents are having trouble negotiating the developmental tasks of the transition to adulthood. In Chapter 13, Cobb and Bradbury consider the implications of attachment for the prevention of marital distress in newlyweds, and in Chapter 14, Bradley and Palmer outline the implications of attachment theory for understanding and intervening in the problems of older adults. In Chapter 15, Josephson addresses gay relationships, an area that has been neglected and in which there is still very little available in the literature to guide therapists, and discusses how an attachment perspective can help the clinician working with such relationships.

In Part IV, there is an emphasis on how attachment theory provides particular insight into specific clinical issues. Chapter 16, by Whiffen, outlines the attachment perspective on depression, which is clearly linked to distress in close relationships and has been called the "common cold" of emotional disorders, and shows how this perspective fosters effective intervention for this disorder. In Chapter 17, Alexander offers an attachment orientation to posttraumatic stress disorder (PTSD) and the echoes of traumatic experience in couple relationships. The impact of PTSD on a survivor's relationships and how those relationships can be a crucial part of the healing process are just beginning to be addressed in the literature. In Chapter 18, Mikail discusses how a consideration of attachment can add to the resources of the clinician who is helping couples cope with chronic pain. From its inception, attachment was considered a physiological process. The essence of attachment theory is that proximity to those we love calms the nervous system, produces a felt sense of well-being, and provides an antidote to stress.

Finally, in Chapter 19, in Part V, Whiffen provides a postscript and a commentary on the book as a whole.

This book would not have been written without the creative leadership of Celia Falicov, the President of AFTA, who initially encouraged the first editor to chair a conference on attachment for the leaders of couple and family therapy; the amazing staff at AFTA; and the other members of AFTA who attended the conference that initiated this volume. We would also like to thank the staff at The Guilford Press, especially Jim Nageotte, Senior Editor, whose editorial guidance made sure the project actually took off. All of the authors patiently went through the arduous process of revising and sometimes reformulating their chapters, and for this we sincerely thank them. We, the editors, found working on this book a fascinating though sometimes difficult process, and one in which we, too, had to work on the bond between us. Secure attachment, a sense of being supported and valued, really matters if people are to work together effectively. We would also like to thank our own attachment figures, our spouses and children in particular, for enduring from us any of the inaccessibility and unresponsiveness that tend to erode secure bonds, and for staying with us throughout this project. We would like to thank as well our students and colleagues at the University of Ottawa and the Ottawa Couple and Family Institute for many stimulating insights, especially in the ongoing clinical supervision of cases. We acknowledge, in particular, Caroline Andrews, the Dean of Social Sciences at the University of Ottawa, who has been more than supportive. Lastly, we would like to thank our clients, who continue to teach us and to show us how hard human beings will fight to stay connected with each other, and how those connections can transform lives.

Contents

xv

PART II
MODELS OF CLINICAL INTERVENTION

PART III
USING AN ATTACHMENT PERSPECTIVE IN INTERVENTIONS
WITH PARTICULAR POPULATIONS

PART IV
SPECIFIC ATTACHMENT INTERVENTIONS
FOR PARTICULAR PROBLEMS

PART V
CONCLUSION

ATTACHMENT PROCESSES IN COUPLE AND FAMILY THERAPY

PART I

RELEVANCE OF ATTACHMENT THEORY FOR CLINICAL PRACTICE

1

Introduction to Attachment

A Therapist's Guide to Primary Relationships and Their Renewal

SUSAN M. JOHNSON

Couple and family therapists spend their professional lives helping people change the nature of their primary attachment relationships. Our clients come to us wanting to put an end to difficult recurring conflicts, to learn how to persuade their child or their spouse to cooperate with them, to deal with the depression and anxiety that arise when the relationships they count on become ambiguous or painful, or, even worse, begin to disintegrate. This is a challenging task. There are many different facets and levels in these relationships and many different lenses through which we can view them. How do we decide what goals are worth pursuing, what to target in therapy, and what in-session events have the potential to redefine a relationship? How do we make sense of the complex patterns of interaction that constitute a close relationship and the sometimes extreme responses that partners and family members display in such relationships?

This book is built on the premise that couple and family therapists need a broad integrative theory of relationships, one that captures the essence of the nature of our bonds of love, if we are to understand, predict, and explain such relationships and so know how to change them for the better. We need to know what really matters, so we can help clients articulate goals and make more than peripheral, transient changes. In other words, we need to know what to focus on so we can change the landscape of intimate relationships, not just the weather. We need a theory that helps the couple and family therapist stay focused and agentic in the baffling, multilayered, and intricate drama called love and belonging.

The contributors to this book believe that one of the most primary human needs is to have a secure emotional connection—an *attachment*—with those who are closest to us: our parents, children, lovers, and partners. It is this need, and the fears of loss and isolation that accompany this need, that provide the script for the oldest and most universal of human dramas that couple and family therapists see played out in their offices every day.

Our focus on attachment does not fit in many ways with the dominant culture in Western societies, which has also influenced the culture of couple and family therapy. This culture has pathologized dependency and exalted the concepts of separateness and self-sufficiency. As Mackay (1996) noted, family therapy has generally neglected the dimension of nurturance in favor of a focus on issues of power, control, and autonomy. John Bowlby, the originator of attachment theory (1969, 1973, 1980), and arguably the first family therapist, questioned this pathologizing view of dependency. As early as 1944 Bowlby wrote what is perhaps the first family therapy professional article, called "Forty-Four Juvenile Thieves: Their Characters and Home Life." He also studied institutionalized children for the World Health Organization and was struck by how they developed into individuals who lacked feeling, had superficial relationships, and were hostile to others. He was struck too by the effects of separation from parents on young children who were hospitalized; in those days parents were allowed to visit their children for just 1 hour a week. When he put all his insights on these phenomena into a theory, developmentalists grasped it and began to use it to examine mother and infant interactions. However, until the late 1980s when the first articles on adult attachment emerged (Hazan & Shaver, 1987; Johnson, 1986), the nature of the love between family members and partners was essentially the purview of literature and the popular press. Bowlby's emphasis on emotional accessibility and responsiveness and the necessity for soothing interactions in all attachment relationships, once so unfashionable, is now supported by empirical work such as studies on the nature of distress in marital relationships (Gottman, 1994). In the last decade, attachment research, including an extensive body of research on adult attachment, has become, "one of the broadest, most profound, and most creative lines of research in 20th-century psychology" (Cassidy & Shaver, 1999, p. x). Each author in this text will offer his or her perspective on this theory and focus on different aspects of the body of work associated with it.

THE TENETS OF ATTACHMENT THEORY

It seems appropriate at the beginning of such a book to briefly outline the central tenets of the theory, offering the reader an overview of the attachment perspective. The 10 central tenets of attachment theory are as follows:

Attachment Is an Innate Motivating Force

Seeking and maintaining contact with significant others is an innate, primary motivating principle in human beings across the lifespan. Dependency, which has been pathologized in our culture (Bowlby, 1988), is an innate part of being human rather than a childhood trait that we outgrow. This perspective has also now been articulated by feminist writers (Miller & Stiver, 1997).

Secure Dependence Complements Autonomy

According to attachment theory, there is no such thing as complete independence from others or overdependency (Bretherton & Munholland, 1999). There is only effective or ineffective dependency. Secure dependence fosters autonomy and self-confidence. Secure dependence and autonomy are thus two sides of the same coin, rather than dichotomies. Research tells us that secure attachment is associated with a more coherent, articulated, and positive sense of self (Mikulincer, 1995). The more securely connected we are, the more separate and different we can be. Health in this model means maintaining a felt sense of interdependency, rather than being self-sufficient and separate from others.

Attachment Offers a Safe Haven

The presence of attachment figures, which usually means parents, children, spouses, and lovers, provides comfort and security, while the perceived inaccessibility of such figures creates distress. Proximity to a loved one tranquillizes the nervous system (Schore, 1994). It is the natural antidote to feelings of anxiety and vulnerability. Positive attachments create *a safe haven* that offers a buffer against the effects of stress and uncertainty (Mikulincer, Florian, & Weller, 1993) and an optimal context for the continuing development of the personality.

Attachment Offers a Secure Base

Secure attachment also provides a *secure base* from which individuals can explore their universe and most adaptively respond to their environment. The presence of such a base encourages exploration and a cognitive openness to new information (Mikulincer, 1997). It promotes the confidence necessary to risk, learn, and continually update models of self, others, and the world so that adjustment to new contexts is facilitated. Secure attachment strengthens the ability to stand back and reflect on oneself, one's behavior, and one's mental states (Fonagy & Target, 1997). When relationships offer a sense of felt security, individuals are better able to reach out to and provide support for others and deal with conflict and stress positively. These relationships tend then to be happier, more stable, and more satisfying.

Accessibility and Responsiveness Build Bonds

The building blocks of secure bonds are emotional accessibility and responsiveness. An attachment figure can be physically present but emotionally absent. Separation distress results from the appraisal that an attachment figure is inaccessible. Emotional engagement and the trust that this engagement will be there when needed are crucial. In attachment terms, any response (even anger) is better than none. If there is no engagement, no emotional responsiveness, the message from the attachment figure reads as "Your signals do not matter to me, and there is no connection between us." Emotion is central to attachment. This theory provides a guide for understanding and normalizing many of the extreme emotions that accompany distressed relationships. Attachment relationships are where our strongest emotions arise and where they seem to have most impact. Emotions tell us and communicate to others what our motivations and needs are; they are the music of the attachment dance (Johnson, 1996). As Bowlby suggests, "The psychology and psychopathology of emotion is . . . in large part the psychology and psychopathology of affectional bonds" (1979, p. 130).

Fear and Uncertainty Activate Attachment Needs

When the individual is threatened, whether by traumatic events, by the negative aspects of everyday life such as illness, or by an assault on the security of the attachment bond itself, powerful affect arises, attachment needs for comfort and connection become particularly salient and compelling, and attachment behaviors, such as proximity seeking, are activated. A sense of connection with a loved one is a primary inbuilt emotional regulation device. Attachment to key others is our "primary protection against feelings of helplessness and meaninglessness" (McFarlane & van der Kolk, 1996, p. 24).

The Process of Separation Distress Is Predictable

If attachment behaviors fail to evoke comforting responsiveness and contact from attachment figures, a prototypical process of angry protest, clinging, depression, and despair occurs, culminating eventually in detachment. Depression is a natural response to loss of connection. Bowlby (1969, 1973, 1980) viewed anger in close relationships as often being an attempt to make contact with an inaccessible attachment figure, and distinguished between the anger of hope and the anger of despair which becomes desperate and coercive. In secure relationships, protest at inaccessibility is recognized and accepted (Holmes, 1996).

A Finite Number of Insecure Forms of Engagement Can Be Identified

The number of ways that human beings have to deal with the unresponsiveness of attachment figures is limited. There are only so many ways of coping with a negative response to the question "Can I depend on you when I need you?" Attachment responses seem to be organized along two dimensions, anxiety and avoidance (Fraley & Waller, 1998). When the connection with an irreplaceable other is threatened but not yet severed, the attachment system may become hyperactivated or go into overdrive. Attachment behaviors become heightened and intense as anxious clinging, pursuit, and even aggressive attempts to obtain a response from the loved one escalate. The second strategy for dealing with the lack of safe emotional engagement, especially when hope for responsiveness has been lost, is to deactivate the attachment system and suppress attachment needs, focusing on tasks, and limiting or avoiding distressing attempts at emotional engagement with attachment figures. These two basic strategies, anxious preoccupied clinging and detached avoidance, can develop into habitual styles of engagement with intimate others. A third insecure strategy has been identified that is essentially a combination of seeking closeness and then responding with fearful avoidance of closeness when it is offered. This strategy is usually referred to as *disorganized* in the child literature and *fearful–avoidant* in the adult literature (Bartholomew & Horowitz, 1991). This strategy is associated with chaotic and traumatic attachments where others are, at the same time, the source of and the solution to fear (Johnson, 2002; Alexander, 1993).

The anxious and avoidant strategies were first identified in experimental separations and reunions with mothers and infants (Ainsworth, Blehar, Waters & Wall, 1978). Some infants were able to modulate their distress on separation, to give clear signals, and so make reassuring contact with the mother when she returned, and then, confidant of her responsiveness if she was needed, to return to exploration and play. They were viewed as *securely attached*. Others became extremely distressed on separation and clung to or expressed anger at the mother on reunion. They were difficult to soothe and were viewed as preoccupied with making contact with the mother and *anxiously attached*. Another group showed signs of physiological distress but showed little emotion at separation or reunion. They focused on tasks and activities and were seen as *avoidantly attached*. These styles are "self-maintaining patterns of social interaction and emotion regulation strategies" (Shaver & Clarke, 1994, p. 119). They echo the display rules for emotion that Ekman and Friesen identified (1975), namely, exaggerating; substituting one feeling for another, as when we focus on anger rather than fear; and minimizing.

While these habitual forms of engagement can be modified by new relationships, they can also mold current relationships and so become self-perpetuating. They involve specific behavioral responses to regulate emotions and protect the self from rejection and abandonment, and cognitive schemas, or working models, of self and other. In the attachment literature the term *styles*, which implies an individual characteristic, is often used interchangeably with the term *strategies*, which implies behavior that is more context-specific. The use of a third term, *forms of engagement*, a term coined by Sroufe (1996), further stresses the interpersonal nature of this concept. These forms of engagement can and do change when relationships change and are best thought of as continuous, not absolute (one can be more secure or less secure). People also seem to use more than one strategy; someone can be habitually secure but move into a more preoccupied anxious mode when threatened. Attachment strategies will also play out differently depending on the attachment characteristics of a partner. Thus attachment style affects marital satisfaction. Individuals with insecurely attached spouses report lower satisfaction; couples where both are securely attached report better adjustment than couples in which either or both partners are insecurely attached (Feeney, 1994; Lussier, Sabourin, & Turgeon, 1997). When we consider these habitual responses and self-perpetuating patterns of interaction, it is easy to see that attachment is a systemic theory (Johnson & Best, 2002), and is concerned with "a reality-regulating and reality-creating not just a reality-reflecting system" (Bretherton & Munholland, 1999, p. 98).

Attachment Involves Working Models of Self and Other

As stated above, attachment strategies reflect ways of processing and dealing with emotion. Some spouses catastrophize and complain when they feel rejected, some become silent for days. Bowlby (1969, 1973, 1980) outlined the cognitive content of the representations of self and other that are inherent in these responses. Secure attachment is characterized by a working model of self that is worthy of love and care and is confident and competent, and indeed research has found secure attachment to be associated with greater self-efficacy (Mikulincer, 1995). Securely attached people, who believe others will be responsive when needed, also tend to have working models of others as dependable and worthy of trust. These models of self and other, distilled out of a thousand interactions, become expectations and biases that are carried forward into new relationships. They are not one-dimensional cognitive schemas; rather, they are procedural scripts for how to create relatedness. A person may have more than one model but one may be more accessible and dominant in a given context. These models involve goals, beliefs, and strategies, and they are heavily infused with emotion. *Working models are formed, elaborated, maintained, and, most important for the couple and family therapist, changed through emotional communication.*

Isolation and Loss Are Inherently Traumatizing

Lastly, it is important to recognize that attachment is essentially a theory of trauma (Atkinson, 1997; Johnson, 2002). Bowlby began his career as a health professional by studying maternal deprivation and separation and its effects on children. Attachment theory describes and explains the trauma of deprivation, loss, rejection, and abandonment by those we need the most and the enormous impact it has on us. Bowlby viewed these traumatic stressors, and the isolation that ensued, as having tremendous impact on personality formation and on a person's ability to deal with other stresses in life. He believed that when someone is confident that a loved one will be there when needed, "a person will be much less prone to either intense or chronic fear than will an individual who has no such confidence" (1973, p. 406). The couple and family therapist knows about the stress of deprivation and separation well. It is an essential part of the ongoing drama of "ordinary" marital distress. Clients often speak of such distress in terms of trauma, that is, in life-and-death terms, and it is clearly related to individual symptoms such as depression and anxious hypervigilance.

ATTACHMENT AS AN INTEGRATIVE PERSPECTIVE

Attachment theory is an integrative perspective. It is a systemic theory that focuses on behavior in context and patterns of communication (Kobak & Duemmler, 1994; Erdman & Caffery, 2002). This theory takes an evolutionary perspective and sets out a control system designed to maintain proximity and care between primary caregivers and children (Bowlby, 1988). It can also be seen as an individual dynamic theory, one that focuses on internal models and ways of perceiving others (Holmes, 1996). Even when attachment is considered as a state of mind associated with key attachment relationships with parents, it is still able to be connected to interpersonal patterns. In a fascinating piece of research Fonagy and his colleagues (Fonagy, Steele, & Steele, 1991) found that women's state of mind about attachment when pregnant predicted their child's attachment behaviors at 12 months. It is important to note, then, that the chapters in this book focus on attachment from different points of view. For example, couple and family therapists tend to see attachment and attachment styles from a transactional perspective, that is, as being continually constructed and reconstructed in interactions with loved ones. An infant may have qualitatively different relationships with different caregivers. Adult attachment styles can and do change as people learn and grow in relationships (Davila, Burge, & Hammen, 1997; Davila, Karney, & Bradbury, 1999). However, other authors may emphasize the relative stability of attachment styles across time and across relationships and focus more on intrapsychic realities and states of mind about relationships. The foci and the words particular authors use may also differ. Some will talk about "attachment styles," some about "attachment strategies," and others about "habitual forms of engagement with attachment figures." Some may focus on how attachment is continually constructed and can be confirmed or modified in present interactions with others. Others tend to focus on how past attachment relationships help to organize perceptions and responses with present attachment figures. Some focus on the universal aspects of attachment and how they help us understand the reality of relationships, others focus more on individual differences predicted by this theory. All, however, struggle with how inner realities and outer interactional patterns intersect and reflect each other. All struggle with how the nature of our relationships shape our inner world, our ways of viewing and responding to others, and also how our inner world plays a part in creating our most important interactions.

Attachment is such a rich theory that the reader may be confused sometimes by the different labels authors place on attachment strategies or forms of engagement. These differences often reflect the fact that authors are dealing with people of different ages or using different measures of attachment. Social psychologists who study current adult attachment relationships by means of questionnaires, for example, will use slightly different language from that used by developmental researchers, who attempt to access how people think about attachment by interviewing people about their own parents (Shaver, Belsky, & Brennen, 2000). All authors refer to "secure attachment" and the "hyperactivation" or "deactivation" of the attachment system as ways to deal with insecurity. All are attempting to capture individual differences across two dimensions that can be described as expressing anxiety over relationships and the avoidance of or discomfort with closeness (Brennen, Clark, & Shaver, 1998). When Ainsworth first identified different patterns in children's responses to separation from their mothers, she identified these patterns as *secure*, *avoidant*, and *ambivalent* (Ainsworth et al., 1978). To help the reader, there follows a list of the different but equivalent terms used to characterize attachment responses by the different authors in this book and in the literature in general:

- *Secure*: A secure state of mind or free to evaluate as assessed by the Adult Attachment Interview (George, Kaplan, & Main, 1996).

- *Anxious*: Hyperactivated attachment, anxious–ambivalent attachment, preoccupied attachment. The "ambivalent" aspect refers to the angry responses that are part of this pattern.
- *Avoidant*: Deactivated attachment, dismissing attachment, dismissing–avoidant attachment.
- *Both Anxious and Avoidant*: Alternately hyperactivated and deactivated attachment, fearful avoidant attachment, disorganized attachment, unresolved attachment (with respect to trauma and loss).

In the secure strategy, we see appropriate, context-sensitive attachment system activation and deactivation. In fearful avoidant or disorganized attachment, we see the collapse of any coherent strategy as a result of opposing tendencies to seek and avoid connection.

Although authors have attempted to integrate the work on attachment across the lifespan, attachment theory has not been investigated equally across all age levels. Investigations into attachment in infancy and childhood, and more recently, into adult partnerships have taken precedence. Less is known about adolescence and old age. However, some seminal work has been completed. For example, in a study of adolescents dealing with conflict with their mothers Kobak and colleagues (Kobak, Cole, Ferenz-Gillies, Fleming, & Gamble, 1993) found that secure adolescents expressed less dysfunctional anger and avoidance and maintained more assertiveness than dismissing adolescents. The basis tenet of attachment theory is that the accessibility and responsiveness of a trusted other leads to greater social and emotional adjustment at any age. Important new work is also being done on key transitions in family relationships, such as the transition to parenthood (Feeney, Hohaus, Noller, & Alexander, 2001), and on the specific implications of different attachment relationships, such as attachment to mother and to father in childhood. Attachment to father, in some studies, has been found to be more consistently related to children's peer relationships than attachment to mother (Kerns & Barth, 1995).

CHANGES IN ATTACHMENT

Changes in attachment can be considered on the level of changes in behavioral responses—for example, becoming more open and empathic, modifying ways of regulating emotion, or changes in relationship-specific and more general cognitive models of self and of other. These cognitive models contain not just specific contents but also rules for the organization of information in attachment relationships. Changes can occur, then, on different levels, in specific contexts with particular partners or on more global, general levels. In his writings, Bowlby focused on how a therapist might help to create insight for an individual client, and so help to change that client's general negative models of attachment. These general models are considered to be the main source of continuity between earlier and later relationships and are seen as consisting of memories, beliefs, expectations, and goals regarding attachment, as well as the strategies discussed above. However, many more recent interventions that seek to change attachment, such as those presented in this book, focus on the processing of emotion and emotional experience. Many of the authors in this volume suggest that creating compelling emotional experiences in ongoing attachment relationships that are inconsistent with existing models is the main route to change in attachment responses and models. These new emotional experiences can then disconfirm past fears and biases (Collins & Read, 1994), allow models to be elaborated and expanded, and enable new behaviors to be constructed and integrated (Johnson & Whiffen, 1999). Presumably, this process may be orchestrated by a therapist or may occur naturally over time as a result of relationship experiences. Indeed spouses' models of their partners, specifically their beliefs about trust, have been found to predict changes in their own attachment models over 2 years (Fuller & Fincham, 1995). Relationship breakups can also shift people from security to insecurity (Kirkpatrick & Hazan, 1994).

From a systemic perspective, it seems useful to think of changes in attachment in terms of constriction and flexibility. Health in systemic terms is about flexibility and the ability to adapt inner models of the world and behavioral responses to new contexts. Bowlby (1969) stressed that to be useful, working models of attachment had to be open to revision and kept up to date, and that restricted or defensive processing of experience could interfere with this process. The attachment-oriented therapist will focus on expanding a client's attachment behaviors and exploring how new experiences and responses are understood and dealt with and whether they revise basic views of self and other. He or she will also focus on how clients internally make sense of their relationships and relationship events and how this then cues specific behaviors. For example, does a mother interpret her child's behavior in a way that promotes an empathic response? If not, can she make new interpretations when aided by the therapist, and can these new ways of seeing translate into new responses and new dyadic interactions? Change happens in the head and in the heart, but also in interactions. For an anxiously attached spouse to become more secure she may have to look at her propensity to be vigilant and easily disappointed and will also have to have new experiences of being able to ask for and achieve secure connection. Many models of couple and family therapy have tended to focus on behavior or on inner realities. An attachment perspective on change argues for integrating both of these foci. Attachment realities are created by how individuals interact and how they grasp and internally attune to that interaction style.

THE SIGNIFICANCE OF ATTACHMENT THEORY
FOR COUPLE AND FAMILY THERAPY

Attachment theory is still growing and developing. There are many unanswered questions. For example, how exactly does attachment fit with the other two key aspects of love that have been identified in the literature, sexuality and caregiving (Fraley & Shaver, 2000)? Some specific answers are emerging to such questions. For example, avoidant attachment seems to be related to promiscuous sexuality (Brennen & Shaver, 1995), whereas secure individuals are less likely to have sex outside their primary relationship (Hazan, Zeifman, & Middelton, 1994). However, the great promise of attachment theory is that it offers answers to some of the most, as Karen (1998, p. 7) puts it, "fundamental questions of human emotional life." Questions such as: How do we learn what to expect from others? How do patterns of behavior get transmitted across generations? How does the marital relationship specifically have an impact on the emotional life of children? (Benoit & Parker, 1994; Cowan, Cowan, Cohn, & Pearson, 1996). How do we become caught in futile strategies that rob us of the love we desire from our partners and family members? Why do we become most angry and violent with the people we love the most at times when we need them the most? Why does distancing fail to cool down difficult emotions or transform conflictual interactions with attachment figures? Why do certain events define the nature of relationships more than others? How does the self get constructed in interactions with significant others, and how can we best repair the bonds with those we love?

Couple and family therapy, having emerged from many different theoretical points of view and clinical trends, is now coming of age. It is developing the coherence and sophistication of a mature discipline (Johnson & Lebow, 2000). There appears, at last, to be a convergence of theory, research, and practice. For example, the data on the nature of distress in couple partnerships, the nature of love as outlined by attachment theory and research, and the writing of feminist scholars (Millar & Stiver, 1997; Fishbane, 2001), as well as the research on outcomes in therapy for models such as emotionally focused therapy, all point in the same direction. The emotional bond between parents and children and between adult lovers is the heart of the matter—the frame that defines these key relationships. Attachment theory offers clinicians a way to grasp and so to help clients shape this bond, transforming their marriages and their families. As there is more and more emphasis on relatively short, efficient, and verifiably effective interventions in the field of psychotherapy, attachment theory also addresses the urgent need for a framework or lens that allows the therapist to hone in on and bring into focus the leading, organizing elements in the drama of relationships and the definition of self. As David Mace (1987, p. 180) suggests, the hope for the future would seem to lie not in an endless succession of technological developments, but in a "grappling with the fundamental quality of human relationships" so that deeply satisfying relationships become not a romantic dream or an ideal but an everyday possibility for more and more individuals and families.

REFERENCES

Ainsworth, M. D. S., Blehar, M. C., Waters, E., & Wall, S. (1978). *Patterns of attachment: A psychological study of the Strange Situation.* Hillsdale, NJ: Erlbaum.

Alexander, P. C. (1993). Application of attachment theory to the study of sexual abuse. *Journal of Consulting and Clinical Psychology, 60,* 185–195.

Atkinson, L. (1997). Attachment and psychopathology: From laboratory to clinic. In L. Atkinson & K. J. Zucker (Eds.), *Attachment and psychopathology* (pp. 3–16). New York: Guilford Press.

Bartholomew, K., & Horowitz, L. (1991). Attachment styles among young adults. *Journal of Personality and Social Psychology, 61,* 226–244.

Benoit, D., & Parker, K. C. (1994). Stability and transmission of attachment across three generations. *Child Development, 65,* 1444–1456.

Bowlby, J. (1944). Forty-two juvenile thieves: Their character and home life. *International Journal of Psychoanalysis, 25,* 19–52, 107–127.

Bowlby, J (1969). *Attachment and loss: Vol I. Attachment.* New York: Basic Books.

Bowlby, J. (1973). *Attachment and loss: Vol II. Separation: Anxiety and anger.* New York: Basic Books.

Bowlby, J. (1979). *The making and breaking of affectional bonds.* London: Tavistock.

Bowlby, J. (1980). *Attachment and loss: Vol III. Loss: Sadness and depression.* New York: Basic Books.

Bowlby, J. (1988). *A secure base.* New York: Basic Books.

Brennen, K. A., Clarke, C. L., & Shaver, P. R. (1998). Self-report measurement of adult attachment: An integrative overview. In J. A. Simpson & W. S. Rholes (Eds.), *Attachment theory and close relationships* (pp. 46–76). New York: Guilford Press.

Brennen, K. A., & Shaver, P. R. (1995). Dimensions of adult attachment, affect regulation, and romantic relationship functioning. *Personality and Social Psychology Bulletin, 21,* 267–283.

Bretherton, I., & Munholland, K. A. (1999). Internal working models in attachment relationships: A construct revisited. In J. Cassidy & P. R. Shaver (Eds.), *Handbook of attachment: Theory, research, and clinical applications* (pp. 89–111). New York: Guilford Press.

Cassidy, J., & Shaver, P. R. (Eds.). (1999). *Handbook of attachment: Theory, research, and clinical applications.* New York: Guilford Press.

Collins, N., & Read, S. (1994). Cognitive representations of attachment: The structure and function of working models. In K. Bartholomew & D. Perlman (Eds.), *Attachment processes in adulthood* (pp. 53–92). London: Jessica Kingsley.

Cowan, P. A., Cowan, C. P., Cohn, D. A., & Pearson, J. L. (1996). Parent's attachment histories and children's externalizing and internalizing behaviors: Exploring family systems models of linkage. *Journal of Consulting and Clinical Psychology, 64*, 53–63.

Davila, J., Burge, D., & Hammen, C. (1997). Why does attachment style change? *Journal of Personality and Social Psychology, 73*, 826–838.

Davila, J., Karney, B. R., & Bradbury, T. N. (1999). Attachment change processes in the early years of marriage. *Journal of Personality and Social Psychology, 76*, 783–802.

Ekman, P., & Friesen, W. (1975). *Unmasking the face.* Englewood Cliffs, NJ: Prentice-Hall.

Erdman, P., & Caffery, T. (Eds.). (2002). *Attachment and family systems: Conceptual, empirical and therapeutic relatedness.* New York: Springer.

Feeney, J. A. (1994). Attachment style, communication patterns and satisfaction across the life cycle of marriage. *Personal Relationships, 4*, 333–348.

Feeney, J. A., Hohaus, L., Noller, P., & Alexander, R. P. (2001). *Becoming parents: Exploring the bonds between mothers, fathers and their infants.* Cambridge, UK: Cambridge University Press.

Fishbane, M. D. (2001). Relational narratives of self. *Family Process, 40*, 273–291.

Fonagy, P., Steele, H., & Steele, M. (1991). Maternal representations of attachment during pregnancy predict the organization of infant mother attachment at one year of age. *Child Development, 62*, 891–905.

Fonagy, P., & Target, M. (1997). Attachment and reflective function: Their role in self-organization. *Development and Psychopathology, 9*, 679–700.

Fraley, C. R., & Shaver, P. R. (2000). Adult romantic attachment: Theoretical developments, emerging controversies and unanswered questions. *Review of General Psychology, 4*, 132–154.

Fraley, R. C., & Waller, N. G. (1998). Adult attachment patterns: A test of the typological model. In J. A. Simpson & W. S. Rholes (Eds.), *Attachment theory and close relationships* (pp. 77–114). New York: Guilford Press.

Fuller, T. L., & Fincham, F. D. (1995). Attachment style in married couples: Relation to current marital functioning stability over time and method of assessment. *Personal Relationships, 2*, 17–34.

George, C., Kaplan, N., & Main, M. (1996). *The Adult Attachment Interview.* Unpublished manuscript, University of California at Berkeley.

Gottman, J. (1994). *What predicts divorce?* Hillsdale, NJ: Erlbaum.

Hazan, C., & Shaver, P. (1987). Romantic love conceptualized as an attachment process. *Journal of Personality and Social Psychology, 52*, 511–524.

Hazan, C., Zeifman, D., & Middelton, K. (1994). *Adult romantic attachment, affection and sex.* Paper presented at seventh International Conference on Personal Relationships, Groningen, The Netherlands.

Holmes, J. (1996). *Attachment, intimacy and autonomy: Using attachment theory in adult psychotherapy.* Northdale, NJ: Jason Aronson.

Johnson, S. M. (1986). Bonds as bargains: Relationship paradigms and their significance for marital therapy. *Journal of Marital and Family Therapy, 12*, 259–267.

Johnson, S. M. (1996). *The practice of emotionally focused marital therapy: Creating connection.* New York: Brunner/Mazel.

Johnson, S. M. (2002). *Emotionally focused couple therapy with trauma survivors: Strengthening attachment bonds.* New York: Guilford Press.

Johnson, S. M., & Best, M. (2002). A systemic approach to restructuring attachment: The EFT model of couple therapy. In P. Erdman & T. Caffery (Eds.), *Attachment and family systems: Conceptual, empirical and therapeutic relatedness* (pp. 165–192). New York: Brunner/Routledge.

Johnson, S. M., & Lebow, J. (2000). The coming of age of couple therapy: A decade review. *Journal of Marital and Family Therapy, 26*, 23–38.

Johnson, S. M., & Whiffen, V. (1999). Made to measure: Adapting emotionally focused couple therapy to partner's attachment styles. *Clinical Psychology: Science and Practice, 6*, 366–381.

Karen, R. (1998). *Becoming attached: First relationships and how they shape our capacity to love.* New York: Oxford University Press.

Kerns, K. A., & Barth, J. M. (1995). Attachment and play: Convergence across components of parent–child relationships and their relations to peer relations. *Journal of Social and Personal Relationships, 60*, 861–869.

Kirkpatrick, L. A., & Hazan, C. (1994). Attachment styles and close relationships: A four year prospective study. *Personal Relationships, 1*, 123–142.

Kobak, R., Cole, H. E., Ferenz-Gillies, R., Fleming, W. S., & Gamble, W. (1993). Attachment and emotion regulation during mother–teen problem solving: A control theory analysis. *Child Development, 64*, 231–245.

Kobak, R., & Duemmler, S. (1994). Attachment and conversation: Towards a discourse analysis of adolescent and adult security. In K. Bartholomew & D. Perlman (Eds.), *Attachment processes in adulthood* (pp. 121–150). London: Jessica Kingsley.

Lussier, Y., Sabourin, S., & Turgeon, C. (1997). Coping strategies as moderators of the relationship between attachment and marital adjustment. *Journal of Social and Personal Relationships, 14*, 777–791.

Mace, D. (1987). Three ways of helping married couples. *Journal of Marital and Family Therapy, 13*, 179–185.

Mackay, S. K. (1996). Nurturance: A neglected dimension in family therapy with adolescents. *Journal of Marital and Family Therapy, 22*, 489–508.

McFarlane, A. C., & van der Kolk, B. A. (1996). Trauma and its challenge to society. In B. A. van der Kolk, A. C. McFarlane, & L. Weisaeth (Eds.), *Traumatic stress* (pp. 211–215). New York: Guilford Press.

Mikulincer, M. (1995). Attachment style and the mental representation of self. *Journal of Personality and Social Psychology, 69*, 1203–1215.

Mikulincer, M. (1997). Adult attachment style and information processing: Individual differences in curiosity and cognitive closure. *Journal of Personality and Social Psychology, 72*, 1217–1230.

Mikulincer, M., Florian, V., & Weller, A. (1993). Attachment styles, coping strategies and post-traumatic psychological distress. *Journal of Personality and Social Psychology, 64*, 817–826.

Miller, J. B., & Stiver, I. P. (1997). *The healing connection: How women form relationships in therapy and in life.* Boston: Beacon Press.

Schore, A. (1994). *Affect regulation and the organization of self.* Hillsdale, NJ: Erlbaum.

Shaver, P. R., Belsky, J., & Brennen, K. A. (2000). The Adult Attachment Interview and self-reports of romantic attachment: Associations across domains and methods. *Personal Relationships, 7*, 25–43.

Shaver, P., & Clark, C. L. (1994). The psychodynamics of adult romantic attachment. In J. Masling & R. Bornstein (Eds.), *Empirical perspectives on object relations theory* (pp. 105–156). Washington, DC: American Psychological Association.

Sroufe, L. A. (1996). *Emotional development: The organization of emotional life in the early years.* Cambridge, UK: Cambridge University Press.

2

Adult Attachment Theory, Psychodynamics, and Couple Relationships

An Overview

DORY A. SCHACHNER
PHILLIP R. SHAVER
MARIO MIKULINCER

What is love? Countless answers have been offered by philosophers, theologians, creative writers, and—in recent times—psychiatrists and psychologists. In the late 1980s, Hazan and Shaver suggested extending Bowlby and Ainsworth's attachment theory, which was designed to characterize human infants' love for and attachment to their caregivers, to create a framework for studying romantic love and adult couple relationships (Ainsworth, Blehar, Waters, & Wall, 1978; Bowlby, 1982; Hazan & Shaver, 1987; Shaver, Hazan, & Bradshaw, 1988). The core assumption was that romantic relationships—or *pair bonds*, as evolutionary psychologists call them (Hazan & Zeifman, 1999)—involve a combination of three innate behavioral systems described by Bowlby (1982): attachment, caregiving, and sex. Each of these behavioral systems has its own evolutionary functions, and although the systems affect each other in various ways, they are conceptualized as distinct.

Unlike mother–infant relationships, love relationships between adults involve two fairly equal partners, both of whom are sometimes threatened, frightened, or injured and in need of protection or comfort. Both are sometimes sympathetic, supportive caregivers to partners in need; and both are sometimes sexually aroused and seeking sexual gratification. In such relationships, qualities of both partners and their unique combination influence emotions, behavior, and outcomes. As Feeney (2003) says, "The couple system involves two mutually regulatory partners, each serving as the other's environment and having an active role in shaping couple interactions." From the standpoint of attachment theory, love is a dynamic state involving both partners' needs and capacities for attachment, caregiving, and sex. The profound joy and gratitude, deep affection, self-protective anxiety, deadening boredom, corrosive anger, uncontrollable jealousy, and intense sorrow experienced in romantic relationships are reflections of the crucial nature of these three behavioral systems.

In order to study the attachment aspects of adult relationships, Hazan and Shaver (1987) created a simple categorical measure of what has come to be called "attachment style" (see Table 2.1). The three relational styles assessed by that measure—avoidant, anxious, and secure—were modeled on the three major patterns of infant–mother attachment described by Ainsworth et al. (1978). Infants and adults with a *secure* attachment style are ones who find it relatively easy to trust others, open up emotionally, and commit themselves to a long-term intimate relationship. Those with an *anxious* style are uncertain that they are loved, worthy of love, and likely to be protected. This fearful uncertainty explains their excessive vigilance, reassurance seeking, frequent angry protests, and jealousy. Those with an *avoidant* style have learned that in order to feel relatively secure they have to rely heavily on themselves and not openly seek support from a partner, even when (especially in the case of infants) such support is necessary for survival and optimal development. For a number of years, researchers who studied adult romantic attachment used the three-category measure of adult attachment style (see Shaver & Hazan, 1993; Shaver & Clark, 1994).

Ainsworth et al.'s (1978) book contained an important diagram show-

---

TABLE 2.1. Original Three-Category Measure of Romantic Attachment Style (Hazan and Shaver, 1987)

I am somewhat uncomfortable being close to others; I find it difficult to trust them completely, difficult to allow myself to depend on them. I am nervous when anyone gets too close and often, others want me to be more intimate than I feel comfortable being. *(Avoidant)*

I find that others are reluctant to get as close as I would like. I often worry that my partner doesn't really love me or won't want to stay with me. I want to get very close to my partner and this sometimes scares people away. *(Anxious)*

I find it relatively easy to get close to others and am comfortable depending on them and having them depend on me. I don't worry about being abandoned or about someone getting too close to me. *(Secure)*

ing how the three attachment patterns could be arrayed in a two-dimensional space, defined by scores on several 9-point behavior rating scales. (The term *attachment style* was not used by Ainsworth and her colleagues; it was coined later by Levy & Davis, 1988.) The two dimensions underlying the three-category classification scheme were unlabeled, but they clearly corresponded to anxiety and avoidance. Over time, researchers in both the infant–parent attachment field and the adult romantic attachment field moved from a three-category to a four-category classification scheme, with the four categories used by personality/social psychologists corresponding to the four quadrants of a two-dimensional space defined by anxiety and avoidance (e.g., Bartholomew, 1990; Shaver & Clark, 1994; see Fraley & Spieker, in press, for a two-dimensional analysis of infant attachment patterns).

Today, adult attachment researchers (e.g., Brennan, Clark, & Shaver, 1998) are moving toward a consensus on two continuous dimensions, anxiety and avoidance, partly because these are consistently obtained in factor analyses of attachment measures and partly because Fraley and Waller (1998) showed convincingly that dimensional representations of adult attachment style are more accurate than categorical representations. Figure 2.1 shows the two-dimensional space and the four type names proposed by

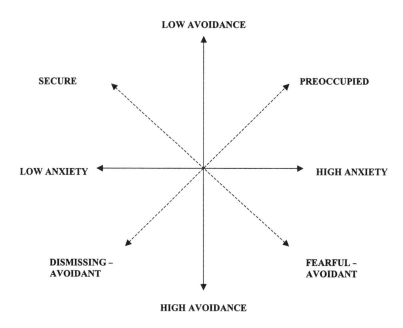

FIGURE 2.1. Diagram of the two-dimensional space defined by attachment anxiety and attachment avoidance. The terms in the four quadrants are Bartholomew's (1990) names for the four major attachment styles.

Bartholomew (1990): secure, preoccupied (anxious), dismissing–avoidant, and fearful–avoidant. Table 2.2 contains examples of the items used to assess people's location in the two-dimensional space (based on Brennan et al., 1998).

Because Hazan and Shaver (1987) included a simple self-report measure of attachment style in their first paper on the topic of adult romantic attachment, researchers subsequently conducted numerous studies focused on individual differences in attachment style without paying much attention to either the underlying attachment behavioral system itself or to the other behavioral systems involved in adult romantic love (i.e., sex and caregiving). More recently this imbalance has begun to be corrected. In the present chapter we provide a brief overview of what has been learned about the attachment system itself as it functions in adulthood; about individual differences in attachment style as they play themselves out in the context of adult relationships; and about the role of caregiving and sexuality in adult relationships as they are conceptualized and measured by attachment researchers. Along the way and in a final section we offer brief suggestions about applying the research findings to couple therapy, the main concern of many of the other chapters in this volume.

ATTACHMENT SYSTEM ACTIVATION IN ADULTS

A basic assumption of Bowlby's theory (1982) is that physical or psychological threats automatically activate the attachment system. Bowlby argued that human infants are born with a repertoire of behaviors (*attachment behaviors*) designed to assure proximity to supportive others (*attachment figures*) as a means of protecting themselves from physical and psychologi-

TABLE 2.2. Sample Items from the Experiences in Close Relationships Scale (ECR), a Measure of Attachment Avoidance and Anxiety (Based on Brennan, Clark, and Shaver, 1998)

Avoidance
1. I prefer not to show a partner how I feel deep down.
2. I try to avoid getting too close to my partner.
3. I feel comfortable depending on romantic partners. (reverse-scored)
4. I turn to my partner for many things, including comfort and reassurance. (reverse-scored)

Anxiety
1. I do not often worry about being abandoned. (reverse-scored)
2. I need a lot of reassurance that I am loved by my partner.
3. I get frustrated if romantic partners are not available when I need them.
4. I resent it when my partner spends time away from me.

cal threats. These proximity-seeking behaviors are organized into an attachment behavioral system. This adaptive system emerged over the course of evolution to increase the likelihood of survival and reproduction on the part of primates born with immature capacities for locomotion, feeding, and defense. Although the attachment system is most critical during the early years of life, Bowlby (1988) claimed that it is active over the entire lifespan and is manifested in thoughts and behaviors related to proximity seeking in times of need. We assume that it is an important component of romantic love and marital commitment, and that meeting needs for a felt sense of security is one of the primary reasons for marriage.

Based on an extensive review of adult attachment studies, Shaver and Mikulincer (2002) proposed a model of the activation and dynamics of the attachment system. This model integrates recent findings with earlier theoretical proposals by Bowlby (1973, 1982), Ainsworth (1991), and Cassidy and Kobak (1988), and is a conceptual extension of previous diagrams of the attachment system created by Shaver et al. (1988) and Fraley and Shaver (2000).

The model (see Figure 2.2) includes three major components (indicated by the gray boxes in the figure). One component concerns the monitoring and appraisal of threatening events and is responsible for activation of the attachment system. The second component includes monitoring and appraisal of the availability and responsiveness of attachment figures who might provide support and relief, satisfy attachment needs, build up the individual's own inner resources, and broaden his or her thought–action repertoire. This second component is responsible for variations in the sense of attachment security; it distinguishes between securely and insecurely attached people, whether anxious, avoidant, or a combination of the two (fearful avoidance). The third component includes monitoring and appraising of the viability of proximity seeking as a means of coping with attachment insecurity and distress. This component is responsible for variations in the use of what attachment theorists call *hyperactivating or deactivating strategies* of affect regulation and distinguishes between anxious and avoidant individuals. (*Hyperactivation* refers to intensification of attachment behaviors; *deactivation* refers to down-regulation of the attachment system.) The model also includes hypothetical excitatory and inhibitory neural circuits (shown as arrows on the left side of the diagram) that result from the recurrent use of hyperactivating or deactivating strategies, which in turn affect the monitoring of threatening events and attachment figures' availability.

Following Bowlby's (2002) analysis, Shaver and Mikulincer (2002) assume that the monitoring of unfolding events results in activation of the attachment system when a potential or actual threat is perceived. Although this part of the model deals mainly with the normal activation of the attachment system, which occurs regardless of individual differences in at-

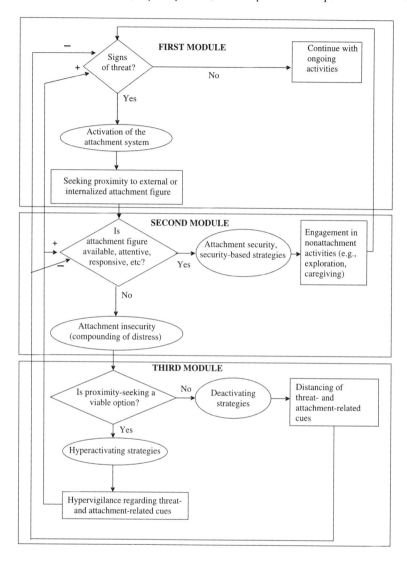

FIGURE 2.2. Shaver and Mikulincer's (2002) integrative model of the activation and dynamics of the attachment system.

tachment history, it is still affected by the excitatory circuits associated with hyperactivating affect-regulation strategies and inhibitory circuits associated with deactivating strategies. Once the attachment system is activated, an affirmative answer to the question about attachment figures' availability results in a "broaden-and-build" cycle of attachment security (Fredrickson, 2001; Shaver & Mikulincer, 2002). This cycle includes distress alleviation and increased personal adjustment as well as facilitation of other behavioral systems, such as exploration and caregiving, which broaden a person's perspectives and capacities. Through this process, individuals move toward optimal development of their unique interests and capacities, and they become not only more satisfied as individuals but also more effective attachment figures for their relationship partners.

Perceived unavailability of an attachment figure results in attachment insecurity, which compounds the distress arising from the appraised threat. This state of insecurity forces a decision about the viability of proximity seeking as a protective strategy. When proximity seeking is appraised as viable or essential—because of attachment history, self-concept, temperamental factors, or contextual cues—people adopt hyperactivating attachment strategies, which include intense appeals to attachment figures and continued reliance on others as a source of comfort. Hyperactivation of the attachment system involves excitatory neural circuits that increase vigilance to threat-related cues and reduce the threshold for detecting cues of attachment figures' unavailability—the two kinds of cues that activate the attachment system (Bowlby, 1973). As a result, minimal threat-related cues are easily detected, the attachment system is chronically activated, psychological pain related to the unavailability of attachment figures is exacerbated, and doubts about one's ability to achieve relief and attain a sense of security are heightened. These excitatory circuits account for many of the psychological correlates of attachment anxiety.

Appraising proximity seeking as unlikely to alleviate distress results in the adoption of deactivating strategies, manifested in distancing oneself from stimuli and events that activate the attachment system and making attempts to handle distress alone. These strategies involve inhibitory circuits that lead to the dismissal of threat- and attachment-related cues, the suppression of threat- and attachment-related thoughts and emotions, and the repression of threat- and attachment-related memories. These inhibitory circuits are further reinforced by the adoption of a self-reliant attitude that decreases dependence on others and acknowledgment of personal faults or weaknesses. These inhibitory circuits account for the psychological manifestations of avoidant attachment.

To give a concrete research example, Mikulincer, Gillath, and Shaver (2002) recently conducted a series of studies that examine the effects of subliminal threats on the cognitive availability of representations of attachment figures. As predicted, threat contexts (even subliminally presented threatening words, such as "failure" and "separation") automatically and unconsciously activated cognitive representations of attachment figures, confirming the theoretical notion that the attachment system becomes activated under conditions of threat. In other words, representations of people who are a source of comfort may be neurologically active and influence mental processes during an encounter with a threat, even if the threat seems irrelevant to interpersonal relationships or to the frustration of attachment needs. In addition, individual differences in attachment style affected attachment system activation: attachment anxiety heightened the accessibility of representations of attachment figures even in nonthreatening contexts, while attachment avoidance inhibited this accessibility in the context of an attachment-related threat (e.g., separation).

Applying these findings to marriage, we would expect that when a person is threatened, either consciously or unconsciously, the person's mind will turn automatically to thoughts of an attachment figure—often a spouse. This is normally the first step in seeking contact with and support from the spouse. Anxious individuals are likely to have their attachment systems activated frequently and for extended periods, to feel threatened by events that would not normally threaten other adults, and to be highly vigilant about their partner's availability and responsiveness. Under these conditions it is easy for one spouse to become dissatisfied and angry about insufficient support, and for the other spouse to become irritated or demoralized about the constant calls for support. Avoidant individuals are likely to downplay threats and wish not to focus on them, to attempt to cope with threats without relying on spousal support, and to disapprove of a partner's "weakness" and need for support. It is not difficult to see how these insecure tendencies might create problems in a marriage. People who are both anxious and avoidant—the ones Bartholomew (1990) called *fearful avoidants*, who often have a history of psychological, physical, or sexual abuse—are likely to long for closeness and support while acting as if they do not want them, a situation almost guaranteed to create problems for a spouse.

In another recent series of studies, Mikulincer, Birnbaum, Woddis, and Nachmias (2000) primed research participants with various threatening words (e.g., "failure," "illness," "death") and measured how quickly they recognized positive attachment-related words such as "love," "hug," and "closeness," and negative words such as "separation," "rejection," and "abandonment." For people with a secure attachment style, the subliminal threat words automatically activated security- or closeness-related words (and presumably the thoughts and images associated with those words); the threatening stimuli did not activate words related to insecurity or interpersonal distance. For people with an anxious attachment style, both kinds of words were automatically activated by threats, suggesting that when their minds turned automatically to representations of attachment figures they encountered both comforting and distressing thoughts and images. Avoidant individuals responded more like secure than like anxious individuals—until a "cognitive load" (an extra attention-demanding task) was added. Then they responded like their anxious counterparts, again suggesting that avoidance involves inhibition of separation-related ideation.

Applied to the marital context, these findings suggest that it may be difficult to bolster an anxious spouse's sense of security because whenever he or she is reminded of seemingly desirable experiences of love and closeness, negative concepts and memories related to past hurts and "attachment injuries" (Johnson, Makinen, & Millikin, 2001) will also become mentally active, whether consciously or unconsciously. Moreover, avoidant spouses are likely to be concerned about separation and abandonment but in a completely unconscious way. Helping them acknowledge their vulnerable thoughts and feelings about close relationships may meet with a great deal of resistance.

INDIVIDUAL DIFFERENCES IN ATTACHMENT STYLE IN THE CONTEXT OF ROMANTIC RELATIONSHIPS

What is known about the actual effects of individual differences in attachment-related anxiety and avoidance in the context of romantic and marital relationships? People who are securely attached (i.e., low in anxiety and avoidance) tend to have long, stable, and satisfying relationships characterized by high investment, trust, and friendship (e.g., Collins & Read, 1990; Hazan & Shaver, 1987; Simpson, 1990). They describe their style of love as relatively selfless and devoid of game playing. In the realm of sexuality, they are open to sexual exploration but usually with a single long-term partner; their intimate relationships are characterized more by mutual initiation of sexual activity and enjoyment of physical contact (Hazan, Zeifman, & Middleton, 1994).

People who are insecurely attached exhibit different patterns in their intimate relationships. Those high in anxiety and low in avoidance tend to become vigilant toward and preoccupied with their romantic partners (Hazan & Shaver, 1987) and experience low relationship satisfaction and a high breakup rate (Collins & Read, 1990; Carnelley, Pietromonaco, & Jaffe, 1996; Collins, 1996). They are more likely than secure or avoidant individuals to experience passionate love (Hatfield, Brinton, & Cornelius, 1989) and to exhibit an obsessive, dependent style of love (Collins & Read, 1990; Shaver & Hazan, 1988; Feeney & Noller, 1990). People high in attachment anxiety show a greater preference for the affectionate and intimate aspects of sexuality than for the genital aspects (Hazan et al., 1994). Anxiety is also associated with less safe sexual practices, as a result of ineffective communication about safe sex (Feeney, Kelly, Gallois, Peterson, & Terry, 1999).

A different pattern of insecure attachment exists among people who are high in avoidance. In comparison with secure and anxious people, predominantly avoidant individuals are less interested in romantic relationships, especially long-term committed ones (Shaver & Brennan, 1992). Like anxious people, their relationships are characterized by low satisfaction and a high breakup rate (Kirkpatrick & Davis, 1994; Hazan & Shaver, 1987), but these relationships are also characterized by relatively low intimacy (Fraley, Davis, & Shaver, 1998; Levy & Davis, 1988). Priming avoidant individuals' insecurity increases their accessibility of negative memories and negative expectations of close relationships (Madsen, 2000).

Avoidant individuals are less likely than secure or anxious people to fall in love (Hatfield et al., 1989) and their love style is characterized by game playing (Levy & Davis, 1988). Although avoidant individuals express dislike for much of sexuality, especially the affectionate and intimate aspects (Hazan et al., 1994), they also hold more accepting attitudes toward casual sex and tend to have more "one-night stands" than secure and anxious people (Brennan & Shaver, 1995; Feeney, Noller, & Patty, 1993; Fraley et al., 1998).

People who are high on both the anxiety and the avoidance dimensions, the people Bartholomew (1990) called *fearful,* show some of the emotional vulnerability and pining for closeness characteristic of their *preoccupied* (highly anxious but nonavoidant) counterparts, but they also back away from closeness behaviorally. For them, this backing away is more consciously motivated by fear of negative outcomes (e.g., rejection and abuse) than is the avoidant behavior of *dismissing* individuals (those who are avoidant but not consciously anxious). As mentioned earlier, research (e.g., Brennan, Shaver, & Tobey, 1991; Shaver & Clark, 1994) suggests that fearful avoidance is, at least in part, a consequence of parental alcoholism and abuse.

ATTACHMENT STYLE AND COUPLE DYNAMICS

Although much of adult attachment research focuses on relatively stable characteristics of individuals, including their conscious and unconscious mental processes, attachment theory is also a theory of individual–couple dynamics. This is explained by Feeney (1999b):

> On one hand, adult attachment style can be conceptualized as an enduring, trait-like characteristic of an individual that influences functioning in close relationships. On the other hand, it can be conceptualized as reflecting recent relationship experiences—that is, experiences specific to particular relationships. (p. 373)

Several research teams are attempting to understand attachment-related processes in long-term dating and marital couples (see Feeney, 2003, for a review). Here we provide a brief summary of recent couple-oriented research that is especially relevant to the issues of marital functioning and marital therapy.

Caregiving and Support

The caregiving system is one of the three behavioral systems, along with attachment and sex, thought to constitute romantic love (Fraley & Shaver, 2000; Shaver et al., 1988). As research with couples has consistently shown, the attachment system, which emerges first in the course of personal development, can affect the later developing caregiving system.

Collins and Feeney (2000) found in a laboratory experiment that avoidant attachment was associated with ineffective support seeking, and anxious attachment was associated with poor caregiving. Furthermore, partners' perceptions of their interactions were biased by attachment style and relationship quality (another variable strongly affected by attachment; see below). Similarly, Simpson, Rholes, and Nelligan (1992) conducted a support-seeking experiment in which the female members of dating couples were told that they would be subjected to a stressful, painful experience later in the study. During a subsequent waiting period, when couple members' interactions were unobtrusively videotaped, high levels of observer-rated anxiety were associated with high levels of support seeking for secure women, but, for more avoidant women, high levels of anxiety were associated with physical and emotional withdrawal from their partners. For secure men, high levels of partner anxiety were associated with high levels of support giving, while for avoidant men, high partner anxiety was associated with low levels of support provision (Simpson et al., 1992)—avoidants thus withdrew precisely when their partner expressed anxiety and needed them the most. This is one of many findings in the attachment literature suggesting that couples in which the wife is anxious and the husband is avoidant—a pattern consistent with predominant sex-role stereotypes—may be especially troubled and perhaps more difficult to work with in therapy.

Attachment anxiety and avoidance also predict how people talk about experiences of caring for their spouses in times of need. According to Feeney and Hohaus (2001), high anxiety is associated with the use of a demeaning or belittling tone in describing needy spouses' problems and behaviors. Laboratory studies have shown that wives of secure husbands are less rejecting and more supportive during problem-solving tasks, and husbands of secure wives listen more effectively in confiding tasks (Kobak & Hazan, 1991). Findings like these suggest that relationship repair may be easier in cases where at least one spouse is relatively secure. In a study of long-term dating couples (Feeney, 2003), the highest levels of friendly touch occurred when the man was anxious but the woman was secure, suggesting that secure women recognize their partners' insecurities and try to be especially warm and supportive. This might provide a point of leverage in marital therapy.

Perceiving one's partner as supportive is especially important to people who score high on attachment anxiety. In a study of pregnant women and their husbands (Rholes, Simpson, Campbell, & Grich, 2001), wife's attachment anxiety interacted with perceived support from husband to determine later postpartum depression (PPD) and relationship dissatisfaction. Anxious women who felt inadequately supported by their husband were especially vulnerable to PPD, while those who felt well supported were no more likely than secure women to become depressed or dissatisfied after giving birth. (For discussion of the uses of attachment theory in the treatment of PPD, see Whiffen & Johnson, 1998.)

The good effects of perceived support extend even to group sources of support. Rom and Mikulincer (in press) studied male and female army recruits in Israel while they were going through a series of training missions. Among those high on attachment anxiety, subjective feelings about performance as well as actual performance (rated by leaders and fellow recruits) were no different from those of secure recruits in highly supportive, cohesive groups, but were deficient when groups seemed less cohesive and supportive.

These recent studies have obvious implications for marital therapy. As one of the hypothesized components of romantic love, caregiving plays an essential role in a successful marriage. A therapist working with an anxious member of a couple should be sensitive to this person's intense need for support and affection, from both the therapist and the spouse. A therapist working with an avoidant member of a couple should be aware of this person's difficulty in providing support, especially when a partner is anxious and needy. It may also be useful to know that the anxious person is likely to exaggerate threats and injuries while the avoidant person seeks to minimize them (as shown earlier in Figure 2.2).

Relationship Quality and Satisfaction

Attachment security (of the individual partners) is associated with relationship satisfaction, and insecurity is associated with relationship deterioration and personal dissatisfaction. Attachment security influences satisfaction by promoting open expression of positive and negative emotions (Feeney, 1995, 1999a), high levels of *facilitative disclosure* (self-disclosure plus the ability to elicit disclosure from one's partner; Keelan, Dion, & Dion, 1998), and mutual expression and negotiation during conflicts (Feeney, 1994). Attachment security is also associated with ability and willingness to give a spouse the benefit of the doubt when interpreting potentially troubling comments or behavior. In contrast, attachment insecurity is associated with destructive "tracking" of recent partner behaviors that might be interpreted as threatening (Feeney, 2002; Jacobson, Follette, & McDonald, 1982).

For both recent and established marriages, and for both men and women, a person's own attachment security predicts greater satisfaction. When examining couple dynamics, however, gender differences are often important. Wives' security predicts husbands' satisfaction. In the early years of marriage, husbands' avoidance and wives' anxiety interact, such that wives' anxiety is related to dissatisfaction for both spouses, but only when husbands are high in avoidance (Feeney, 1994). Apparently, avoidant husbands fail to provide the reassurance that anxious wives crave, and anxious wives are unable to accept the emotional distance desired by avoidant husbands, creating a vicious cycle in which the wife's need for reassurance and the husband's need for distance aggravate each other (Feeney, 2003; Minuchin, 1985).

Relationship quality is predicted most strongly by men's low avoidance and women's low anxiety, implying mutual androgyny or a softening of gender-role stereotypes (Collins & Read, 1990; Kirkpatrick & Davis, 1994; Shaver et al., 1996). Men's avoidance and women's anxiety are associated with negative ratings of a relationship by both partners, and men with highly anxious partners tend to rate their relationships as lower in love, satisfaction, and commitment (Kirkpatrick & Davis, 1994; Simpson, 1990).

Some researchers have categorized couples, rather than each partner, in terms of attachment style. In their studies, secure couples (those in which both partners are secure) show better adjustment than other couples, in terms of self-reports of marital intimacy, partners' relationship functioning, and partners' responses to conflict. It is less clear how mixed couples—those in which one partner is secure and the other insecure—fare. Senchak and Leonard (1992) found mixed couples to be generally similar to insecure couples (those in which both partners are insecure) regardless of whether the secure partner was male or female. A study of dating couples, however, found that mixed couples scored between those of secure and insecure couples on measures of negative emotion and emotion control (Feeney, 1995). A third study, using a small sample of married couples, found that both secure and mixed couples were rated as lower in conflict and better in overall functioning than insecure dyads (Cohn, Silver, Cowan, Cowan, & Pearson, 1992). As discussed in more detail below, a secure partner can sometimes buffer the negative effects of an insecure partner, but, alternately, an insecure partner can sometimes erode his or her partner's sense of security (Feeney, 2003; Hazan & Shaver, 1987; Rothbard & Shaver, 1994).

Sexuality

The sexual behavior system, along with attachment and caregiving, is a central component of romantic love (Shaver et al., 1988). The quality of a couple's sex life is an important contributor to relationship satisfaction, and is affected by attachment security or insecurity. Securely attached people are open to sexual exploration in the context of a stable relationship; if both partners are secure, initiation of sexual activity is mutual and physical closeness is enjoyed. Secure individuals engage in sex primarily to show love for their partners (Tracy, Shaver, Albino, & Cooper, 2003).

As mentioned previously, many anxious individuals prefer the affectionate and intimate aspects of sexuality, such as hugging and cuddling, over the genital aspects, while avoidant people tend not to get as much pleasure from sex as nonavoidant people (Hazan et al., 1994). Research with adolescents has shown that anxious individuals engage in sex primarily to please their partners, feel accepted, and avoid abandonment, while avoidant adolescents have sex for reasons such as losing their virginity, and generally have less sexual experience than secure or anxious adolescents (Tracy et al., 2003).

In spite of their generally low ratings on sexual pleasure and satisfaction, avoidant individuals are more likely than secure or anxious individuals to approve of casual sex and "one-night stands" (Brennan & Shaver, 1995; Feeney et al., 1993; Fraley et al., 1998). Consistent with this notion, Schachner and Shaver (2002) found that both *mate poaching*, or attempting to attract someone who is already in a relationship, and being open to being *poached* by others—in the context of short-term, but not long-term relationships—are associated with avoidance. "Relationship exclusivity," an attitude measured by a scale designed by Schmitt and Buss (2000), is highly negatively correlated with attachment avoidance, suggesting that avoidant people tend to be more promiscuous and nonexclusive in their relationships (Schachner & Shaver, 2002). Anxious individuals tend to worry about losing their partners; indeed, the ones in our recent studies (Schachner & Shaver, 2002) actually had lost their partners more often than less anxious individuals. Even if they try to "poach" other people's partners, as many avoidant individuals do, they do not succeed as often as less anxious individuals.

If these findings extend to couples who enter marital therapy, therapists can expect to see differences between anxious and avoidant individuals' wishes and preferences about physical affection and sexual intercourse as well as differences in the likelihood of extramarital sexual encounters.

Conflict

Couple conflict is affected by attachment styles. Both partners' anxiety levels are important in explaining conflict behavior in dating and married couples. Men's and women's anxiety levels interact to predict women's self-reported coercion, distress, and avoidance (in married couples) and observer ratings of women's power assertion, avoidance, and touch (in dating couples). Feeney (2003) found that couples with two anxious partners functioned especially poorly, engaging in high levels of emotional manipulation and power assertion. Anxious individuals tend to feel misunderstood and underappreciated, become demanding and coercive, and focus on their own concerns at the expense of their partner's needs (Noller, Feeney, Bonnell, & Callan, 1994). (This, incidentally, is the kind of parenting that seems to create the anxious attachment pattern in children; see Ainsworth et al., 1978; Cassidy & Berlin, 1994.)

On the other hand, physical aggression among cohabiting and married couples tends to be predicted by an interaction between the perpetrator's anxiety and the partner's avoidance. Anxiety is linked to aggression only if the partner is avoidant, establishing the pattern mentioned earlier in which one partner's fear of abandonment and the other partner's fear of intimacy exacerbate each other (Roberts & Noller, 1998). A study of hurt feelings in couple relationships revealed that anxiety is linked to more severe long-term effects on the victim (e.g., loss of confidence and self-esteem), while avoidance is linked to more severe long-term effects on the relationship (e.g., distrust and dislike of partner, permanent weakening of the bond) (Feeney, 2001).

More generally, insecure attachment seems to be associated with less favorable reports of spouse behavior. Insecure individuals' evaluations of their relationships are more reactive to recent spouse behavior (Feeney, 2002). More anxious men and women report feeling more distress and hostility during problem-centered discussions, while avoidant men are rated as engaging in lower quality interactions (Simpson, Rholes, & Phillips, 1996).

Some of insecure individuals' misperceptions may be understandable in terms of the clinical concept *projection*. Mikulincer and Horesh (1999) found that avoidant individuals' perceptions of others are colored by defensive projection of their own unwanted traits ("unwanted-self" traits) onto others and then distancing themselves from others partly because of these projected traits. This has two effects: maintenance of interpersonal distance and enhancement of the avoidant person's self-esteem. If this happens in the context of marriage, avoidant partners can be expected to project their own unwanted traits onto their spouse and then to criticize and reject their spouse while boosting their own self-image. Mikulincer and Horesh (1999) also found that anxious individuals tend to project their own "actual-self" traits onto others and then view themselves as overly similar to these others. This has two effects: it allows anxious individuals to feel closer and more similar to others and it provides an imagined basis for sharing each other's pain. If this happens in the context of marriage, it might cause a spouse, especially one with avoidant tendencies, to feel uncomfortable, suffocated, and misunderstood.

Attachment Stability and Dynamics within Couples

Most people prefer secure partners (Chappell & Davis, 1998). When research subjects were asked to imagine themselves in relationships with hypothetical partners, secure subjects reported less positive feelings about relationships with either type of insecure partner, while insecure subjects (especially those classified as avoidant) responded less favorably to an avoidant partner than to a preoccupied partner (Pietromonaco & Carnelley, 1994).

A secure partner may buffer the negative effects of insecurity (Cohn et al., 1992) and foster the sense of security of the couple: if the other partner already has a sense of security, this experience of warm and responsive interaction confirms existing models; if the other partner is insecure, the experience disconfirms existing models and may gradually reshape them (Feeney, 2003; Rothbard & Shaver, 1994). In other words, when a secure partner consistently encourages openness and mutual expression, the insecure partner can modify maladaptive behaviors associated with insecurity.

However, a couple containing at least one insecure partner can also erode the sense of security of both of its members. The insecurities in one individual can be perpetuated or even exacerbated by the responses of his or her partner, and even secure individuals can become anxious about loss and rejection in the face of emotionally distant partners—for example, an avoidant partner might prompt a secure person to feel and act anxious (Feeney, 2003; Hazan & Shaver, 1987).

The couple system contains homeostatic features that tend to maintain a relatively stable state; when behavior departs from the expected range, it is controlled via corrective feedback loops, which can involve rigid patterns and considerable distress in the case of dysfunctional couples. Destructive pursuer–distancer cycles (a struggle to regulate proximity and control the emotional climate of the relationship) can be maintained in part by negative perceptions of intention (Feeney, 2003; Byng-Hall, 1999).

CAN ATTACHMENT SECURITY BE ENHANCED AND INFLUENCE OTHER BEHAVIORS?

During most of the history of research on romantic attachment, investigators have been busy documenting associations between measures of attachment style and a variety of potential causes and consequences. Only recently have we begun to ask whether it might be possible to intervene experimentally to enhance people's sense of attachment security (through exposure to security primes) and foster the outcomes associated with it. Much of this research has been done in Israel, against a background of war in the Middle East rather than conflict within marriages, so we will have to extrapolate findings to the marital domain for present purposes.

Mikulincer, Gillath, Sapir-Lavid, et al. (2001) found that *security primes* (recollections of personal memories and pictorial representations of supportive others) increased the priority people placed on *self-transcendent values*, or values that reflect a concern for the welfare of both close and distant others, at the expense of more *selfish values* such as "social recognition" and "an exciting life." If a sense of security causes people to endorse values that are associated with supportive, caring behaviors, then it follows that the activation of attachment security should lead to less selfishness and greater kindness and support within the context of a marriage.

In another series of studies, Mikulincer, Gillath, Halevy, et al. (2001) found that exposing individuals to attachment security primes (in the form of recollections of personal memories, pictorial representations of supportive others, and subliminal presentations of proximity-related words) strengthens empathy and inhibits personal distress in reaction to others' needs. In other words, a sense of attachment security leads people to adopt a more empathic attitude toward both strangers and close relationship partners through means of altruistic motivations (rather than egoistic motivations aimed at reducing one's own distress). These findings suggest that the activation of images of attachment security might promote greater empathy and altruism between marital partners.

Mikulincer and Arad (1999) examined attachment style differences in the revision of knowledge about a relationship partner following behavior on the part of the partner that seemed inconsistent with this knowledge. Compared to secure persons, both anxious and avoidant individuals changed their perception of their partner less after being exposed to expectation-incongruent information about their partner's behavior. They were also less capable of recalling this information. This finding was replicated when relationship-specific attachment orientations were assessed: the higher the level of attachment anxiety or avoidance toward a specific partner, the fewer the revisions people made in their perception of this partner upon receiving expectation-incongruent information (Mikulincer & Arad, 1999, Study 2). Moreover, the activation of a sense of attachment security (visualizing a supportive other) increased cognitive openness and led even chronically anxious and avoidant people to revise their conception of a partner based on new information (Mikulincer & Arad, 1999, Study 3). These studies suggest that increasing the momentary sense of security of marital partners in a therapeutic setting could help the partners alter their mental representations of each other in a helpful way, allowing them to abandon destructive models based on past betrayals and "attachment injuries."

Conscious and unconscious security primes also can be related to hostility to members of particular outgroups (in Israel) (Mikulincer & Shaver, 2001). Across a series of different groups that were viewed as outgroups by secular, heterosexual Jewish students (e.g., Israeli Arabs, ultra-Orthodox Jews, Russian immigrants, and homosexuals), security primes were found to decrease hostility to outgroup members, even when participants thought that a particular member of the outgroup whom they were evaluating had made negative comments about secular Jewish students. Attachment anxiety scores were related to greater outgroup hostility in these studies, but the positive effects of security enhancement worked equally well regardless of attachment style, suggesting that security primes might alleviate hostility and contempt between marital partners regardless of attachment style. Given the importance of corrosive emotions such as contempt and disgust for marital dissolution and divorce (Gottman, 1994), any procedure that reduces those emotions and increases spouses' tolerance toward each other should be welcome to therapists.

IMPLICATIONS FOR THERAPY

Although neither of us is a therapist or even a clinical researcher, we suspect that research on romantic attachment provides useful leads for individual and marital therapy. As Johnson et al. (2001) have explained, one of the primary problem areas for couples in therapy is trust, which can easily be eroded by attachment injuries. An attachment injury occurs when one partner violates the expectation that the other will offer comfort and caring in times of danger or distress (Johnson et al., 2001). The expectations of a secure individual can be summarized in the form of a secure-base script: "If I encounter an obstacle or become distressed, I can approach a significant other for help; he or she is likely to be available and supportive; I will experience relief and comfort as a result of proximity to this person and can then return to other activities" (Mikulincer & Shaver, 2001; Waters, Rodrigues, & Ridgeway, 1998). The expectations of an avoidant individual are based on past violations of this script, leading eventually to the belief that self-reliance is the only safe foundation for security. The expectations of an anxious individual are based on repeatedly finding that attachment figures failed to come through in times of need. Rather than turn away and adopt a self-reliant stance, anxious individuals become more vigilant and clingy. To move insecure individuals toward security, a therapist would have to help clients feel secure, partly as a result of trusting the therapist to serve as a "secure base" (Bowlby, 1988), and partly as a result of maneuvering them into situations where they can feel and accept their partners' forgiveness and support.

The research we have reviewed suggests that, on an individual level, even momentary increases in security (including ones induced subliminally) can cause corresponding increases in altruism, empathy, the willingness to change negative impressions of one's partner, and other supportive and caring behaviors that may help overcome insecure individuals' negative perceptions of their relationships. In dealing with avoidant individuals, therapists must somehow break through and restructure negative working models and expectations regarding relationships. Anxious clients, on the other hand, need to feel that their therapist approves of them and provides a secure base from which they can open up emotionally, without fear of rejection.

Regarding change at the level of the couple, research suggests that attachment injuries are a major block to relationship repair (Johnson et al., 2001). Small disappointments often remind an insecure, "injured" spouse of more important, unresolved injuries from the past. The model in Figure 2.2 shows how this kind of raw vulnerability can make a person even more sensitive to threats and slights and more critically observant of a partner's lack of optimal support. In many cases, the "offending" partner may not even notice or recall the injurious event, in effect compounding the injury. As Johnson et al. (2001) explain, situations in which an attachment figure is both a source of pain and fear and also a potential soother and caregiver sometimes lead to a breakdown in the attachment system—perhaps the state that infancy researchers (e.g., Main & Solomon, 1986) call "disorganized/disoriented" behavior and an extreme form of what Bartholomew (1990) calls "fearful avoidance"—causing the injured partner to swing between hyperactivating and deactivating strategies, alternately accusing and clinging, begging and withdrawing.

Therapy in these situations involves identifying and delineating the problematic cycles and emotions, and then encouraging communication of the needs and hurts of the injured partner in ways that simultaneously encourage the spouse's empathy and responsiveness. The couple can then complete a positive bonding interaction where each can risk, share, and find a safe haven in the other (Johnson et al., 2001). Research on emotionally focused couple therapy (EFT) has shown that "bonding interactions" such as "softenings" (Johnson & Greenberg, 1988), in which an angry, blaming spouse is able to ask for and receive reassurance (both spouses being accessible and responsive to each other), are associated with decreases in marital distress. At present, EFT, which specifically focuses on creating secure bonds between spouses, has the best outcomes of all forms of couple therapy tested (Johnson, Hunsley, Greenberg, & Schindler, 1999), and the outcomes appear to be stable across time.

Following repeated iterations of this process, perhaps alternately focusing on one person's injuries and then the other's, the therapist can work toward a consolidation in which both partners construct positive models of the relationship and work to solve ongoing problems (Johnson, 1999). The experimental work in which we and our colleagues have documented positive effects of even very short-term increases in people's sense of security causes us to be optimistic about the prospects for therapeutic enhancement of spouses' security. On the other hand, the hundreds of studies showing that long-term, fairly stable differences in attachment style profoundly affect perceptions, emotions, and behaviors in all kinds of social relationships cause us to wonder how successful therapy can be in altering well-established working models of self and relationship partners.

In this chapter, we have provided a review of recent research related to attachment theory as it applies to couple relationships, and in several places we have pointed out ways in which the findings may be relevant to marital therapy. We have also touched on a range of measures and experimental techniques used in such research (e.g., unconscious priming of security-related images or names), in hopes that some of these techniques may prove useful in therapy. We realize, however, that it is a long way from the laboratory to the marriage clinic, and we do not view ourselves as competent to span that gap. We therefore eagerly look forward to reading the other chapters in this book, especially the ones by authors with extensive experience as marital therapists.

ACKNOWLEDGMENTS

Preparation of this chapter was facilitated by a grant from the Fetzer Institute.

REFERENCES

Ainsworth, M. D. S. (1991). Attachment and other affectional bonds across the life cycle. In C. M. Parkes, J. Stevenson-Hinde, & P. Marris (Eds.), *Attachment across the life cycle* (pp. 33–51). New York: Routledge.

Ainsworth, M. D. S., Blehar, M. C., Waters, E., & Wall, S. (1978). *Patterns of attachment: Assessed in the Strange Situation and at home.* Hillsdale, NJ: Erlbaum.

Bartholomew, K. (1990). Avoidance of intimacy: An attachment perspective. *Journal of Social and Personal Relationships, 7,* 147–178.

Bowlby, J. (1973). *Attachment and loss: Vol. II. Separation: Anxiety and anger.* New York: Basic Books.

Bowlby, J. (1982). *Attachment and loss: Vol. I. Attachment* (2nd ed.). New York: Basic Books. (First edition published in 1969)

Bowlby, J. (1988). *A secure base: Clinical applications of attachment theory.* London: Routledge.

Brennan, K. A., Clark, C. L., & Shaver, P. R. (1998). Self-report measurement of adult attachment: An integrative overview. In J. A. Simpson & W. S. Rholes (Eds.), *Attachment theory and close relationships* (pp. 46–76). New York: Guilford Press.

Brennan, K. A., & Shaver, P. R. (1995). Dimensions of adult attachment, affect regulation, and romantic relationship functioning. *Personality and Social Psychology Bulletin, 21,* 267–283.

Brennan, K. A., Shaver, P. R., & Tobey, A. E. (1991). Attachment styles, gender and parental problem drinking. *Journal of Social and Personal Relationships, 8,* 451–466.

Byng-Hall, J. (1999). Family and couple therapy: Toward greater security. In J.

Cassidy & P. R. Shaver (Eds.), *Handbook of attachment: Theory, research, and clinical applications* (pp. 625–645). New York: Guilford Press.

Carnelley, K. B., Pietromonaco, P. R., & Jaffe, K. (1996). Attachment, caregiving, and relationship functioning in couples: Effects of self and partner. *Personal Relationships, 3,* 257–277.

Cassidy, J., & Berlin, L. J. (1994). The insecure/ambivalent pattern of attachment: Theory and research. *Child Development, 65,* 971–991.

Cassidy, J., & Kobak, R. R. (1988). Avoidance and its relationship with other defensive processes. In J. Belsky & T. Nezworski (Eds.), *Clinical implications of attachment* (pp. 300–323). Hillsdale, NJ: Erlbaum.

Chappell, K. D., & Davis, K. E. (1998). Attachment, partner choice, and perception of romantic partners: An experimental test of the attachment-security hypothesis. *Personal Relationships, 5,* 327–342.

Cohn, D. A., Silver, D. H., Cowan, C. P., Cowan, P. A., & Pearson, J. (1992). Working models of childhood attachment and couple relationships. *Journal of Family Issues, 13,* 432–449.

Collins, N. L. (1996). Working models of attachment: Implications for explanation, emotion, and behavior. *Journal of Personality and Social Psychology, 71,* 810–832.

Collins, N. L., & Feeney, B. C. (2000). A safe haven: An attachment theory perspective on support seeking and caregiving in intimate relationships. *Journal of Personality and Social Psychology, 78,* 1053–1073.

Collins, N. L., & Read, S. J. (1990). Adult attachment, working models, and relationship quality in dating couples. *Journal of Personality and Social Psychology, 58,* 644–663.

Feeney, J. A. (1994). Attachment style, communication patterns, and satisfaction across the life cycle of marriage. *Personal Relationships, 1,* 333–348.

Feeney, J. A. (1995). Adult attachment and emotional control. *Personal Relationships, 2,* 143–159.

Feeney, J. A. (1999a). Adult attachment, emotional control and marital satisfaction. *Personal Relationships, 6,* 169–185.

Feeney, J. A. (1999b). Adult romantic attachment and couple relationships. In J. Cassidy & P. R. Shaver (Eds.), *Handbook of attachment: Theory, research, and clinical applications* (pp. 355–377). New York: Guilford Press.

Feeney, J. A. (2001). *Understanding psychological hurt in couple relationships.* Unpublished manuscript, Department of Psychology, University of Queensland, Brisbane, Australia.

Feeney, J. A. (2002). Attachment, marital interaction and relationship satisfaction: A diary study. *Personal Relationships, 9,* 39–55.

Feeney, J. A. (2003). The systemic nature of couple relationships: An attachment perspective. In P. Erdman & T. Caffery (Eds.), *Attachment and family systems: Conceptual, empirical, and therapeutic relatedness* (pp. 139–163). New York: Brunner/Mazel.

Feeney, J. A., & Hohaus, L. (2001). Attachment and spousal caregiving. *Personal Relationships, 8,* 21–39.

Feeney, J. A., Kelly, L., Gallois, C., Peterson, C., & Terry, D. J. (1999). Attachment style, assertive communication, and safer-sex behavior. *Journal of Applied Social Psychology, 29,* 1964–1983.

Feeney, J. A., & Noller, P. (1990). Attachment style as a predictor of adult romantic relationships. *Journal of Personality and Social Psychology, 58,* 281–291.

Feeney, J. A., Noller, P., & Patty, J. (1993). Adolescents' interactions with the opposite sex: Influence of attachment style and gender. *Journal of Adolescence, 16,* 169–186.

Fraley, R. C., Davis, K. E., & Shaver, P. R. (1998). Dismissing-avoidance and the defensive organization of emotion, cognition, and behavior. In J. A. Simpson & W. S. Rholes (Eds.), *Attachment theory and close relationships* (pp. 249–279). New York: Guilford Press.

Fraley, R. C., & Shaver, P. R. (2000). Adult romantic attachment: Theoretical developments, emerging controversies, and unanswered questions. *Review of General Psychology, 4,* 132–154.

Fraley, R. C., & Spieker, S. J. (in press). Are infant attachment patterns continuously or categorically distributed?: A taxometric analysis of strange situation behavior. *Developmental Psychology.*

Fraley, R. C., & Waller, N. G. (1998). Adult attachment patterns: A test of the typological model. In J. A. Simpson & W. S. Rholes (Eds.), *Attachment theory and close relationships* (pp. 77–114). New York: Guilford Press.

Fredrickson, B. L. (2001). The role of positive emotions in positive psychology: The broaden-and-build theory of positive emotions. *American Psychologist, 56,* 218–226.

Gottman, J. M. (1994). *What predicts divorce?* Hillsdale, NJ: Erlbaum.

Hatfield, E., Brinton, C., & Cornelius, J. (1989). Passionate love and anxiety in young adolescents. *Motivation and Emotion, 13,* 271–289.

Hazan, C., & Shaver, P. R. (1987). Romantic love conceptualized as an attachment process. *Journal of Personality and Social Psychology, 52,* 511–524.

Hazan, C., & Zeifman, D. (1999). Pair bonds as attachments: Evaluating the evidence. In J. Cassidy & P. R. Shaver (Eds.), *Handbook of attachment: Theory, research, and clinical applications* (pp. 336–354). New York: Guilford Press.

Hazan, C., Zeifman, D., & Middleton, K. (1994, July). *Adult romantic attachment, affection, and sex.* Paper presented at the seventh International Conference on Personal Relationships, Groninger, The Netherlands.

Jacobson, N. S., Follette, W. C., & McDonald, D. W. (1982). Reactivity to positive and negative behavior in distressed and nondistressed married couples. *Journal of Consulting and Clinical Psychology, 50,* 706–714.

Johnson, S. M. (1999). Emotionally focused couple therapy: Straight to the heart. In J. M. Donovan (Ed.), *Short-term couple therapy* (pp. 12–42). New York: Guilford Press.

Johnson, S. M., & Greenberg, L. S. (1988). Relating process to outcome in marital therapy. *Journal of Marital and Family Therapy, 14,* 175–183.

Johnson, S. M., Hunsley, J., Greenberg, L., & Schindler, D. (1999). Emotionally focused couples therapy: Status and challenges (a meta-analysis). *Journal of Clinical Psychology: Science and Practice, 6,* 67–79.

Johnson, S. M., Makinen, J. A., & Millikin, J. W. (2001). Attachment injuries in couple relationships: A new perspective on impasses in couples therapy. *Journal of Marital and Family Therapy, 27,* 145–155.

Keelan, J. P. R., Dion, K. K., & Dion, K. L. (1998). Attachment style and relationship satisfaction: Test of a self-disclosure explanation. *Canadian Journal of Behavioural Science, 30,* 24–35.

Kirkpatrick, L. E., & Davis, K. E. (1994). Attachment style, gender, and relationship stability: A longitudinal analysis. *Journal of Personality and Social Psychology, 66,* 502–512.

Kobak, R. R., & Hazan, C. (1991). Attachment in marriage: Effects of security and accuracy of working models. *Journal of Personality and Social Psychology, 60,* 861–869.

Levy, M. B., & Davis, K. E. (1988). Lovestyles and attachment styles compared: Their relations to each other and to various relationship characteristics. *Journal of Social and Personal Relationships, 5,* 439–471.

Madsen, L. B. (2000). *Cognitive processes and attachment: The structure and function of working models.* Unpublished master's thesis, University of Queensland, Brisbane, Australia.

Main, M., & Solomon, J. (1986). Discovery of a new, insecure disorganized/disoriented attachment pattern. In T. B. Brazelton & M. Yogman (Eds.), *Affective development in infancy* (pp. 95–124). Norwood, NJ: Ablex.

Mikulincer, M., & Arad, D. (1999). Attachment, working models, and cognitive openness in close relationships: A test of chronic and temporary accessibility effects. *Journal of Personality and Social Psychology, 77,* 710–725.

Mikulincer, M., Birnbaum, G., Woddis, D., & Nachmias, O. (2000). Stress and accessibility of proximity-related thoughts: Exploring the normative and intra-individual components of attachment theory. *Journal of Personality and Social Psychology, 78,* 509–523.

Mikulincer, M., Gillath, O., Halevy, V., Avihou, N., Avidan, S., & Eshkoli, N. (2001). Attachment theory and reactions to others' needs: Evidence that activation of the sense of attachment security promotes empathic responses. *Journal of Personality and Social Psychology, 81,* 1205–1224.

Mikulincer, M., Gillath, O., Sapir-Lavid, Y., Yaacovi, E., Arias, K., Tal-Aloni, L., & Bor, G. (2001). *Attachment theory and concern for others' welfare: Evidence that the sense of secure base promotes self-transcendence values.* Unpublished manuscript, Department of Psychology, Bar-Ilan University, Israel.

Mikulincer, M., Gillath, O., & Shaver, P. R. (2002). Activation of the attachment system in adulthood: Threat-related primes increase the accessibility of mental representations of attachment figures. *Journal of Personality and Social Psychology, 83,* 881–895.

Mikulincer, M., & Horesh, N. (1999). Adult attachment style and the perception of others: The role of projective mechanisms. *Journal of Personality and Social Psychology, 76,* 1022–1034.

Mikulincer, M., & Shaver, P. R. (2001). Attachment theory and intergroup bias: Evidence that priming the secure base schema attenuates negative reactions to outgroups. *Journal of Personality and Social Psychology, 81,* 97–115.

Minuchin, P. (1985). Families and individual development: Provocations from the field of family therapy. *Child Development, 56,* 289–302.

Noller, P., Feeney, J. A., Bonnell, D., & Callan, V. J. (1994). A longitudinal study of conflict in early marriage. *Journal of Social and Personal Relationships, 11*, 233–252.

Pietromonaco, P. R., & Carnelley, K. B. (1994). Gender and working models of attachment: Consequences for perceptions of self and romantic relationships. *Personal Relationships, 1*, 63–82.

Rholes, W. S., Simpson, J. A., Campbell, L., & Grich, J. (2001). Adult attachment and the transition to parenthood. *Journal of Personality and Social Psychology, 81*, 421–435.

Roberts, N., & Noller, P. (1998). The associations between adult attachment and couple violence: The role of communication patterns and relationship satisfaction. In J. A. Simpson & W. S. Rholes (Eds.), *Attachment theory and close relationships* (pp. 317–350). New York: Guilford Press.

Rom, E., & Mikulincer, M. (in press). Attachment theory and group processes: The association between attachment style and group-related representations, goals, memories, and functioning. *Journal of Personality and Social Psychology.*

Rothbard, J. C., & Shaver, P. R. (1994). Continuity of attachment across the lifespan. In M. B. Sperling & W. H. Berman (Eds.), *Attachment in adults: Theory, assessment, and treatment* (pp. 31–71). New York: Guilford Press.

Schachner, D. A., & Shaver, P. R. (2002). Attachment style and human mate poaching. *New Review of Social Psychology, 1*, 122–129.

Schmitt, D. P., & Buss, D. M. (2000). Sexual dimensions of person description: Beyond or subsumed by the Big Five? *Journal of Research in Personality, 34*, 141–177.

Senchak, M., & Leonard, K. E. (1992). Attachment styles and marital adjustment among newlywed couples. *Journal of Social and Personal Relationships, 9*, 51–64.

Shaver, P. R., & Brennan, K. A. (1992). Attachment styles and the "Big Five" personality traits: Their connections with each other and with romantic relationship outcomes. *Personality and Social Psychology Bulletin, 18*, 536–545.

Shaver, P. R., & Clark, C. L. (1994). The psychodynamics of adult romantic attachment. In J. M. Masling & R. F. Bornstein (Eds.), *Empirical perspectives on object relations theories* (pp. 105–156). Washington, DC: American Psychological Association.

Shaver, P. R., & Hazan, C. (1988). A biased overview of the study of love. *Journal of Social and Personal Relationships, 5*, 473–501.

Shaver, P. R., & Hazan, C. (1993). Adult romantic attachment: Theory and evidence. In D. Perlman & W. Jones (eds.), *Advances in personal relationships* (Vol. 4, pp. 29–70). London: Jessica Kingsley.

Shaver, P. R., Hazan, C., & Bradshaw, D. (1988). Love as attachment: The integration of three behavioral systems. In R. J. Sternberg & M. Barnes (Eds.), *The psychology of love* (pp. 68–99). New Haven, CT: Yale University Press.

Shaver, P. R., & Mikulincer, M. (2002). Attachment-related psychodynamics. *Attachment and Human Development, 4*, 133–161.

Shaver, P. R., Papalia, D., Clark, C. L., Koski, L. R., Tidwell, M., & Nalbone, D. (1996). Androgyny and attachment security: Two related models of optimal personality. *Personality and Social Psychology Bulletin, 22*, 582–597.

Simpson, J. A. (1990). Influence of attachment styles on romantic relationships. *Journal of Personality and Social Psychology, 59*, 971–980.

Simpson, J. A., Rholes, W. S., & Nelligan, J. S. (1992). Support seeking and support giving within couples in an anxiety-provoking situation: The role of attachment styles. *Journal of Personality and Social Psychology, 62,* 434–446.

Simpson, J. A., Rholes, W. S., & Phillips, D. (1996). Conflict in close relationships: An attachment perspective. *Journal of Personality and Social Psychology, 71,* 899–914.

Tracy, J. L., Shaver, P. R., Albino, A. W., & Cooper, M. L. (2003). Attachment styles and adolescent sexuality. In P. Florsheim (Ed.), *Adolescent romance and sexual behavior: Theory, research, and practical implications* (pp. 137–149). Mahwah, NJ: Erlbaum.

Waters, H. S., Rodrigues, L. M., & Ridgeway, D. (1998). Cognitive underpinnings of narrative attachment assessment. *Journal of Experimental Child Psychology, 71,* 211–234.

Whiffen, V. E., & Johnson, S. M. (1998). An attachment theory framework for the treatment of childbearing depression. *Clinical Psychology: Science and Practice, 5,* 478–493.

3

The Essential Nature of Couple Relationships

CINDY HAZAN

If you were to ask a dozen anthropologists for an evolutionary perspective on human mating, you might well get a dozen different answers. But if instead you perused the scientific literature that represents the field of personal relationships, you would find just one: sexual strategies theory (SST; Buss & Schmitt, 1993). This sort of singularity is sometimes an indication that through careful analysis and comparison a particular model has been judged the most valid. However, the prominence of SST in relationship research is the result of its being the *only* evolutionary perspective on human mating thus far proposed.

According to this model, men and women are fundamentally different in their mate preferences and mating behavior. Indeed, it formalizes many common stereotypes regarding differences between the sexes—for example, men look for sex while women seek commitment; men want mates who are young and attractive, whereas women prefer those with money and power. In theory, such differences are not due to gender-biased socioeconomic structures or socialization practices but rather are coded into our genes as a result of selection pressure over tens of thousands of years. In other words, they are hard-wired and not likely to change anytime soon.

I happen to share the view that models of human mating must include the forces that for millennia shaped our brains and behavioral dispositions. However, I think the available evidence tells a very different evolutionary story than the one implied by SST. First, a close examination of the findings reveals that sex differences in mating are much smaller in size and more trivial in significance than is generally claimed. Minor sex differences have been overemphasized while major sex similarities have been downplayed. Second, there are many important and well-documented facts of human mating that SST simply ignores. Several are ones that the theory cannot account for; a few appear to be incompatible with it.

In what follows I provide an overview of SST, address some of its logical and empirical limitations, and then propose an alternative model. The alternative is founded on Bowlby's (1973, 1980, 1982) attachment theory. It takes into account many of the facts overlooked by SST and also offers a more realistic and grounded account of how *Homo sapiens* go about the business of mating.

SEXUAL STRATEGIES THEORY AND EVIDENCE

Sexual strategies theory (SST; Buss & Schmitt, 1993) is based in part on a real feature of human biology. Men are able to reproduce their genes with as little investment as a few minutes and a few sperm. By comparison, the cost to women—including gestation, lactation, and childcare—is years of investment. In theory, this asymmetry between the sexes resulted in different, sex-specific strategies for achieving reproductive success.

The mating behaviors seen today reflect psychological mechanisms that evolved to solve specific adaptive problems faced by each sex in the environment of evolutionary adaptation (EEA). For example, unlike many primate females who have obvious sexual swellings to signal fertility, in human females ovulation is concealed. Thus, ancestral males had to solve the problem of how to identify fertile partners. Given that female fertility declines with age, youth is one possible cue. Another is physical attractiveness, the markers of which are hypothesized to be correlates of health. In theory, then, the ancestral solution to the male problem of identifying fertile partners was an evolved preference for young and attractive mates. In addition, the relatively small investment required for gene replication supposedly resulted in a male preference for multiple partners. In the words of Buss (1989, p. 24), "Men who lack mechanisms such as a desire for a variety of partners . . . would have been out-reproduced" by men who had such preferences.

The situation is different for human females in that every sexual encounter is potentially quite costly. The typical woman produces an average of one egg per month from puberty through middle age, in stark contrast to her male counterparts who produce approximately 500 million tiny sperm cells every day (Zimmerman, Maude, & Moldawar, 1965). And once a woman's egg is fertilized, she has to forgo other reproductive opportunities for a relatively long time. As a consequence, she should be far more sexually cautious and choosy. Because postpubertal males continue to produce sperm throughout their lives, identifying fertile male partners was never difficult. Instead, the problem faced by ancestral females was one of finding a mate who possessed resources and was willing to commit them to her and her offspring. According to SST, the most favorable female strategy for achieving reproductive success is to hold out for one high-status male who will provide for her and the children she has to nurture.

SST acknowledges that the mating behavior of men and women can be similar in certain respects under certain conditions. For example, a man might agree to long-term mating if necessary for obtaining a woman of high mate value (Buss & Schmitt, 1993, p. 214), and a woman might accept a short-term mating arrangement if she can quickly extract needed resources (p. 220). Technically, males and females are free to adopt either strategy, but the costs and benefits differ dramatically for the two sexes. Although SST admits the possibility of sex similarities, above all it emphasizes differences. The clear take-home message is that sex differences are the hallmark of human mating.

Scores of studies have been conducted to test SST. By far the most impressive is a survey of over 10,000 individuals in 37 different cultures located on six continents and five islands (Buss, 1989). The findings show that males worldwide assign greater importance than females to the age and physical appearance of potential mates, preferring those who are young and attractive. In contrast, females report caring more than males about the social status, ambition, and earning power of potential mates. In sum, the sex differences in mate preferences predicted by SST appear to be both statistically reliable and culturally universal.

Another central prediction of SST—sex differences in sexual promiscuity—also appears to have strong empirical support. Buss and Schmitt (1993) asked subjects about the degree to which they seek short-term ("one-night stand") as opposed to long-term (marriage) partners, the estimated likelihood of sexual intercourse after relationships ranging from 1 hour to 5 years, and the ideal number of sexual partners over periods of time extending from 1 month to 30 years. By all measures, males on average were more interested in and more eager to pursue casual sexual liaisons than were females.

QUESTIONS ABOUT THE THEORY AND EVIDENCE

In this section I address some limitations of the empirical and logical evidence upon which SST is based. The section is organized around questions derived from basic tenets of the theory.

Do Men "Naturally" Prefer Short-Term, Multipartner Mating?

According to SST, the gender discrepancy in reproductive costs created a situation in which males, relative to females, stood to gain more from short- versus long-term mating. There is arguably no tenet upon which the standard model depends more than the sex difference in short-term mating proclivity. As an indication of its importance, in the first comprehensive exposition of the theory (Buss & Schmitt, 1993) three separate figures were devoted to demonstrating that, *on average*, males are more sexually promiscuous than females. But averages can be misleading.

In a recent replication, Miller and Fishkin (1997) asked a large group of undergraduates the same question posed by Buss and Schmitt: "Ideally, how many sex partners would you like to have in the next 30 years?" The results were consistent with those reported previously. The mean number for females was two; for males, it was 64. However, another measure of central tendency paints a very different picture. The *median* ideal number of future sexual partners as reported by females was one; for males, the number was also one. Obviously the distribution was grossly skewed, in which case the mean is a poor reflection of the average value. More importantly, the use of a different central tendency statistic leads to the conclusion that the ideal number of future sexual partners is the same for males and for females.

The demographic characteristics of Miller and Fishkin's sample deserve note. The subjects were undergraduate students. The typical undergraduate male is young, single, and has access to the largest pool of potential mates that he likely ever will. Yet he says that over the next three decades what he would "ideally" like is *one* sexual partner. If human males have been programmed by natural selection to want and seek out opportunities for sex with as many females as possible, why is this not reflected in the self-reported desires of men who are at their sexual peak and living in the midst of extraordinary numbers of young and attractive women? This finding seriously undermines a central tenet of SST.

Is "Short-Term" Mating an Effective Human Strategy?

According to SST, short-term (multipartner) mating is the optimal male route to reproductive success and the strategy that men would naturally adopt if only they could get women to go along. This claim is sufficiently central to warrant further analysis.

Nobody knows for sure what life was like in the EEA when our mating behaviors were taking shape. Anthropologists have traditionally used contemporary hunter–gatherer societies as the best available substitute. It has been estimated that in such groups the typical female is either pregnant or lactating (and therefore not ovulating) during approximately 24 of the average 26 years between puberty and menopause (Symons, 1979). As a result, she would be fertile on only about 80 of these 8,000 or so days. In other words, only one out of 100 random copulations could even *potentially* result in conception. Normally, it takes several months of unprotected sex to produce a viable pregnancy. In light of these facts, it seems highly improbable that moving from one-night stand to one-night stand would ever have been an effective human strategy for achieving reproductive success, or that such a strategy would ever have been selected-for.

Was Fertility Detection a "Problem" to Be Solved?

A foundational claim of SST is that men had to surmount the formidable challenge of identifying fertile partners. Again, in the absence of information about early human life, we are left with guesses derived from modern hunter–gatherer societies. According to available estimates (Symons, 1979), more than 90% of postpubescent young people in contemporary hunter–gatherer groups are fertile. If these estimates are even close to representing EEA conditions, fertility detection may not have been an adaptive problem. And if this particular problem never arose, there would not have been any need or selection pressure for the evolution of a specialized fertility-detecting mechanism. It would not have required a rocket scientist or even an unusually clever hominid to identify a fertile mate.

The proposed solution to the alleged fertility detection problem for males was an evolved preference for females who are young and physically attractive. Although youth is a pretty reliable cue of fertility and reproductive capability *in both sexes*, the claim that beauty is a signal of fertility and genetic quality is a proposition that has yet to be tested among humans.

The real "problem" for human males is that human female ovulation is not overt. Her relative youth is a reasonable proxy for her reproductive potential—that is, how many ovulatory cycles she has left, just as a male's relative youth is a reasonable indicator of his sperm quality and erectile capacity—but beauty (or lack thereof) is not a reliable indicator of her present or future health status (Kalick, Zebrowitz, Langlois, & Johnson, 1998) or whether she is able to conceive on any given occasion.

Are Women "Naturally" Attracted to Rich and Powerful Men?

In theory, women's comparatively greater parental investment resulted in a female preference for males with resources and status. Indeed, females worldwide consistently give higher importance ratings to resource- and status-related mate traits than do males (Buss, 1989). This sex difference is nearly universal and supports SST claims that resource/status detection is an innate feature of female mating psychology.

However, if a gender-imbalanced social structure were responsible for female concern about a potential mate's status and resources, then the degree to which women judge men on these qualities should vary as a function of the local financial standing of women. In fact, it does. In 1999,

Kasser and Sharma reanalyzed Buss's 37 cultures data and found that females (but not males) strongly prefer resource-acquisition characteristics in mates when they live in cultures low in both female reproductive freedom and educational equality. From SST research reports, one could easily get the impression that a mate's financial prospects are a priority consideration for women. In fact, it ranked 12th on the international female list of desired attributes (Buss, Abbott, & Angleitner, 1990).

Is Human Mating a "Strategic" Process?

According to SST, human mating behavior is guided by evolved psychological mechanisms compelling men and women not only to *desire* certain qualities but also to *select* mates on the basis of these desires. However, the methods usually employed in tests of the theory do not and cannot directly address the selection part of the prediction. Subjects—typically college students—either generate a list of qualities on which they believe their eventual mate selections will be based or rank/rate the perceived importance of a list of traits provided by researchers. Although male–female differences regarding the relative importance of physical appearance and resources are consistent with SST, practically everyone, regardless of gender, wants a mate who is nice, smart, rich, good-looking, has a winning personality, and so on. But the more important question of whether these are the criteria they will ultimately use to select their mates was left unanswered—until recently.

In an innovative study Lykken and Tellegen (1993) used objective (rather than self-report) measures to examine real-world (as opposed to hypothetical) mate choice. The data came from the Minnesota Twin Registry, which includes personality, achievement, IQ, attitude, occupation, and physical attractiveness information on more than 1,000 twin pairs. The findings indicate that the criteria people *think* they will use to select their mates are *not* the factors that ultimately influence their actual mate choices. In fact, the researchers found no evidence for any strategic process whatsoever.

Do Men and Women Have Fundamentally Different Mate Preferences?

In Buss's (1989) 37-cultures study, it was reported (in both title and text) that males and females universally differ in the qualities they seek in a mate. What gets less press is the fact that the qualities ranked highest by both sexes *are exactly the same*! More than anything, men and women reported wanting a mate who is kind, understanding, and intelligent. It is noteworthy that the study context was a hypothetical scenario in which participants were free to describe their dream mate. Every figure in the report of findings highlighted male–female differences, and yet the results could have been presented as evidence that men and women look for the same qualities in a mate.

Further evidence of sex similarities in mate preferences comes from research on facial attractiveness. Cunningham and colleagues (Cunningham, Druen, & Barbee, 1997) used facialmetric methods and multicultural samples to identify the features that influence attractiveness ratings. They found three distinct types of facial characteristics: *expressive* features (e.g., size of smile area) serve as cues of warmth and sensitivity; *neotenous* features (e.g., large forehead) signal vulnerability; *sexual–maturational* features (e.g., prominent cheekbones) function as markers of reproductive capability. Attractiveness ratings were highest for individuals whose faces included all three types of features. This was true for both sexes.

The findings suggest that human mate preferences are not governed by a single, sex-specific mechanism but rather by multiple species-typical mechanisms. To understand why this might be so and what specific mechanisms might be involved, it is useful to consider what is required for reproductive success in our species. At a minimum, it requires successful negotiation of at least three adaptive challenges: surviving to reproductive age, acquiring and retaining a mate, and providing adequate care to offspring so that they too survive to reproduce. Solving these three different adaptive problems likely necessitated the evolution of three distinct mechanisms: attachment, sexual mating, and parenting/caregiving (Hazan & Shaver, 1994a, 1994b; Hazan & Zeifman, 1999). And given that men and women had to surmount the same three challenges to achieve reproductive success, it is not surprising that the associated mechanisms are reflected in the preferences of both sexes. The faces judged most appealing are those that combine the signal stimuli of all three mechanisms.

Summary

The available evidence is *not* consistent with the claim that men "naturally" prefer short-term mating, that "short-term" mating is or ever was an effective human strategy, that fertility detection was an adaptive "problem" for ancestral males, that women are "naturally" attracted to males with resources, that human mate selection is a "strategic" process, or that men and women have fundamentally different mate preferences. In short, there are some major problems with the logic of and evidence for SST.

AN ATTACHMENT PERSPECTIVE ON HUMAN MATING

Recognizing that all theories about the ancestral nature of human behavior are necessarily speculative, in what follows I attempt to show that the available evidence supports a very different evolutionary perspective on human mating.

The Normative Human Mating Pattern

Imagine that you have been assigned the task of figuring out which of several possible mating strategies characterize a particular species. Your best bet would be to adopt the traditional ethological approach—that is, simply observe what most members of that species actually do. In species where reproductive success requires nothing more than conception, you would likely observe sexual partners going their separate ways as soon as a viable pregnancy had been achieved—in some cases after a single copulatory sequence. But what would you observe if the species you'd been assigned to study were *Homo sapiens*? Variation, surely, but a species-typical pattern nonetheless: most human reproductive partners stay together for an extended period of time (Lancaster & Kaplan, 1994; Van den Berghe, 1979). And if they do eventually separate, the timing corresponds roughly to the duration of the human reproductive cycle including gestation, lactation, and weaning—that is, approximately 4 years (Fisher, 1989, 1992).

It has been hypothesized that the norm of extended associations between human mates evolved in response to a birthing crisis in which the infant's large head could not easily pass through the birth canal of our bipedal female ancestors (Trevathan, 1987; Washbum, 1960). Babies born prematurely, with less developed brains and correspondingly smaller heads, were more likely to survive. However, the effort required to adequately care for extremely dependent offspring during an exceptionally protracted period of immaturity made *paternal* investment an advantage, if not a necessity (Mellen, 1981; Small, 1995). Helpless and vulnerable human infants would have had greatly improved chances of surviving to reproductive age and developing the skills needed for their own eventual mating and parenting roles if fathers shared responsibility for protecting and socializing them. This posed a new adaptive problem: how to keep the parents together.

At the time this adaptive challenge arose, our species already had an evolved mechanism for fostering an enduring bond between two individuals: attachment (Bowlby, 1973, 1979, 1980, 1982, 1988). This mechanism helped ensure a survival-enhancing tie between infants and their mothers and it appears that the same mechanism was "exapted" (Gould & Vrba, 1982) for the new purpose of cementing a bond between reproductive partners. In fact, there is abundant evidence that the bond between mated pairs is a genuine attachment (Hazan & Zeifman, 1999).

The Nature of Pair Bond Relationships

Bowlby was very specific about the type of interpersonal relationship to which his theory applied. According to his definition, attachments have four distinguishing features, all of which are evident in behavior directed toward an attachment figure: seeking and maintaining physical proximity

(*proximity maintenance*), seeking aid or comfort (*safe haven*), being distressed by prolonged separations (*separation distress*), and using an attachment figure as a base of security for engaging in nonattachment activities (*secure base*).

An explicit proposition of attachment theory is that these behaviors, which in infancy are directed toward primary caregivers, are ultimately redirected toward a mate. Two empirical investigations have confirmed this prediction (Fraley & Davis, 1997; Hazan & Zeifman, 1994). Although it is not at all unusual for adults to maintain contact with a variety of individuals or to turn to them for comfort or assistance, most of these relationships do not meet the criteria of attachment. Those that do, by virtue of containing all four defining features, are almost exclusively formed with sexual partners. By this standard, mate relationships qualify as attachments in the technical sense.

Additional evidence that attachment is an integral part of human mating comes from the literature on bereavement. Bowlby's original inspiration for attachment theory was his observation that infants and children separated from their primary caregivers exhibit a universal sequence of responses that unfold over time in an invariant order: *protest* (characterized by crying, clinging, anxiety, and search behavior), followed by *despair* (sleep disruptions, reduced appetite, inactivity, and depression), and eventually *detachment* (evident upon reunion in the form of emotional and/or physical distancing from caregivers). Several studies have documented the same pattern of responses in adults grieving the loss of a long-term partner, but not the loss of other kinds of social connections (Fraley & Shaver, 1999; Hazan & Shaver, 1992; Parkes & Weiss, 1983; Weiss, 1975). Even brief, routine marital separations are enough to trigger a less intense but essentially identical pattern of reactions (Vormbrock, 1993). Thus, in this sense also, pair bonds qualify as attachments.

It is well documented that attachments have unique and powerful effects on overall functioning. Human infants, like the young of many other primate species, suffer lasting consequences if they are not given an opportunity to bond with an attachment figure or if an established bond is disrupted (Harlow & Harlow, 1965; Kraemer, 1997; Robertson, 1953; Spitz, 1946; Suomi, 1997). Although adults are clearly less dependent on an attachment figure for basic survival, there is abundant evidence that they also incur benefits from having one and are at significantly increased risk for numerous physical and psychological problems if they do not. For example, divorce is associated with an increased likelihood of admission to a psychiatric facility, suicide, alcoholism and other types of substance abuse, as well as impaired functioning of the cardiac, endocrine, and immune systems (e.g., Goodwin, Hurt, Key, & Sarret, 1987; Lynch, 1977; Uchino, Cacioppo, & Kiecolt-Glaser, 1996). The severing of any valued interpersonal relationship can be quite painful, but such losses have not been found to jeopardize physical and psychological well-being to the same degree as the loss of a mate relationship. Notably, it is *men* who benefit most from an attachment relationship and men who suffer the most ill effects when an attachment is disrupted (Bloom, Asher, & White, 1978).

Further evidence that the attachment mechanism is operative in human mating is the type of physical contact that distinguishes attachments from other kinds of social relationships. Our first experiences of physical intimacy are with caregivers during infancy. That's when we are initiated into the pleasures of cuddling, kissing, nuzzling, sucking, mutual gazing, and skin-to-skin, ventro–ventral contact. The frequency of this type of contact between infant and caregiver decreases over the first few of years of life. As children get older, parents touch them less often and less intimately (McAnarney, 1990). Not until puberty, and in the context of a romantic/sexual relationship, does one again experience such intimate social contact. In fact, this constellation of privileged interpersonal exchanges is universally observed in only two types of relationships: infant–caregiver and adult sexual/romantic pairings (Eibl-Eibesfeldt, 1975). Not coincidentally, this kind of physical contact is known to foster attachment.

The effects of intimate physical contact appear to have the same chemical basis in adult mates and in mother–infant pairs (for a review, see Insel, 2000). Oxytocin, the endogenous hormone that triggers labor in pregnant women and milk letdown in nursing mothers, promotes infant attachment as well as maternal caregiving by inducing a state of contentment and stimulating a desire for continued physical closeness. This hormonal system is also activated by sexual contact. In both male and female lovers, oxytocin builds with sexual stimulation and arousal, and has been implicated in the cuddling or "afterplay" that often follows sexual intercourse (Carter, 1992, 1998). As was famously demonstrated by Harlow (1958), cuddling or contact comfort is crucial for the establishment of attachment bonds. If sexual contact triggers release of a hormone that increases desire for bond-promoting contact, it thereby effectively increases the chances that a mating pair will become emotionally attached.

Several features of human sexuality further enhance the likelihood that an enduring bond will develop between reproductive partners. One of the striking differences between our reproductive physiology and that of most other primates is the absence of outward signs of estrus. In contrast to the vast majority of their mammalian counterparts, human females are able to have sex throughout their cycles despite the fact that conception can occur only during a brief period. Males of many species guard their mates during phases of receptivity so as to ensure paternity. When the fertile period has passed, they can safely move on to the next receptive female. But if ovulation is not overt, making it impossible for them to know just when fertilization is possible, a different strategy is more successful. One obvious solution to the adaptive problem posed by hidden ovulation is for a male to remain with the same female for a more extended period of time (Alcock, 1989).

Genital differences between us and other primates are also consistent with the view that human sexual interaction fosters pair bonding. For example, the exceptional length, thickness, and flexibility of the human penis relative to that of other great apes (Eberhard, 1985, 1991) made possible a wider variety of copulatory positions, including more intimate, face-to-face, bond-promoting ones. The large male penis may also directly enhance reproductive success by heightening female readiness for sexual activity (Miller, 1998).

Penis size alone is not an accurate predictor of monogamous versus polygamous mating patterns among primates, nor is our species unique in such reproductive characteristics as hidden ovulation, female orgasm, or face-to-face copulation (Blaffer-Hrdy, 1988). Nevertheless, multiple features of human sexual anatomy and physiology support the view that we have an evolved propensity to bond with our reproductive partners.

For anyone familiar with SST, facts like these may be somewhat surprising. If men have an innate predisposition to favor one-time sexual encounters with as many different fertile females as they can woo, why would so many evolved features of human mating be so conducive to more extended associations between reproductive partners? The answer, I would argue, is that males and females benefit equally from pair bonding—at least in terms of reproductive success.

Reproductive Advantages of Pair Bonding

One benefit of human mates remaining together and investing in their joint offspring is a lower rate of infant mortality (Hill & Hurtado, 1995). But pair bonding conveys reproductive advantages beyond the survival of infants. For example, women ovulate more often and more regularly within the context of a stable sexual partnership (Cutler, Garcia, Huggins, & Preti, 1986; Veith, Buck, Getzlaf, Van Dalfsen, & Slade, 1983). They also continue ovulating longer and reach menopause significantly later. Thus, female fertility itself is enhanced by pair bonding. As was noted previously, individuals of both sexes who are in long-term mating relationships enjoy more robust physical and mental health. This leaves them better able to function in all of the various reproduction-related roles that adults are called upon to fill, including those of parent and grandparent, thereby enhancing reproductive success.

In addition, there is considerable evidence that the offspring of stable pairs are better equipped to attract and retain their own mates. For example, adolescents from father-absent homes reach sexual maturation earlier and have less interest in long-term relationships than do their counterparts in father-present homes (Draper & Belsky, 1990; Draper & Harpending,

1982; Surbey, 1990). In addition, pair bond instability is associated with lower socioeconomic status (Lillard & Gerner, in press), fears of intimacy, and a lack of achievement orientation in offspring (Wallerstein, 1994). Recall Miller and Fishkin's (1997) study on the ideal number of future sexual partners. The few subjects who skewed the male distribution by reporting a desire for large numbers of sex partners were disproportionately insecure in their attachments, especially to their *fathers*.

Does all this imply that humans are "naturally" monogamous? The answer depends on one's definition of *monogamy*. The term means one thing in colloquial usage and quite another in the science of animal behavior. Monogamy, in the lexicon of human couples, usually implies an agreement not to have sex with other people. By this definition, a significant number of men and women would fail the test. In the field of ethology a species can be classified as monogamous if mates jointly invest in their offspring, spend time in close proximity outside the estrus period, and/or exhibit distress when separated (Dewsbury, 1987). Note that sexual exclusivity is *not* part of the definition. In fact, DNA analyses of offspring provide objective evidence that extra-pair copulations are not uncommon in species that by all criteria qualify as monogamous (Carter et al., 1997; Mendoza & Mason, 1997).

At some point in human evolution, pair bonding became the norm. It is of course possible that this normative pattern is nothing more than a culturally prescribed arrangement, universally preferred because it is so conducive to social stability and so supportive of familial economic interests. I think a far more plausible explanation, based on the available evidence, is that pair bonding evolved as a sex-indifferent pathway to reproductive success for a species whose young fare best with two investing parents.

A Mechanism to Foster Pair Bonding

An enduring emotional bond between any two individuals takes time to develop. In infant–caregiver relationships, it requires an average of 6–8 months of interaction before a full-blown attachment containing all four defining features is in place (Ainsworth, Blehar, Waters, & Wall, 1978; Bowlby, 1982). The infant's immaturity and vulnerability, coupled with the caregiver's nurturing instincts, help ensure that the two will have the kind of intimate physical contact that promotes bonding. But for less vulnerable adults, a different psychological mechanism would have been needed to hold pairs together long enough for an attachment to form.

To function effectively, this mechanism would have to accomplish several things. First, it would need to engender a single-minded focus on the partner at hand, to the exclusion of other potential mates. Second, it would need to be present in both sexes and operate as strongly, if not more so, in males as in females. Third, it would have to promote and sustain a strong desire for the type of physical contact that fosters attachment. In fact, there is a psychological mechanism that has all of these features; it's known as *romantic infatuation*.

In the largest and most systematic investigation of romantic infatuation, Tennov (1979) analyzed the contents of questionnaire and interview responses of hundreds of men and women. Among the more important findings to emerge was that this highly common phenomenon is characterized by a common and distinctive set of features. In addition to a reduction in sleep and appetite, and a paradoxical increase in energy, the symptoms include mental preoccupation, idealization, and intense longing for intimate physical contact with the target person. Leibowitz (1983) hypothesized that the physiological arousal and idealization that typify romantic infatuation are mediated by phenylethylamine (PEA), an endogenous amphetamine that has mild hallucinogenic effects.

Whatever the source of these symptoms, they seem to strike men and women with equal intensity and frequency. This fact poses a serious challenge for SST. If males have a hard-wired preference for and stand to gain substantial reproductive advantage from short-term mating, why would they be so susceptible to falling in love with the female targets of their attraction? It fits easily within a pair-bonding model but is more difficult to explain from an SST perspective.

Infatuation can drastically alter social perceptions. Take, for example, physical attractiveness. This is a quality that can be defined objectively, and has been in several empirical studies. Nevertheless, how physically attractive one perceives another to be depends in large part on how one feels about that person. Murstein (1976) demonstrated this effect in a study in which married couples were asked to rate the physical attractiveness of their respective spouses. Eighty-five percent of the husbands rated their wives as above-average on looks, although fewer than 25% were judged to be above-average in physical attractiveness by a panel of judges using the same rating scales. It is usually assumed that a woman is desired because she is attractive. Murstein's findings show that the causal arrow can actually run in the opposite direction.

Another example of the influence of romantic infatuation on social perception comes from a study by Simpson, Gangestad, and Lerma (1990). Heterosexual subjects with steady dating partners rated opposite-sex age-mates as less physically and sexually attractive than did subjects without steady partners. The two groups did not differ, however, in their ratings of much older or much younger opposite-sex targets, suggesting that the effect was specific to potential mates. Given that the availability of attractive alternative partners constitutes one of the greatest threats to relationship stability (Rusbult, 1980, 1983), the power of idealization to simultaneously inflate perceptions of a mate's appeal and reduce the appeal of potential rivals underscores its importance in maintaining pair bonds.

Although romantic infatuation can explain why two people would engage in the kinds of intimate interaction that could lead them to become attached, it begs the question of how and why one *particular* individual becomes the sole focus of attention and passion. In other words, what triggers romantic infatuation? In one of the few mating studies to use subjects who actually had partners, Aron and colleagues (Aron, Dutton, Aron, & Iverson, 1989) discovered a possible answer. The approach involved asking subjects to provide detailed accounts of their falling-in-love experiences. According to the results, the factor primarily responsible for the shift from attraction to infatuation is reciprocal liking. Whether expressed in a warm smile or a prolonged gaze or any of a number of other flirtation signals, the message is unmistakable: "It's safe to approach. I'll be nice. You're not in danger of being rejected." Recall that when subjects are asked to make lists of their ideal mate qualities, a trait ranked among the highest by both males and females is kindness. In other words, they say they want a mate who will respond positively to them and treat them well. Reciprocal liking is a sign that they have found such a person. This signal of invitation from an attractive other appears to be enough to send most people head over heels. And for a significant number, it is sufficient to hold their interest until a more enduring bond develops. How long does that take? In adult pairs, approximately 2 years, give or take 6 months (Hazan & Zeifman, 1994). Not coincidentally, this time frame corresponds to the average duration of romantic infatuation (Tennov, 1979).

Mate "Selection"

According to SST, human mate selection is inherently strategic. Men and women are equipped with specific mate choice mechanisms that guide them toward the best available mates, adjusted for their own mate value. Other things being equal, a man should pursue the best-looking woman he believes he can get and a woman should go after the man with the highest status or most resources she feels she can attract. As noted previously, tests of SST predictions regarding mate selection typically involve asking subjects to describe the kind of partner they would someday like to have. The finding that males and females reliably differ in their relative rankings of physical appearance and status/resources is taken as support for the theory and, by implication, support for the notion that these are the criteria on which real-world mating decisions are based. But rankings of ideal partners in hypothetical mating scenarios, no matter how consistent within gender or across cultures, do not constitute sufficient evidence that these qualities figure into actual mate selection.

In the twin study described earlier, selection criteria were examined not by asking people what they desired in a mate, or what they thought would influence their choices, but instead by exploring the nature of actual pairings. The findings were not consistent with those from studies based on self-reported ideals, nor did they support predictions derived from SST. In fact, the pattern of pairings observed in this large sample of couples led the study authors to question whether human mate selection is strategic at all.

In the end, they concluded that human mating appears to be more "adventitious" than is generally assumed. That is, the true pool of eligibles may consist not of the individuals who best match some idealized list of qualities but instead those who, by happenstance, are under foot or under nose when one is looking to mate. In other words, *propinquity* could turn out to be a major factor in human mating. It not only affords opportunities for getting together but also provides a context for the kind of repeated exposure and prolonged association that increase *familiarity*, which itself fosters attraction (Rubin, 1973).

As every zookeeper knows, a nearly sure-fire way to get two members of any species to mate is simply to house them in the same cage. Why must it be different for *Homo sapiens*? In fact, it may not be different. One of the more robust findings about human mating is that most people end up with a mate who lives within walking distance (Eckland, 1968). But of course "lives within walking distance" or "conveniently located" are not qualities that people put on their mate wish lists. This is important for what it reveals about the evolution of mate selection processes in our species. The factors that exert the strongest influence may operate completely outside of conscious awareness, and therefore are unlikely to be discovered using self-report methods, no matter how many people from any number of corners of the world are asked.

Buss and Schmitt (1993) consider and then dismiss propinquity and familiarity theories on several grounds, including (1) they cannot be used to make specific predictions about mating; (2) they assume that the processes that guide human mating are the same for males and for females; and (3) they fail to specify the origins or functions of these mating influences.

But what if the processes that guide human mating *are* the same for males and females? It seems unjustified to fault a theory for not presuming sex differences. And what if, as the twin findings strongly suggest, human mate selection is not a strategic process? A theory's "failure" to make specific predictions about mate choice might not be a shortcoming so much as an acknowledgment of reality. And what if, as many anthropologists contend, our mating behaviors evolved in an environment characterized by small and relatively isolated social groups? It could mean that the average EEA dweller would not have had many mate options, and almost certainly not the wide range of options that typify the contemporary college student on whose mate preferences SST is largely based. It is quite possible that there was never strong selection pressure for the development of any specific mate choice mechanism in either sex.

Indeed, one could argue that a highly specific mechanism would actually be *maladaptive*. In human infants, the mental image of a suitable attachment figure is only schematic and can be engaged by almost any conspecific. Although babies are happiest and develop optimally when caregivers are consistently warm and responsive (Ainsworth et al., 1978; Bowlby, 1982), they nevertheless become fully attached to abusive caregivers (Crittenden, 1995) and even other children if adult figures are not available (Freud & Dann, 1951). Both Harlow (1958) and Lorenz (1935) demonstrated rather dramatically just how flexible the attachment mechanism is. And it makes very good sense for it to be flexible. Imagine how survival would be jeopardized if infants rejected any protector who failed to match some ideal of the perfect caregiver!

The search image for a suitable mate may also be inherently flexible. However, logic dictates that mating decisions cannot be completely random. Our species would have expired long ago had we not succeeded in choosing mates who were reproductively capable. But was this, as SST posits, a real *problem*? Earlier I cited evidence for a more than 90% fertility rate in the EEA. Under such conditions, it could have sufficed for our ancestors to avoid mating with those who (1) had not yet reached puberty and (2) showed signs of disease or advanced age (e.g., open sores, gross asymmetries, wrinkled skin, sagging body parts). The markers of puberty are easy enough to recognize to satisfy the first requirement; the innate disgust response could serve to satisfy the second.

What I am suggesting is that evolution equipped us with mate *rejection* as opposed to mate *selection* criteria. That is, our mating system may be designed to steer us away from poor choices rather than toward "ideal" ones. Clear skin and symmetrical features may not be as powerful attractants as open lesions and gross deformities are powerful repellants. To be in the running, a potential mate may simply need to surpass some threshold based on our own mate value and "window" of acceptability (Regan, 1998).

This speaks to the possible origins and functions of propinquity and familiarity. The effects of familiarity on attraction are thought to reflect an evolved tendency to respond favorably to individuals who have passed the friend-versus-foe test. As for propinquity, a cost–benefit evaluation would tend to favor mating with one who is readily accessible. It might be possible to find a marginally more attractive or higher status mate with a longer and wider search, but a small incremental change on either dimension would probably make little difference in the final (reproductive fitness) analysis.

SUMMARY AND CONCLUSIONS

Bonds between human mates and between infants and caregivers share key features that distinguish them from other kinds of social relationships. The time course and processes by which each type of bond develops are essentially the same. Separations evoke a similar emotional dynamic in both. The effects of each on individual physical and psychological well-being are similarly profound and pervasive. And so on. The evidence is abundant and compelling that both kinds of relationships are regulated by the same evolved mechanism: the attachment system.

Human reproductive success depended on solutions to the adaptive problems of surviving to reproductive age, mating, and then providing adequate care to offspring to ensure that they also reached sexual maturity and mated. Attachment was undoubtedly the mechanism that evolved to solve the first problem of survival through infancy and childhood. The second problem (mating) entails identifying and attracting someone fit to serve as a reproductive partner and coparent. For both men and women it forces consideration of a potential mate's suitability as an attachment figure, for self as well as for offspring. The attachment mechanism also helps solve the third adaptive problem by fostering a bond between reproductive partners that gives their progeny an edge in survival and the competition for mates.

That human males are more sexually promiscuous than females cannot be denied. Although strong arguments have been made on both sides of the nature–nurture debate, this appears to be a biologically based, hardwired difference between the sexes. Given that testosterone boosts libido in both, and males on average produce this hormone in much greater quantities than females, it follows that men would be more attuned to sexual cues and more responsive to sexual opportunities. But this difference, which is amplified by cross-cultural socialization practices, may have little if anything to add to our understanding of human mating. *If* we were a species whose parental investment ended with conception *and* the probability of conception following a single act of sexual intercourse was high, then *maybe* this sex difference would have important mating implications. But we are *not* one of those species.

Throughout this chapter I have presented evidence that men and women are more similar in their mating behavior than one would conclude from SST. According to a series of best-selling books, the sexes are so different that they might as well hail from different planets. I think a more accurate description was captured by a recent conference paper title: "Men Are from North Dakota, Women Are from South Dakota." Different? Yes, but not that different.

To understand human mating, we must go beyond fantasies and stereotypes and hypothetical scenarios to a thorough investigation of the processes by which mating relationships are established and what such relationships are really like. Attachment theory is widely accepted as a valid framework for examining parent–child relationships. It also has much to say about the essential nature of mate relationships, and therefore much to offer those wishing to help build, repair, and restore such bonds.

REFERENCES

Ainsworth, M. D. S., Blehar, M. C., Waters, E., & Wall, S. (1978). *Patterns of attachment: Assessed in the Strange Situation and at home.* Hillsdale, NJ: Erlbaum.

Alcock, J. (1989). *Animal behavior: An evolutionary approach.* Boston: Sinauer.

Aron, A., Dutton, D. G., Aron, E. N., & Iverson, A. (1989). Experiences of falling in love. *Journal of Social and Personal Relationships, 6,* 243–257.

Blaffer-Hrdy, S. (1988). The primate origins of human sexuality. In R. Bellig & G. Stevens (Eds.), *The evolution of sex* (pp. 101–131). San Francisco: Harper & Row.

Bloom, B. L., Asher, S. J., & White, S. W. (1978). Marital disruption as a stressor: A review and analysis. *Psychological Bulletin, 85,* 867–894.

Bowlby, J. (1973). *Attachment and loss: Vol. II. Separation: Anxiety and anger.* New York: Basic Books.

Bowlby, J. (1979). *The making and breaking of affectional bonds.* London: Tavistock.

Bowlby, J. (1980). *Attachment and loss: Vol. III. Loss: Sadness and depression.* New York: Basic Books.

Bowlby, J. (1982). *Attachment and loss: Vol. I. Attachment* (2nd ed.). New York: Basic Books. (First edition published in 1969)

Bowlby, J. (1988). *A secure base: Parent–child attachment and healthy human development.* New York: Basic Books.

Buss, D. M. (1989). Sex differences in human mate preferences: Evolutionary hypotheses tested in 37 cultures. *Behavioral and Brain Sciences, 12,* 1–49.

Buss, D. M., Abbott, M., & Angleitner, A. (1990). International preferences in seeking mates: A study of 37 cultures. *Journal of Cross-Cultural Psychology, 21,* 5–47.

Buss, D. M., & Schmitt, D. P. (1993). Sexual strategies theory: An evolutionary perspective on human mating. *Psychological Review, 100,* 204–232.

Carter, C. S. (1992). Oxytocin and sexual behavior. *Neuroscience and Biobehavioral Reviews, 16,* 131–144.

Carter, C. S. (1998). Neuroendocrine perspectives on attachment and love. *Psychoneuroendocrinology, 23,* 779–818.

Carter, C. S., DeVries, A. C., Taymans, S. E., Roberts, R. L., Williams, J. R., & Getz, L. L. (1997). Peptides, steroids, and pair bonding. *Annals of the New York Academy of Sciences, 807,* 260–272.

Crittenden, P. M. (1995). Attachment and psychopathology. In S. Goldberg, R. Muir, & J. Kerr (Eds.), *Attachment theory: Social, developmental, and clinical perspectives* (pp. 367–406). Hillsdale, NJ: Analytic Press.

Cunningham, M. R., Druen, P. B., & Barbee, A. P. (1997). Angels, mentors, and friends: Trade-offs among evolutionary, social, and individual variables in physical appearance. In J. A. Simpson & D. T. Kenrick (Eds.), *Evolutionary social psychology* (pp. 109–140). Mahwah, NJ: Erlbaum.

Cutler, W. B., Garcia, C. R., Huggins, G. R., & Preti, G. (1986). Sexual behavior and steroid levels among gynecologically mature premenopausal women. *Fertility and Sterility, 45,* 496–502.

Dewsbury, D. A. (1987). The comparative psychology of monogamy. In D. W. Leger (Ed.), *Nebraska Symposium on Motivation* (Vol. 35, pp. 6–43). Lincoln: University of Nebraska Press.

Draper, P., & Belsky, J. (1990). Personality development in evolutionary perspective. *Journal of Personality, 58,* 141–161.

Draper, P., & Harpending, H. (1982). A sociobiological perspective on the development of human reproductive strategies. In K. MacDonald (Ed.), *Sociobiological perspectives on human development* (pp. 340–372). New York: Springer-Verlag.

Eberhard, W. G. (1985). *Sexual selection and animal genitalia.* Cambridge, MA: Harvard University Press.

Eberhard, W. G. (1991). Copulatory courtship and cryptic female choice in insects. *Biological Review, 66,* 1–31.

Eckland, B. K. (1968). Theories of mate selection. *Eugenics Quarterly, 15,* 71–84.

Eibl-Eibesfeldt, I. (1975). *Ethology: The biology of behavior.* New York: Holt, Rinehart & Winston.

Fisher, H. E. (1989). Evolution in human serial pair bonding. *American Journal of Physical Anthropology, 73,* 331–354.

Fisher, H. E. (1992). *Anatomy of love.* New York: Norton.

Fraley, R. C., & Davis, K. E. (1997). Attachment formation and transfer in young adults' close friendships and romantic relationships. *Personal Relationships, 4,* 131–144.

Fraley, R. C., & Shaver, P. R. (1999). Loss and bereavement: Attachment theory and recent controversies concerning "grief work" and the nature of detachment. In J. Cassidy & P. R. Shaver (Eds.), *Handbook of attachment: Theory, research, and clinical applications* (pp. 735–759). New York: Guilford Press.

Freud, A., & Dann, S. (1951). An experiment in group upbringing. In R. Eisler et al. (Eds.), *The psychoanalytic study of the child* (Vol. 6, pp. 127–168). New York: International Universities Press.

Goodwin, J. S., Hurt, W. C., Key, C. R., & Sarret, J. M. (1987). The effect of marital status on stage, treatment and survival of cancer patients. *Journal of the American Medical Association, 258,* 3125–3130.

Gould, S. J., & Vrba, E. S. (1982). Exaptation—A missing term in the science of form. *Paleobiology, 8,* 4–15.

Harlow, H. F. (1958). The nature of love. *American Psychologist, 13,* 673–685.

Harlow, H. F., & Harlow, M. K. (1965). The affectional systems. In A. M. Schrier, H. F. Harlow, & F. Stollnitz (Eds.), *Behavior of nonhuman primates* (Vol. 2, pp. 287–334). New York: Academic Press.

Hazan, C., & Shaver, P. R. (1992). Broken attachments. In T. L. Orbuch (Ed.), *Close relationship loss: Theoretical approaches* (pp. 90–108). Hillsdale, NJ: Erlbaum.

Hazan, C., & Shaver, P. R. (1994a). Attachment as an organizational framework for research on close relationships. *Psychological Inquiry, 5,* 1–22.

Hazan, C., & Shaver, P. R. (1994b). Deeper into attachment theory. *Psychological Inquiry, 5,* 68–79.

Hazan, C., & Zeifman, D. (1994). Sex and the psychological tether. *Advances in Personal Relationships, 5,* 151–177.

Hazan, C., & Zeifman, D. (1999). Pair bonds as attachments: Evaluating the evidence. In J. Cassidy & P. R. Shaver (Eds.), *Handbook of attachment theory, research and clinical applications* (pp. 336–354). New York: Guilford Press.

Hill, K., & Hurtado, M. (1995). *Demographic/life history of Ache foragers.* New York: Aldine de Gruyter.

Insel, T. R. (2000). Toward a neurobiology of attachment. *Review of General Psychology, 4,* 176–185.

Kalick, S. M., Zebrowitz, L. A., Langlois, J. H., & Johnson, R. M. (1998). Does human facial attractiveness honestly advertise health?: Longitudinal data on an evolutionary question. *Psychological Science, 9*, 8–13.

Kasser, T., & Sharma, Y. S. (1999). Reproductive freedom, educational equality, and females' preference for resource-acquisition characteristics in mates. *Psychological Science, 10*, 374–377.

Kraemer, G. W. (1997). Psychobiology of early social attachment in rhesus monkeys. In S. Carter, I. Lederhendler, & B. Kirkpatrick (Eds.), *The integrative neurobiology of affiliation: Vol. 807. Annals of the New York Academy of Sciences* (pp. 401–418).

Lancaster, J. B., & Kaplan, H. (1994). Human mating and family formation strategies: The effects of variability among males in quality and the allocation of mating effort and parental investment. In T. Nishida, W. C. McGrew, P. Marler, M. Pickford, & F. B. M. de Waal (Eds.), *Topics in primatology, Vol. 1: Human origins* (pp. 21–33). Tokyo: University of Tokyo Press.

Leibowitz, M. (1983). *The chemistry of love.* New York: Berkeley Books.

Lillard, D., & Gerner, J. (in press). Getting to the Ivy League: How family composition affects college choice. *Journal of Higher Education.*

Lorenz, K. E. (1935). Der Kumpan in der Umvelt des Vogels. In C. H. Schiller (Ed.), *Instinctive behavior.* New York: International Universities Press.

Lykken, D. T., & Tellegen, A. (1993). Is human mating adventitious or the result of lawful choice?: A twin study of mate selection. *Journal of Personality and Social Psychology, 65*, 56–68.

Lynch, J. J. (1977). *The broken heart: The medical consequences of loneliness.* New York: Basic Books.

McAnarney, E. R. (1990). Adolescents and touch. In K. E. Barnard & T. B. Brazelton (Eds.), *Touch: The foundation of experience* (pp. 497–515). Madison, WI: International Universities Press.

Mendoza, S. P., & Mason, W. A. (1997). Attachment relationships in new world primates. In S. Carter, I. Lederhendler, & B. Kirkpatrick (Eds.), *The integrative neurobiology of affiliation: Vol. 807. Annals of the New York Academy of Sciences* (pp. 203–209).

Mellen, S. L. W. (1981). *The evolution of love.* Oxford, UK: Freeman.

Miller, G. F. (1998). How mate choice shaped human nature: A review of sexual selection and human evolution. In C. Crawford & D. L. Krebs (Eds.), *Handbook of evolutionary psychology: Ideas, issues, and applications* (pp. 87–129). Mahwah, NJ: Erlbaum.

Miller, L. C., & Fishkin, S. A. (1997). On the dynamics of human bonding and reproductive success: Seeking windows on the adapted-for human–environment interface. In J. A. Simpson & D. T. Kenrick (Eds.), *Evolutionary social psychology* (pp.197–235). Mahwah, NJ: Erlbaum.

Murstein, B. I. (1976). *Who will marry whom?: Theories and research in marital choice.* New York: Springer.

Parkes, C. M., & Weiss, R. S. (1983). *Recovery from bereavement.* New York: Basic Books.

Regan, P. C. (1998). What if you can't get what you want?: Willingness to compromise ideal mate selection standards as a function of sex, mate value, and relationship context. *Personality and Social Psychology Bulletin, 24*, 1294–1303.

Robertson, J. (1953). Some responses of young children to the loss of maternal care. *Nursing Times, 49*, 382–386.

Rubin, Z. (1973). *Liking and loving*. New York: Holt, Rinehart & Winston.

Rusbult, C. E. (1980). A longitudinal test of the investment model: The development (and deterioration) of satisfaction and commitment in heterosexual involvements. *Journal of Personality and Social Psychology, 45*, 101–117.

Rusbult, C. E. (1983). Commitment and satisfaction in romantic associations: A test of the investment mode. *Journal of Experimental Social Psychology, 16*, 172–186.

Simpson, J. A., Gangestad, S. W., & Lerma, M. (1990). Perception of physical attractiveness: Mechanisms involved in the maintenance of romantic relationships. *Journal of Personality and Social Psychology, 59*, 1192–1201.

Small, M. F. (1995). *What's love got to do with it? The evolution of human mating*. New York: Anchor Books.

Spitz, R. A. (1946). Anaclitic depression. *Psychoanalytic Study of the Child, 2*, 313–342.

Suomi, S. J. (1997). Early determinants of behaviour: Evidence from primate studies. *British Medical Bulletin, 53*, 170–184.

Surbey, M. (1990). Family composition, stress, and human menarche. In F. Bercovitch & T. Zeigler (Eds.), *The socioendocrinology of primate reproduction* (pp. 71–97). New York: Liss.

Symons, D. (1979). *The evolution of human sexuality*. New York: Oxford University Press.

Tennov, D. (1979). *Love and limerence: The experience of being in love*. New York: Stein & Day.

Trevathan, W. (1987). *Human birth*. New York: Aldine de Gruyter.

Uchino, B. N., Cacioppo, J. T., & Kiecolt-Glaser, J. K. (1996). The relationship between social support and physiological processes: A review with emphasis on underlying mechanisms and implications for health. *Psychological Bulletin, 119*, 488–531.

Van den Berghe, P. L. (1979). *Human family systems: An evolutionary view*. Westport, CT: Greenwood Press.

Veith, J. L., Buck, M., Getzlaf, S., Van Dalfsen, P., & Slade, S. (1983). Exposure to men influences the occurrence of ovulation in women. *Physiology and Behavior, 31*, 313–315.

Vormbrock, J. K. (1993). Attachment theory as applied to war-time and job-related marital separation. *Psychological Bulletin, 114*, 122–144.

Wallerstein, J. S. (1994). Children after divorce: Wounds that don't heal. In L. Fenson & J. Fenson (Eds.), *Human development* (Vols. 94–95, pp. 160–165). Guilford, CT: Dushkin.

Washbum, S. L. (1960). Tools and human evolution. *Scientific American, 203*, 3–15.

Weiss, R. S. (1975). *Marital separation*. New York: Basic Books.

Zimmerman, S. J., Maude, M. B., & Moldawar, M. (1965). Frequent ejaculation and total sperm count, motility and forms in humans. *Fertility and Sterility, 16*, 342–345.

4

Stability and Change of Attachment Representations from Cradle to Grave

ELAINE SCHARFE

Tempora mutantur, et nos mutamur in illis [Times change, and we change with them].

—ANONYMOUS

Plus ça change, plus c'est la même chose [The more things change, the more they are the same].

—ALPHONSE KARR

The controversy about whether personality is consistent over time has influenced thought in both popular culture and academic circles (see Epstein, 1980; Mischel, 1969). Recently this controversy has made its way into the field of attachment. Originally, Bowlby (1982) proposed that once formed, internal working models of attachment would remain relatively stable across the lifespan. Subsequently, researchers have expanded the discussion of the properties of relationships and proposed that *lessons* learned in previous relationships often inform the patterns carried forward to current relationships (Caspi & Elder, 1979; Hinde, 1979). Attachment researchers maintain that attachment representations are relatively stable across both time and place, that attachment behavior is organized and coherent, and that it is reasonable to expect particular attachment behaviors to be consistent for particular individuals. However, Bowlby (1982) also discussed changes in attachment. In particular, he highlighted that, when necessary, changes in attachment models and behaviors were not only likely in reaction to particularly traumatic events but also adaptive. Therefore, the processes of stability and change are important to explore to completely understand Bowlby's theory. This chapter summarizes the empirical literature exploring the stability and change of attachment representations across the lifespan. The summary begins with an outline of the work in infancy and continues through to adulthood, concluding with the most recent work exploring stability over decades, a discussion of areas for future research, and the implications of this work for clinicians.

STABILITY IN INFANCY

> What, it may be asked, is the degree of stability of the pattern and of its two components, the child's attachment behaviour and the mother's caregiving behaviour? The answers to these questions are complex.
> —BOWLBY (1982, p. 348)

Although little work has explored the stability of parental caregiving, considerable research has demonstrated that mother–infant attachment categories (i.e., secure, anxious–resistant, avoidant, disorganized) show moderate to high stability when infants' caregiving experiences are stable. Furthermore, many studies have explored the influence of variables that Bowlby (1982) originally suggested might produce change (e.g., negative life events, depression, birth of a sibling). In one of the first studies to explore the stability of infant attachment, Waters (1978) found that 96% of the infants in his sample were judged to have the same attachment category at 12 and 18 months (see Table 4.1 for a summary of stability of infant and child attachment). However, Waters (1978) deliberately chose his sample to demonstrate stability when environments were stable. To date, researchers have reported considerably lower stability in infants experiencing a wide range of circumstances.

Several researchers have found significant associations between caregiving and change in infant attachment categories. For example, Egeland and Sroufe (1981) reported that children who received inadequate care tended to become avoidantly attached. Furthermore, children tended to become secure when their caregiving experiences changed to include a supportive other (e.g., grandmother) or their mothers reported a reduction of stressful life events. Vaughn, Egeland, Sroufe, and Waters (1979) also found that mothers of infants who changed from secure to anxious attachment reported more stressful life events than mothers of infants who remained secure. Similarly, Thompson, Lamb, and Estes (1982) reported that infant at-

TABLE 4.1. Stability of Infant and Childhood Attachment Categories

	n	Ages[a]	% stable
Atkinson et al. (1999)	40	26 and 42 months	62%
Bar-Haim et al. (2000)	42	14 to 24 months	64%
	43	14 to 58 months	42%
	45	24 to 58 months	38%
	42	14, 24, and 58 months	29%
Barnett et al. (1999)[b]	39	12 and 18 months	64%
	36	18 and 24 months	69%
	36	12 and 24 months	69%
Belsky et al. (1996)			
Mother–infant	125	12 and 18 months	52%
Father–infant	120	13 and 20 months	46%
Depressed mothers	90	12 and 18 months	46%
Egeland & Farber (1984)	189	12 and 18 months	60%
Egeland & Sroufe (1981)			
Excellent care	32	12 and 18 months	81%
Inadequate care	25	12 and 18 months	48%
Goossens et al. (1986)			
Lab–lab	9	17.6 and 18.7 months	100%
Home–home	10	17.5 and 18.6 months	90%
Home–lab	9	18.4 and 19.3 months	33%
Lab–home	11	17.9 and 18.9 months	55%
Howes and Hamilton (1992)	106	12 and 48 months	71%
Main and Cassidy (1988)			
Mother–child[c]	32	12 and 72 months	84%
Father–child	33	12 and 72 months	61%
Test–retest sample	50	72 and 73 months	76%
Main and Weston (1981)			
Mother–infant	15	12 and 20 months	73%
Father–infant	15	12 and 20 months	87%
NICHD Early Child Care Research Network (2001)	1060	15 and 36 months	46%
Owen et al. (1984)			
Mother–infant	59	12 and 20 months	78%
Father–child	53	12 and 20 months	62%
Rauh et al. (2000)	70	12 and 21 months	64%
Thompson et al. (1982)	43	12.5 and 19.5 months	53%
Touris et al. (1993)			
Transition group	20	16.3 and 21 months	40%
Nontransition group	20	17.6 and 21.5 months	80%
Vaughn et al. (1979)	100	12 and 18 months	62%

(continued)

TABLE 4.1. (*continued*)

	n	Ages[a]	% stable
Vondra et al. (1999)[d]	90	12 and 18 months	54%
Vondra et al. (2001)	195	12 and 18 months	45%
	145	12/18 and 24 months	45%
Wartner et al. (1994)[e]	40	12 and 72 months	88%
Waters (1978)	50	12 and 18 months	96%

Note. Unless indicated all studies assessed mother–infant attachment, used Ainsworth's Strange Situation, and scored attachment behavior according to Ainsworth's original three-category model (secure, anxious–avoidant, anxious–resistant).
[a]Ages represent average age of children during each assessment of attachment.
[b]Results are based on a four-category system. Stability of three categories was lower (64% vs. 54%).
[c]Stability results including the disorganized category were considerably lower (62%).
[d]Stability results including the disorganized category were similar (50%).
[e]Stability results including the disorganized category were similar (82%).

tachment was likely to change when infants experienced a change in caregiving (e.g., maternal employment and/or change in childcare). These infants, however, were just as likely to change from secure to insecure as from insecure to secure, thereby suggesting that both the event and how infants' caregivers dealt with the event were important variables to understand the direction of change.

Egeland and Farber (1984) and Vondra, Hommerding, and Shaw (1999) continued the examination of the influence of maternal characteristics on change of attachment. Both groups assessed mother–infant attachment at 12 and 18 months, as well as a number of maternal and infant characteristics and life experiences. The researchers compared infants who remained stable with infants who had changed and found that some changes could be explained. In both studies, mothers of infants who were judged to have stable security reported significantly lower scores on aggression and suspicion and fewer disruptions in the family than the other groups. Both studies emphasized the effect of parents' negative emotions (e.g., aggression, suspiciousness, anger) on the development and maintenance of attachment insecurity. For example, mothers of children who changed from secure to insecure (either avoidant or anxious–resistant) reported higher scores on pre- and/or postnatal assessments of aggression, anger expression and control, and suspiciousness. Vondra et al. (1999) included the disorganized category and found that mothers of infants who were classified as disorganized at 18 months reported the highest scores on aggression and suspiciousness. Interestingly, mothers of infants who changed toward disorganization reported the most disruption to the family; however, despite their chaotic lives, these mothers reported the least expressed anger and the most anger control, and insisted that they were "people who do not get angry" (p. 138).

Consistent with previous research, both studies also found that change in caregiving ability and living arrangements were also found to be predictive of change in infant attachment. Mothers of infants who changed toward security were more likely to report that this was their first child, that they were living with a romantic partner, and that they had relatively high relationship satisfaction, with few disruptions to the family (Egeland & Farber, 1984; Vondra et al., 1999). Vondra et al. suggested that these primarily first-time mothers were adjusting, albeit successfully, to parenthood over their children's first 18 months. Egeland and Farber summarized that "in almost every instance of change from anxious to secure attachment, there was some indication of the mother becoming more relaxed, 'less anxious and depressed,' and in general, more confident in dealing with her infant" (1984, pp. 766–767). Together these results clearly support Bowlby's proposal that life events, in particular events that influence parents' ability to care for the infant, may be important predictors of change. Consequently, researchers have begun to explore changes in security during common family life events.

It is increasingly more common for children to experience nonfamilial care in their first few years of life. Owen, Easterbrooks, Chase-Lansdale, and Goldberg (1984) explored the influence of maternal employment on the stability of attachment for both mothers and fathers. They reported moderate to high stability and, with one exception, found no evidence that maternal employment disrupted the quality of parent–child attachment. The one exception was that changes toward insecure father–infant attachment were most likely to occur when mothers returned to work for the first time during children's second year. The authors proposed that this interesting, but unexplained, finding suggests that the manner in which the parent(s) prepare for family transitions may be associated with stability or change of attachment. Recently, two studies have found support for this proposal (NICHD Early Child Care Research Network, 2001; Rauh, Ziegenhain, Müller, & Wignroks, 2000). Rauh et al. (2000) reported moderate to high stability. Furthermore, they found that, without exception, all children who changed from secure at 12 months to insecure at 21 months experienced an abrupt introduction to daycare at about 12 months. Further support was recently reported in a larger study of the effects of childcare on attachment (NICHD Early Child Care Research Network, 2001). Researchers found that maternal sensitivity, not childcare experience, was a predictor of change toward security or insecurity. Clearly these studies provide support for the proposal that stability or change in attachment following a relatively common life event (i.e., mothers returning to work) can be explained by examining how sensitively families manage the new situation.

Both Bowlby (1982) and Ainsworth and colleagues (Ainsworth, Blehar,

Waters, & Wall, 1978) proposed that maternal sensitivity was linked to the development of attachment (see Atkinson et al., 2000, for recent meta-analysis); however, to date, only one study has simultaneously explored the stability of both mother–infant attachment and maternal sensitivity. Vereijken, Riksen-Walraven, and Kondo-Ikemura (1997) rated both maternal sensitivity and security of attachment in a sample of Japanese mothers and their infants (at 14 and 24 months). They found a significant association between maternal sensitivity and attachment within time (e.g., sensitivity at 14 months was significantly associated with attachment at 14 months). However, these relationships were not consistently significant across time (e.g., sensitivity at 14 months was not associated with attachment at 24 months). Furthermore, they determined that maternal sensitivity, but not infant attachment security, was stable over time. Their results provide further support that changes in maternal sensitivity may directly influence change in attachment and suggest that changes in maternal sensitivity are more powerful predictors of change of attachment than perhaps currently believed. This interpretation is supported by recent work implementing attachment-based interventions to at-risk insecure parents (see Lieberman & Zeanah, 1999, for a review).

Although little work has explored the stability of parental sensitivity, a few studies have explored change of attachment during common family life transitions in which one might expect changes in the level of sensitivity. Touris, Kromelow, and Harding (1993) explored changes in firstborn children's attachment to their mother after the arrival of a sibling. Attachment was assessed 2–3 months before and 6–10 weeks after the birth of a sibling. Touris et al. found a high degree of change in the transition group. Interestingly, infants were just as likely to change from secure to insecure as from insecure to secure, suggesting that the birth of the second child may bring positive or negative effects for the mother–firstborn child relationship. Teti, Sakin, Kucera, and Eiden (1996) replicated these findings in a larger sample ($n = 188$). Although they reported a high correlation between time 1 and time 2 security scores ($r = .71$), they noted a significant effect for age: children older than 24 months experienced more distress and greater decrease in attachment security than children younger than 24 months. Mothers of children who scored below the average security score at both time points ($n = 20$) functioned poorly on indices of psychosocial functioning. Furthermore, mothers of children who experienced a decrease in security ($n = 23$) reported increasing psychiatric symptoms over the transition. Mothers of children who maintained their attachment security after the birth of a sibling (n = 48) consistently reported low levels of psychiatric symptoms and high levels of marital harmony and affective involvement with the firstborn child. In summary, both studies found that mother–infant attachment was likely to change soon after the birth of the second child. In each study, attachment was assessed soon after the birth and it is yet to be determined if these observed changes in attachment are temporary or permanent; some firstborns may have been temporarily stressed by the arrival of their sibling.

Compared to the number of studies exploring the stability of mother–infant attachment, the stability of father–infant attachment has been virtually ignored. In a small sample, Main and Weston (1981) reported high stability of father–infant attachment and moderate concordance with mother–infant attachment categories. As discussed above, Owen et al. (1984) reported moderate stability. In a larger sample of father–son dyads, Belsky, Campbell, Cohn, and Moore (1996) reported low to moderate stability. Therefore, the degree of stability (ranging from 46% to 87%) is consistent with work examining stability of mother–infant attachment; however, much more work is needed to explore the variables that influence change of father–infant attachment.

To date, only one study has explored the stability of attachment in different contexts. However, the results suggest that context is an important consideration when interpreting stability results. Goossens, van IJzendoorn, Tavecchio, and Kroonenberg (1986) found that stability of attachment classification over 1 month was influenced by the context in which the Strange Situation was administered. Mother–infant dyads who were tested in the same context (i.e., home or lab) twice over 1 month were found to be highly stable, whereas dyads who were tested in different contexts displayed low to moderate stability. The results of this study suggest that changes in methodology might dramatically reduce observed stability. For example, with repeated administrations of the Strange Situation, how might the use of different *strangers* or *rooms* influence stability findings? Interestingly, although this study was published almost two decades ago, the hypothesis that changes in procedure might greatly influence stability has yet to be fully explored.

In summary, research exploring mother–infant attachment has found that approximately 65% of infants are classified in the same category at two points in time. Several studies have found that increased quality of care was associated with changes from insecure to secure attachment (e.g., Egeland & Farber, 1984; Rauh et al., 2000; Vondra et al., 1999). Correspondingly, decreases in quality of care have been found to be associated with changes from secure to insecure attachment (Egeland & Sroufe, 1981; Vaughn et al., 1979; Vondra et al., 1999). Despite many studies examining the stability of mother–infant attachment and the variables that influence change, research is required to determine which factors influence stability of father–infant attachment. Furthermore, discordance of attachment over time with one parent may be better understood if researchers examined the influence of both parents (cf. Fonagy, Steele, & Steele, 1991). For example, Owen et al. (1984) found that for some families the mothers' decision to return to work influenced father–infant attachment. Finally, researchers have yet to determine how life events influence the reorganization of attachment and whether particular events have more or less impact depending on when they occur. For example, older children were more distressed at the birth of a sibling and more likely to experience a drop in security scores (Teti et al., 1996). Perhaps changes in attachment are more likely during the acquisition of developmental milestones (e.g., increased cognitive abilities). It is likely that these co-occurring interpersonal and developmental changes may increase children's stress to a level that is unmanageable, resulting in a decrease of observed security.

STABILITY FROM INFANCY TO CHILDHOOD

Initially, research exploring stability of attachment beyond the second year was delayed due to the lack of valid coding systems for older children. But several new coding schemes have been developed for children, and to date a few studies have explored stability from infancy to childhood. This work, however, is limited by the fact that different coding systems may not overlap, thereby underestimating degree of stability. For example, Vondra, Shaw, Swearingen, Cohen, and Owens (2001) assessed attachment in mother–infant dyads at 12, 18, and 24 months. Using different systems at 12 and 18 months versus at 24 months, they found that only 16% of the sample had the same classification at three points in time and that 26% of the sample changed classifications at each point in time. However, several studies have reported moderate to high stability. In a sample of children with Down syndrome (Atkinson et al., 1999) and a sample of maltreated and comparison infants (Barnett, Ganiban, & Cicchetti, 1999) researchers reported moderate stability from over 16 to 18 months. Main and Cassidy (1988) and Wartner, Grossman, Fremmer-Bombik, and Suess (1994) studied the stability of attachment from infancy to 6 years of age and reported moderate to high stability. In general, these studies have replicated the findings from infancy: attachment is moderately stable, but, there is opportunity for change. Recent work has begun to explore variables that may evoke change.

In a study designed to replicate infancy results demonstrating the influence of life events on change of attachment, Bar-Haim, Sutton, Fox, and Marvin (2000) studied change of attachment in a middle- to upper-middle-class sample. They reported low to moderate stability and found that mothers of children who remained secure reported fewer negative and more positive life events than mothers of children who changed. Children who remained secure also exhibited higher levels of emotional openness at 58 months when discussing a hypothetical child's reaction to separation from her or his parents.

In a pair of longitudinal studies, Howes and Hamilton (1992) expanded the search for variables that influence stability and change. Mothers, fathers, and teachers of 47 children enrolled in a child-centered daycare participated in the first study. The researchers observed parent–child interactions during arrivals to daycare and reunions as well as teacher–child interactions at 18, 24, 30, 36, and 42 months. At each time, for each relationship, the sample was predominantly secure. The average correlation across time between mothers' reports of children's security scores was .25, thereby demonstrating low to moderate stability. Unexpectedly, as in Teti et al. (1996), results indicated that attachment was more likely to change depending on the age of the child. Age-related changes of attachment need to be studied further to determine if the findings are merely an anomaly or if particular developmental milestones provide opportunity for change of attachment. In their second study, Howes and Hamilton (1992) explored the stability of attachment and the effect of nonmaternal childcare in 106 mother–child dyads at ages 12 and 48 months. Mother–infant attachment was relatively stable (71% overall). While age of entry to childcare was not associated with stability, children who entered daycare part-time had more stable attachments than children who were enrolled more than 20 hours per week.

Consistent with research on stability of infant attachment, the average stability in early childhood is approximately 65%. This percentage must be considered in light of the problem that the infancy and childhood attachment systems do not overlap and stability from infancy to childhood is likely to be underestimated. The research also provides further support that life events continue to influence change of attachment in childhood.

STABILITY IN ADULTHOOD

> [The] model proposed postulates that the psychological
> processes that result in personality structure are endowed with
> a fair degree of sensitivity to environment, especially to family
> environment, during the early years of life, but a sensitivity
> that diminishes throughout childhood and is already very
> limited by the end of adolescence. Thus the developmental
> process is conceived as able to vary its course, more or less
> adaptively, during the early years, according to the
> environment in which development is occurring: and
> subsequently, with the reduction of environmental sensitivity,
> as becoming increasingly constrained to the particular pathway
> already chosen.
>
> —BOWLBY (1973, pp. 415–416)

Bowlby (1973) proposed that internal working models would be well developed in late adolescence and early adulthood, and therefore that one might expect higher stability in adulthood than childhood. In the last decade, several studies have explored the stability of adult attachment and researchers have demonstrated that attachment representations are moderately to highly stable over times ranging from 2 weeks to 30 years (see Table 4.2 for stability of continuous measures; Brennan & Shaver, 1995; Collins & Read, 1990; Hammond & Fletcher, 1991; Keelan, Dion, & Dion, 1994). These studies measure either attachment dimensions (e.g., security, avoidance, preoccupiedness) or related constructs (e.g., comfort with closeness, anxiety) using 5- to 7-point Likert scales. Furthermore, when participants are asked to choose their predominant attachment category, 80% of participants reported the same category over time (see Table 4.3). Feeney, Noller, and Callan (1994), who reported moderate stability of their measures of closeness and anxiety over 9 months, were one of the first group of researchers to consider instrument reliability when interpreting stability. They demonstrated that when the unreliability of the scales was considered, correlations (.79 for closeness and .84 for anxiety) suggested relatively high stability. In summary, research has demonstrated that the magnitude of the correlations are similar over varying periods of time and, when the unreliability of the measures is considered, the degree of stability is quite high.

A few studies have also demonstrated that stability of attachment self-reports remains high over much longer time spans. For example, Asendorpf and Wilpers (2000) assessed attachment in 171 university students three times over 18 months. They found that test–retest correlations of attachment measures were high for all relationships. As expected, they found that

TABLE 4.2. Stability of Continuous Ratings of Attachment in Adulthood

	Time lapse	Average stability coefficient
Brennan and Shaver (1995)	8 months	.57
Collins and Read (1990)	2 months	.64[a]
Davila et al. (1999)	24 months[b]	.70 women and .61 men
Feeney et al. (1994)	9 months	.63[c]
Fuller and Fincham (1995)	24 months	.60 women and .63 men
Hammond and Fletcher (1991)	4 months	.47
Keelan et al. (1994)	4 months	.60[d]
Klohnen and Bera (1998)	9 years	.71
	27 years	.55
Levy and Davis (1988)	2 weeks	.57
Scharfe and Bartholomew (1994)	8 months	.64 women and .73 men
Scharfe and Cole (2002)	7 months	.68

[a]Stability of closeness, dependence, and anxiety scales.
[b]Stability coefficients are from time 1 and time 5 only.
[c]Stability of closeness and anxiety scales.
[d]Stability of Simpson (1990) closeness and anxiety scales.

TABLE 4.3. Stability of Attachment Categories in Adulthood

	n	Time lapse	% reporting same category
Self-reports			
Baldwin and Fehr (1995)	517	1 to 40 weeks	72%
Davila et al. (1997)	155	6 months/ 24 months	72%/66%
Fuller and Fincham (1995)	44	24 months	64% women and 68% men
Iwaniec and Sneddon (2001)[a]	31	20 years	61%
Keelan et al. (1994)	105	4 months	80%
Kirkpatrick and Hazan (1994)	172	4 years	70%
Scharfe and Bartholomew (1994)	72	8 months	63% women and 56% men
Scharfe and Cole (2002)	73	7 months	47%
Interviews			
Bakersman-Kranenburg and van IJzendoorn (1992)	83	2 months	78%
Benoit and Parker (1994)	84	12 months	90%
Hamilton (2000)[a]	30	16 to 18 years	63%
Lewis et al. (2000)[a]	84	17 years	42%
Sagi et al. (1994)	59	3 months	90%
Scharfe and Bartholomew (1994)	72	8 months	75% women and 80% men
Waters et al. (2000)[a]	50	19 to 21 years	64%
Weinfield et al. (2000)[a]	57	18 years	39%

[a]First assessment was during infancy using the Strange Situation.

stability of attachment to parents was higher than stability to peers. Given that young adults have long relationship histories with their parents, it is not surprising that this relationship was less likely to change. Future work needs to explore whether length of relationship with peers is likely to influence change. For example, if a new peer relationship does not meet previously learned expectations, it is likely that the relationship may end or, if the relationship endures, the attachment representations of one or both of the individuals may change. Further research is needed to explore this hypothesis and to determine the length of time necessary for change.

In a sample of 44 married couples, Fuller and Fincham (1995) reported moderate stability of categorical and dimensional measures of attachment over 2 years. Kirkpatrick and Hazan (1994) found similar results in a sample of adults over 4 years. To date, Klohnen and Bera (1998) have explored stability of attachment over the longest time span (i.e., over 25 years). Women completed the Hazan and Shaver (1987) three-category measure (e.g., participants chose which category best describes their relationships: secure, avoidant, or preoccupied) at age 52 and the researchers derived a measure of attachment at ages 27 and 43 using an adjective checklist. They reported stability correlations ranging from .49 to .75 over 25 years. Unfortunately, Klohnen and Bera did not test specifically why some participants changed, but the degree of stability was similar to that reported in previous studies.

Consistent with Bowlby's proposal that attachment would change to adapt to experiences, researchers examining short-term stability in adulthood have consistently demonstrated that approximately 70% of samples are stable. This finding has been reported even when researchers set out to demonstrate that attachment was not stable (see Baldwin & Fehr, 1995). Although considerable work has gone into the reasons for change in childhood, only a handful of studies have examined reasons for change in adulthood. Davila, Burge, and Hammen (1997) tested two hypotheses regarding change of attachment in 155 women who had recently graduated from high school. First, they tested whether change occurred in reaction to stress experienced during this life event. Second, they tested the hypothesis that people who changed were vulnerable in other ways (i.e., personality disturbance, history of personal and family psychopathology, and likelihood of growing up in a nonintact family). Using Hazan and Shaver's (1987) self-report assessment of attachment, they reported moderate stability over 6 months and 2 years. They found weak support for the hypothesis that change occurred in reaction to stressful life events. Both stable insecurity and changes in insecurity were associated with higher reports of symptomology than stable security. There was strong support for the hypothesis that people who changed were vulnerable in other ways. They found that personal or family history psychopathology, personality disturbance, and history of family breakup was associated with both attachment insecurity and instability.

Davila and her colleagues then expanded their examination of stability in a sample of newlyweds (Davila, Karney, & Bradbury, 1999). Participants were interviewed in person or completed mailed questionnaires once every 6 months for 2.5 years. Davila et al. reported relatively high levels of stability over time for women (correlations of attachment scores across time ranging from .62 to .80) and men (scores ranging from .50 to .81). Consistent with their previous research, people who changed toward insecurity reported vulnerabilities such as personality disturbance, past or family history of psychopathology, and a nonintact family of origin.

In an attempt to further explore how life transitions may influence changes in adult attachments, Scharfe and Cole (2002) explored stability and change in students undergoing the transition from university. They found that the stable secure participants, as well as participants moving toward security, consistently reported higher scores on self-esteem, trust, and life satisfaction and lower scores on anxiety, depression, and loneliness than the insecure participants. The insecure participants seemed to be vulnerable to the stress of leaving university for the real world. For example, those individuals who reported stress and remained insecure did not respond to the transition in positive ways. Their scores on anxiety, depression, and loneliness were high before the transition and remained high approximately 7 months later. These results provide support for Bowlby's suggestion that change was not only likely in response to stressful situations but in some cases positive and healthy. Specifically, the participants who changed from insecure to secure over the transition seemed to adjust better to the transition than their stable insecure peers. The stable insecure participants may have had a biased negative interpretation of this stressful event (see Collins, 1996; Simpson, Rholes, & Nelligan, 1992), resulting in their resistance to change. Each of the above studies asked participants to rate their attachment style on continuous Likert scales or to choose an attachment category that was most like themselves. Recent work has also explored stability of attachment using interview measures of attachment.

Stability of Attachment Using Interviews

In 1985, Main and her colleagues introduced the Adult Attachment Interview (AAI; Main, Kaplan, & Cassidy, 1985). This interview was the first published method of assessing attachment representations. Several researchers have since examined the stability of the AAI. Bakermans-Kranenburg and van IJzendoorn (1993) interviewed a sample of mothers 2 months apart and found moderate to high stability. Sagi et al. (1994) reported high stability over 3 months in a sample of university students. Although Sagi et al. reported higher stability proportions for secure participants, examination of the base rates across categories indicated that each of the categories showed higher stability than expected.

Several studies examining the intergenerational transmission of attachment have reported data to support the hypothesis of stability. Fonagy et al. (1991) reported that prenatal maternal AAI categories (either secure or insecure) predicted mother–infant attachment security (and insecurity), as evidenced by infant behaviors in the Strange Situation, 75% of the time. Using the 3-category system to classify attachment for both mothers and infants, the concordance was 66%. Benoit and Parker (1994) explored the intergenerational transmission of attachment across three generations. Mothers were interviewed twice (prenatal and 11 months postnatal); 90% of these mothers were judged to have the same attachment category (using Main's three-category system) during pregnancy and when their infant was approximately 11 months old. The concordance between mothers' and grandmothers' attachment categories was 75%; it was 81% between mothers' prenatal AAI and infant categories at 12 months, 82% between mothers' postnatal AAI and infant categories, and 68% between maternal grandmother and infant. Furthermore, 65% of the triads were found to have the same attachment model. In summary, each of the above studies provided support for the intergenerational transmission, hence stability, of attachment from caregivers to infants. However, approximately 20% of mother–infant attachments were discordant; to date, researchers have not explained these findings. Perhaps, as first suggested by Fonagy et al. (1991), this discordance may be better understood if the attachment of the father and father–infant attachment were assessed.

In a comprehensive study of stability of adult attachment representations, Scharfe and Bartholomew (1994) explored the stability of self-report, partner report, and interview assessments of attachment in a sample of young established couples. Each partner completed questionnaires and were administered the Peer Attachment Interview (Bartholomew & Horowitz, 1991) twice over 8 months. Similar to Waters's (1978) initial explorations of stability in childhood, they deliberately chose a stable sample and found that attachment representations were moderately to highly stable (category stability ranged from 63% to 80% and correlations ranged from .37 to .82). They also outlined how the reliability of the assessment tool was particularly important to consider when examining stability. For example, by controlling for unreliability of measures (using structural equation modeling), they were able to demonstrate high stability of the interview assessments (ranging from .72 to .85). In conclusion, studies examining stability of attachment using interview assessments have consistently demonstrated that attachment representations are highly stable over periods ranging from 2 to 12 months.

In summary, research examining the stability of self-report and interview assessments of attachment (and attachment-related constructs) have demonstrated that adult attachment representations are at least moderately stable. Studies using categorical assessments consistently report that approximately 70% of participants report the same attachment category over time. Studies using continuous attachment ratings have also reported moderate stability, typically reporting correlations between scores ranging from .40 to .70. These findings provide some support for the proposal that the attachment construct is quite stable over varying periods of time and that stability may be underestimated due to the low reliability of the self-report measures (Feeney et al., 1994; Scharfe & Bartholomew, 1994). Several authors (Davila et al., 1999; Kirkpatrick & Hazan, 1994; Feeney et al., 1994) have reported higher security over time, although, as discussed, there is no evidence of increased security over time if base rates or mean differences are considered (Scharfe & Bartholomew, 1994). More importantly, researchers using interviews have not reported higher stability of security.

STABILITY FROM INFANCY TO YOUNG ADULTHOOD

The first generation of Strange Situation participants has grown up. To date, five studies have explored stability from infancy to adolescence or young adulthood. The results provide promising support for Bowlby's proposition that attachment is relatively stable across the lifespan (Hamilton, 2000; Iwaniec & Sneddon, 2001; Lewis, Feiring, & Rosenthal, 2000; Waters, Merrick, Treboux, Crowell, & Albersheim, 2000; Weinfield, Sroufe, & Egeland, 2000). Three of the five studies reported categorical stability over time ranging between 61% and 64% (Hamilton, 2000; Iwaniec & Sneddon, 2001; Waters et al., 2000). Conversely, Lewis et al. (2000) and Weinfield et al. (2000) reported considerable changes in attachment (42% and 39% stability, respectively). Although there was variability in degree of change, each of the five studies consistently demonstrated that change was not random. Specifically, maintenance of insecurity or change toward insecurity was associated with attachment-related negative life events such as maternal depression, parental divorce, illness, or abuse (Hamilton, 2000; Lewis et al., 2000; Waters et al., 2000; Weinfield et al., 2000), and change toward security was associated with improved caregiving arrangements (Iwaniec & Sneddon, 2001) and better family functioning (Weinfield et al., 2000). The variability of stability findings has yet to be explained. Perhaps, as suggested by Waters et al. (2000), change toward security may be observed in samples in which participants did not experience stressful events, whereas higher stability of insecurity may be observed in samples experiencing considerably more stress.

CLINICAL SIGNIFICANCE OF THIS RESEARCH

Much of the research exploring stability of attachment during the first few decades of life has demonstrated that attachment is moderately to highly stable. Furthermore, there is considerable support that, after the first year, change of attachment tends to occur together with changes in the environment. Specifically, research has found that change in attachment is likely during transitions; depending on how these transitions are handled, there may be changes toward security or toward insecurity. Davila and her colleagues (Davila et al., 1997, 1999) suggested that individuals who experienced stressful childhood events (and who were presumably insecure) may be more likely to change. Alternatively, it is equally likely that these predominately insecure individuals would be resistant to change. Insecure individuals may distort positive information that would elicit change. For example, they may be reluctant to request or accept support when it is offered, as this support may be viewed as unnecessary, manipulative, or malicious. An interesting future direction would be to explore whether some degree of security is necessary to reevaluate and reorganize insecure models. If you compare two predominantly insecure individuals (e.g., one who has no security and one who has a small degree—or healthy dose—of security), an insecure individual with a healthy dose of security may be more likely to request or accept support and may not view this support negatively. Examination of stability and change in adults experiencing psychotherapy or a stressful but relatively successful life transition may provide insights into how attachment changes.

Furthermore, a few researchers have found that emotions may play a key role in change. Caregivers who report high levels of anger, anxiety, or depression tend to react to infant requests for proximity in insensitive and/or rejecting ways, increasing the likelihood that their child will develop an insecure representation. Children who develop these insecure styles are more likely to respond insensitively to future attempts of support seeking or caregiving, thus transmitting their insecure ways to family and peer relationships. Couple or family therapy that highlights learning to act in a consistent and responsive manner to others' requests for support should prove to be beneficial in changing attachment representations (cf. Lieberman & Zeanah, 1999). Fonagy et al. (1991) and Benoit and Parker (1994) found that attachment during pregnancy predicted children's attachment behavior at 12 months, suggesting that these parent–child interventions can begin as early as pregnancy.

Therapists are also cautioned to consider developmental issues. For example, Davila et al. (1997) found that romantic stress was predictive of changes over 2 years in a group of young women. Based on their age, it is likely that this sample was resolving developmental issues pertaining to intimacy (Erikson, 1950). It may be that the attachment stability of older adults who are influenced by generativity or integrity concerns is predicted by variables such as efficacy in parenting and not relationship stress.

There are several limitations in methodology that may have implications for clinical work. First, in childhood, it is well established that stability of attachment is higher in low-risk, middle-class samples as compared to high-risk poverty samples. To date, most of the research exploring stability of adult attachment has studied stability in privileged samples. Stability of attachment in nonuniversity, non-middle-class samples is necessary. Second, researchers exploring adult attachment must ensure that they are assessing *attachment relationships* and not merely short-term affectional, nonattachment bonds (Ainsworth, 1989). Finally, to date, researchers have not explored stability of attachment in adults who have experienced traumatic events (e.g., war, natural disaster).

The empirical question of how and when attachment representations change remains to be addressed. To date, researchers have determined that change of attachment is not random. Studies using participants of different ages, over varying period of time, and using very different assessments tools report that an average of 30% of participants change attachment over time. Although predictors of change are well documented in childhood, considerable work is yet to be completed to understand why adults continue to show the same degree of change. Furthermore, researchers and clinicians need to explore why some individuals seem to be open to change and other individuals seem to be resistant to change. It is possible that security provides the individual with the ability to be open to experience (Bar-Haim et al., 2000) and the flexibility to change aspects of his or her life when change is necessary. However, it is likely that insecure individuals may attempt to revise insecure models if provided with a secure base (i.e., a base from which to explore) and a safe haven (i.e., a place to return to for comfort and support). Both a secure base and a safe haven may be found in successful client–therapist relationships.

ACKNOWLEDGMENTS

Preparation of this chapter was supported in part by a Social Science and Humanities Research Council of Canada research grant. My sincere thanks to Sue Johnson and Valerie Whiffen who commented on previous versions of this chapter and to Hilary Adams, Michelle Beckman, Andrea D'Addario, Lesley Dale, Steve Renner, Natalie Séguin, and Heather Smith who assisted with library research.

REFERENCES

Ainsworth, M. D. S. (1989). Attachments beyond infancy. *American Psychologist, 44,* 709–716.

Ainsworth, M. D. S., Blehar, M. C., Waters, E., & Wall, S. (1978). *Patterns of attachment: A psychological study of the Strange Situation.* Hillsdale, NJ: Erlbaum.

Asendorpf, J. B., & Wilpers, S. (2000). Attachment security and available support: Closely linked relationship qualities. *Journal of Social and Personal Relationships, 17,* 115–138.

Atkinson, L., Chisholm, V. C., Scott, B., Goldberg, S., Vaughn, B. E., Blackwell, J., Dickens, S., & Tam, F. (1999). Maternal sensitivity, child functional level, and attachment in Down syndrome. In J. I. Vondra & D. Barnett (Eds.), Atypical attachment in infancy and early childhood among children at developmental risk. *Monographs of the Society for Research in Child Development,* 64(3, Serial No. 258), 45–66.

Atkinson, L., Niccols, A., Paglia, A., Coolbear, J., Parker, K. C. H., Poulton, L., Guger, S., & Sitarenios, G. (2000). A meta-analysis of time between maternal sensitivity and attachment assessments: Implications for internal working models in infancy/toddlerhood. *Journal of Social and Personal Relationships,* 17, 791–810.

Bakermans-Kranenburg, M. J., & van IJzendoorn, M. H. (1993). A psychometric study of the adult attachment interview: Reliability and discriminant validity. *Developmental Psychology, 29,* 870–879.

Baldwin, M. W., & Fehr, B. (1995). On the instability of attachment style ratings. *Personal Relationships, 2,* 247–261.

Bar-Haim, Y., Sutton, D. B., Fox, N. A., & Marvin, R. S. (2000). Stability and change of attachment at 14, 24, and 58 months of age: Behavior, representation, and life events. *Journal of Child Psychology and Psychiatry, 41,* 381–388.

Barnett, D., Ganiban, J., & Cicchetti, D. (1999). Maltreatment, negative expressivity, and the development of type D attachment from 12 to 24 months of age. In J. I. Vondra & D. Barnett (Eds.), Atypical attachment in infancy and early childhood among children at developmental risk. *Monographs of the Society for Research in Child Development, 64*(3, Serial No. 258), 97–118.

Bartholomew, K., & Horowitz, L. (1991). Attachment styles among young adults: A test of a four-category model. *Journal of Personality and Social Psychology, 61*, 226–244.

Belsky, J., Campbell, S. B., Cohn, J. F., & Moore, G. (1996). Instability of infant–parent attachment security. *Developmental Psychology, 32*, 921–924.

Benoit, D., & Parker, K. C. H. (1994). Stability and transmission of attachment across three generations. *Child Development, 65*, 1444–1456.

Bowlby, J. (1973). *Attachment and loss: Vol. II. Separation: Anger and anxiety.* New York: Basic Books.

Bowlby, J. (1982). *Attachment and loss: Vol. I. Attachment.* New York: Basic Books. (First edition published in 1969)

Brennan, K. A., & Shaver, P. R. (1995). Dimensions of adult attachment, affect regulation, and romantic relationship functioning. *Personality and Social Psychology Bulletin, 21*, 267–283.

Caspi, A., & Elder, G. H. (1988). Emergent family patterns: The intergenerational construction of problem behavior and relationships. In R. A. Hinde & J. Stevenson-Hinde (Eds.), *Relationships within families* (pp. 218–240). Oxford, UK: Clarendon Press.

Collins, N. L. (1996). Working models of attachment: Implications for explanation, emotion, and behavior. *Journal of Personality and Social Psychology, 71*, 810–832.

Collins, N. L., & Read, S. J. (1990). Adult attachment, working models, and relationship quality in dating couples. *Journal of Personality and Social Psychology, 58*, 644–663.

Davila, J., Burge, D., & Hammen, C. (1997). Why does attachment style change? *Journal of Personality and Social Psychology, 73*, 826–838.

Davila, J., Karney, B. R., & Bradbury, T. N. (1999). Attachment change processes in the early years of marriage. *Journal of Personality and Social Psychology, 76*, 783–802.

Egeland, B., & Farber, E. A. (1984). Infant–mother attachment: Factors related to its development and changes over time. *Child Development, 55*, 753–771.

Egeland, B., & Sroufe, L. A. (1981). Attachment and early maltreatment. *Child Development, 52*, 44–52.

Epstein, S. (1980). The stability of behavior: II. Implications of psychological research. *American Psychologist, 35*, 790–806.

Erikson, E. H. (1950). *Childhood and society.* New York: Norton.

Feeney, J. A., Noller, P., & Callan, V. J. (1994). Attachment style, communication and satisfaction in the early years of marriage. In K. Bartholomew & D. Perlman (Eds.), *Advances in personal relationships: Vol. 5. Attachment processes in adulthood* (pp. 269–308). London: Jessica Kingsley.

Fonagy, P., Steele, H., & Steele, M. (1991). Maternal representations of attachment during pregnancy predict the organization of infant–mother attachment at one year of age. *Child Development, 62*, 891–905.

Fuller, T. L., & Fincham, F. D. (1995). Attachment style in married couples: Relation to current marital functioning, stability over time, and method of assessment. *Personal Relationships, 2,* 17–34.

Goossens, F. A., van IJzendoorn, M. H., Tavecchio, L. W. C., & Kroonenberg, P. M. (1986). Stability of attachment across time and context in a Dutch sample. *Psychological Reports, 58,* 23–32.

Hamilton, C. E. (2000). Continuity and discontinuity of attachment from infancy through adolescence. *Child Development, 71,* 690–694.

Hammond, J. R., & Fletcher, G. J. O. (1991). Attachment styles and relationship satisfaction in the development of close relationships. *New Zealand Journal of Psychology, 20,* 56–62.

Hazan, C., & Shaver, P. R. (1987). Romantic love conceptualized as an attachment process. *Journal of Personality and Social Psychology, 52,* 511–524.

Hinde, R. A. (1979). *Towards understanding relationships.* London: Academic Press.

Howes, C., & Hamilton, C. (1992). Children's relationship with child care teachers: Stability and concordance with parental attachments. *Child Development, 63,* 867–878.

Iwaniec, D., & Sneddon, H. (2001). Attachment style in adults who failed to thrive as children: Outcomes of a 20 year follow-up study of factors influencing maintenance or change in attachment style. *British Journal of Social Work, 31,* 179–195.

Keelan, J. P. R., Dion, K. L., & Dion, K. K. (1994). Attachment style and heterosexual relationships among young adults: A short-term panel study. *Journal of Social and Personal Relationships, 11,* 201–214.

Kirkpatrick, L. A., & Hazan, C. (1994). Attachment styles and close relationships: A four-year prospective study. *Personal Relationships, 1,* 123–142.

Klohnen, E. C., & Bera, S. (1998). Behavioral and experiential patterns of avoidantly and securely attached women across adulthood: A 31–year longitudinal perspective. *Journal of Personality and Social Psychology, 74,* 211–223.

Levy, M. B., & Davis, K. E. (1988). Lovestyles and attachment styles compared: Their relations to each other and to various relationship characteristics. *Journal of Social and Personal Relationships, 5,* 439–471.

Lewis, M., Feiring, C., & Rosenthal, S. (2000). Attachment over time. *Child Development, 71,* 707–720.

Lieberman, A. F., & Zeanah, C. H (1999). Contributions of attachment theory to infant–parent psychotherapy and other interventions with infants and young children. In J. Cassidy & P. R. Shaver (Eds.), *Handbook of attachment: Theory, research, and clinical applications* (pp. 555–574). New York: Guilford Press.

Main, M., & Cassidy, J. (1988). Categories of response to reunion with the parent at age 6: Predictable from infant attachment classifications and stable over a 1–month period. *Developmental Psychology, 24,* 415–426.

Main, M., Kaplan, N., & Cassidy, J. (1985). Security in infancy, childhood, and adulthood: A move to the level of representation. In I. Bretherton & E. Waters (Eds.), Growing points in attachment theory and research. *Monographs of the Society for Research in Child Development, 50*(1–2), 66–104.

Main, M., & Weston, D. R. (1981). The quality of the toddler's relationship to mother and to father: Related to conflict behavior and the readiness to establish new relationships. *Child Development, 52,* 932–940.

Mischel, W. (1969). Continuity and change in personality. *American Psychologist, 24,* 1012–1018.

NICHD Early Child Care Research Network. (2001). Child-care and family predictors of preschool attachment and stability from infancy. *Developmental Psychology, 37,* 847–862.

Owen, M. T., Easterbrooks, M. A., Chase-Lansdale, L., & Goldberg, W. A. (1984). The relation between maternal employment status and the stability of attachments to mother and to father. *Child Development, 55,* 1894–1901.

Rauh, H., Ziegenhain, U., Müller, B., & Wignroks, L. (2000). Stability and change in infant–mother attachment in the second year of life: Relations to parenting quality and varying degrees of day-care experience. In P. Crittenden (Ed.), *The organization of attachment relationships: Maturation, culture, and context* (pp. 251–276). Cambridge, UK: Cambridge University Press.

Sagi, A., van IJzendoorn, M. H., Scharf, M., Koren-Karie, N., Joels, T., & Mayseless, O. (1994). Stability and discriminant validity of the Adult Attachment Interview: A psychometric study in young Israeli adults. *Developmental Psychology, 30,* 771–777.

Scharfe, E., & Bartholomew, K. (1994). Reliability and stability of adult attachment patterns. *Personal Relationships, 1,* 23–43.

Scharfe, E., & Cole, V. (2002). *Stability and change of attachment representations during the transition from university.* Unpublished manuscript.

Simpson, J. A. (1990). The influence of attachment styles on romantic relationships. *Journal of Personality and Social Psychology, 59,* 971–980.

Simpson, J. A., Rholes, W. S., & Nelligan, J. S. (1992). Support-seeking and support-giving within couple members in an anxiety-provoking situation: The role of attachment styles. *Journal of Personality and Social Psychology, 62,* 434–446.

Teti, D. M., Sakin, J. W., Kucera, E., & Eiden, R. D. (1996). And baby makes four: Predictors of attachment security among preschool-age firstborns during the transition to siblinghood. *Child Development, 67,* 579–596.

Thompson, R. A., Lamb, M. E., & Estes, D. (1982). Stability of infant–mother attachment and its relationship to changing life circumstances in an unselected middle-class sample. *Child Development, 53,* 144–148.

Touris, M., Kromelow, S., & Harding, C. (1993). Mother–firstborn attachment and the birth of a sibling. *American Journal of Orthopsychiatry, 65,* 293–297.

Vaughn, B., Egeland, B., Sroufe, A., & Waters, E. (1979). Individual differences in infant–mother attachment at twelve and eighteen months: Stability and change in families under stress. *Child Development, 50,* 971–975.

Vereijken, C. M. J. L., Riksen-Walraven, M., & Kondo-Ikemura, K. (1997). Maternal sensitivity and infant attachment security in Japan: A longitudinal study. *International Journal of Behavioral Development, 21,* 35–49.

Vondra, J. I., Hommerding, K. D., & Shaw, D. S. (1999). Stability and change in infant attachment in a low income sample. In J. I. Vondra & D. Barnett (Eds.), Atypical attachment in infancy and early childhood among children at developmental risk. *Monographs of the Society for Research in Child Development, 64*(3, Serial No. 258), 119–144.

Vondra, J. I., Shaw, D. S., Swearingen, L., Cohen, M., & Owens, E. B. (2001). Attachment stability and emotional and behavioral regulation from infancy to preschool age. *Development and Psychopathology, 13,* 13–33.

Wartner, U. G., Grossman, K., Fremmer-Bombik, E., & Suess, G. (1994). Attachment patterns at age six in south Germany: Predictability from infancy and implications for preschool behavior. *Child Development, 65,* 1014–1027.

Waters, E. (1978). The reliability and stability of individual differences in infant–mother attachment. *Child Development, 49,* 483–494.

Waters, E., Merrick, S., Treboux, D., Crowell, J., & Albersheim, L. (2000). Attachment security in infancy and early adulthood: A twenty-year longitudinal study. *Child Development, 71,* 684–689.

Weinfield, N. S., Sroufe, A. L., & Egeland, B. (2000). Attachment from infancy to early adulthood in a high-risk sample: Continuity, discontinuity, and their correlates. *Child Development, 71,* 695–702.

5

Alternate Pathways to Competence

Culture and Early Attachment Relationships

VIVIAN J. CARLSON
ROBIN L. HARWOOD

The importance of early attachment relationships and their role in guiding future socioemotional development has been widely documented in recent decades (Cassidy & Shaver, 1999). Investigations of the role of culture in early attachment formation have been less numerous, but are now providing a growing body of evidence highlighting the need for careful consideration of cultural meanings in attachment research (van IJzendoorn & Sagi, 1999). Combining cultural issues with attachment theory requires a multidisciplinary approach that includes a common definition of "culture," one that is accepted across disciplines.

Cultural psychologists and anthropologists often characterize *culture* as shared knowledge about how the world works (e.g., Cole, 1996; Dunn, 1988; Handwerker, in press). The simplicity of this definition belies its underlying complexity. Because culture is the medium in which all development takes place, our efforts to investigate it are perhaps best described by the time-honored analogy of a school of fish attempting to study water. We are immersed in cultural knowledge that we use to interpret and respond to events and experiences in our lives. We acquire cultural knowledge through our social interactions and life experiences. Culture is ever-changing because it exists within individuals and is continuously modified in the context of social interactions. This shared cultural knowledge thus provides a framework of expectations and values upon which we base our social interactions, structure our daily lives, and interpret our experiences. As we encounter new experiences and interact with new people, we may come to share new knowledge, new social expectations, and new interpretations of our experiences. It is this fluid, changeable aspect of culture that defies simplistic definition and necessitates complex multimethod research designs and therapeutic considerations.

Many overly simplistic conceptualizations tend to reify culture by defining it as a "thing," such as a set of facts about a particular group. Such static definitions deny the richness and complexity of our multicultural society as well as our individual uniqueness (Garcia Coll & Magnuson, 1999; Harwood, Handwerker, Schöoelmerich, & Leyendecker, 2001). Current cultural research avoids this type of oversimplification and promotes awareness of the fluid nature of cultural communities (Falicov, 1998; Harwood, Schöoelmerich, Schulze, & Gonzalez, 1999; Leyendecker & Lamb, 1999; Posada et al., 1995). One individual may be a member of a number of different groups, each of which shares a common body of knowledge, expectations, and rules for interactions. As individuals, we may identify with a particular religious community, with one or more sporting or hobby groups, with others who share our educational or professional backgrounds, and with members of our specific ethnic group. When meeting new acquaintances we instinctively seek areas of cultural commonality, using these various subgroup affiliations to explore educational, occupational, religious, sport, ethnic, social class, or cohort similarities in conversation. The discovery of some area of commonality enables comfortable conversation with a new acquaintance. When commonalities are not immediately apparent, communication becomes more difficult, and may end rather abruptly.

The challenge for professionals lies in learning to understand group commonalities as well as individual differences and needs without resorting to stereotypic assumptions and inferences. How can we use cultural understanding to learn about nonshared values and beliefs, maintain individual responsiveness, and identify and respect alternate pathways to developmental competence?

CULTURAL RECIPROCITY

One answer to this question involves the cultivation of cultural reciprocity in professional relationships. *Cultural reciprocity* denotes the ability to engage others in interactions designed to explore and negotiate cultural issues while maintaining ongoing awareness of personal cultural values and beliefs (Kalyanpur & Harry, 1997). Cultural reciprocity requires two ongoing processes: self-awareness of one's own cultural assumptions and beliefs, and a willingness to explore the cultural beliefs of others in the full context of their personal and shared histories, assumptions, goals, and practices. Developing self-awareness of our own cultural assumptions and beliefs is a lifelong process requiring an open and inquiring approach to self and others.

Until we develop awareness of our own shared knowledge and assumptions, we are not prepared to explore culturally different values and beliefs. Most cultural assumptions remain unconscious until they are violated. Shared knowledge about interactive behaviors, such as maintaining the appropriate distance between conversational partners or the use of a handshake versus a hug in greeting acquaintances, do not enter conscious thought unless our expectations are not met. Violated interactive assumptions often stimulate strong emotional reactions, leading to communicative difficulties or breakdowns. Failure to examine personal assumptions and beliefs may thus lead to frequent communicative difficulties in interactions with individuals with whom we do not share a common cultural heritage.

Examination of personal values and beliefs is best undertaken in the context of reflective consultations with a trusted group of colleagues. Although personal reflection may lead to some increased awareness, the contrasts and insights provided through honest, open-ended discussions with others often offer invaluable insights into both shared and individual beliefs and values. Examining our interactive assumptions and our responses to violations of these expectations enables conscious consideration of the sources of our cultural knowledge and the variety inherent in human development. Why are we uncomfortable in social situations with some people, but not with others? What roles do body language, eye contact, and response timing play in our assumptions about interactions? What interactive qualities make us feel most relaxed and gregarious? How are my answers to these questions similar to or different from others' answers? Just as cultural knowledge exists in the context of interactions with others, so must our most effective explorations of this knowledge occur in the context of interactive experiences.

In a recent workshop exploring these issues, participants were surprised to find strong disagreements among the group regarding the appropriate rules for interactions in parent–professional conversations. Some felt that a simple greeting, such as "Hi, how are you?," should be immediately followed by "getting down to business" discussing the issues at hand. Others felt that several minutes of social interaction including conversation about the parents' activities and the family as a whole should precede the main topic, and that the lack of this interval would be perceived as very rude and result in parental inattention to the professional's comments. Such disagreements clearly signal differing expectations and rules for social interactions. Listening carefully to the feelings and beliefs of participants on both sides of this discussion led to increased understanding of the need for sensitivity to the social expectations of others.

Sharing personal reflections in the context of a supportive group also highlights the need for continuous vigilance in distinguishing group tendencies from individual variations. Although information regarding group tendencies provides us with some ideas that may be useful in initiating cultural discussions with individuals, we must constantly guard against the temptation to generalize from groups to individuals. If culture is viewed as fluid, modified in the context of interactions, and based on both individual and shared experiences, then we would expect variations *within* any given group to be at least as great as variations *between* groups. Effective working relationships with diverse individuals require proactive efforts to elicit information about personal goals, beliefs, values, and experiences. Only after a mutual understanding has been reached regarding assumptions and expectations can the negotiation of meaningful therapeutic goals take place.

For example,[1] the mothers of two toddlers with Down syndrome express very different goals and values. Maria hopes that her daughter will always be attractive, appealing, well-behaved, and friendly. Kathy hopes that her daughter will learn to communicate clearly and effectively and become fully independent in daily activities. Two different therapeutic goals, one that reflect Maria's interest in social skills and another that reflects Kathy's interest in communication and self-help, will best serve the needs of these two children and their families. The skilled clinician will be able to focus on a variety of developmental and/or parenting skills by first recognizing and working toward the family's needs and priorities, then, if necessary, gradually introducing his or her own perspectives and negotiating mutually acceptable goals and activities.

Many articles about cultural differences have focused on differences in practices without providing contextual understanding of background beliefs, values, and goals developed through shared history and individual experiences. Knowledge of differences in practices does not lead to the kind of comprehensive understanding needed to make judgments about which differences should be respectfully accepted, and which might present risks to development. For example, knowing that Latina mothers usually continue to spoonfeed their toddlers and preschoolers while Anglo ("Anglo" is used herein with its Spanish meaning, i.e., non-Hispanic white) mothers encourage early self-feeding as soon as possible does not give a clinician enough information to begin negotiating intervention goals based on the developmental needs of Maria's daughter with Down syndrome. This level of knowledge might lead one to think of Maria's spoonfeeding as an annoy-

---

[1]All case examples included in this chapter are entirely fictional and generic in nature, based upon the first author's many years of experience working with families of young children with special needs.

ing, old-fashioned tradition that has little relevance to the current situation instead of understanding that it is an indication of the importance she attributes to making sure that her daughter is well-cared-for, attractive, and socially acceptable. If, however, the therapist is skilled in questioning the parents about their childrearing goals, beliefs, experiences, and practices, and sharing her or his own perspectives, a mutually satisfactory compromise becomes increasingly likely.

Cultural reciprocity in practice enables mutually respectful understandings of similarities and differences in perspectives between professionals and the families they serve. Culturally reciprocal relationships are a necessary first step in the journey toward recognition of a variety of pathways to developmental competence.

LONG-TERM SOCIALIZATION GOALS

An understanding of cultural meanings, socialization goals, and their roles in the everyday lives of families is another important part of this journey. *Cultural meanings* represent our understanding of the world, help us to interpret events and experiences, direct behavior, and evoke particular feelings (D'Andrade, 1984). The cultural meaning systems of caregivers would thus be expected to include mental representations of ideal parent and child behaviors and desirable child developmental end points, as well as to direct daily caregiving behaviors, and to evoke strong emotions in relation to childrearing beliefs and practices. Adults use their understandings of these cultural meaning systems to construct long-term childrearing goals. Childrearing goals provide a very useful window into basic cultural beliefs. These goals are shaped by the life experiences, beliefs, and values of parents. Parents use socialization goals to guide their participation in social networks, to shape their expectations for attainment of developmental milestones, and to define their parenting practices in the context of everyday life (Harwood, Miller, Carlson, & Leyendecker, 2002; Harwood et al., 1999).

Socialization goals provide a foundation for childrearing beliefs that adults tend to assume are shared by all or are universally correct. Research among a variety of cultural groups negates this assumption. Americans tend to assume that a competent adult is assertive and autonomous, whereas the Japanese find such an adult to be immature and poorly educated (Rothbaum, Weisz, Pott, Miyake, & Morelli, 2000). Many American mothers emphasize happiness, confidence, and independence; but Latina mothers often emphasize respect, obedience, and interdependence (Harwood, Miller, & Irizarry, 1995). Professionals who have not explored the childrearing goals of the families in their care risk creating inappropriate and ineffective goals and interventions. Indeed, clinicians who assume that individual well-being and psychological independence are universal goals may alienate service recipients from a wide variety of cultural backgrounds. For example, a physical therapist who stated her assumption that Maria's family wanted their daughter to be as independent as possible seriously damaged her relationship with the family. Maria's husband was deeply offended: "What kind of family does she think we are? We will always care for our daughter! She is God's special gift to our family. When Maria and I are gone, her brothers and sisters will care for her!" Maria's family no longer wanted to work with this therapist because they were hurt and offended by her assumption that family members would not always protect and care for this child throughout her lifespan.

PARENTING STYLES

What parenting strategies best predict children's long-term developmental competence? This apparently straightforward question becomes increasingly complex when diverse cultural groups are included in the search for definitions of optimal parenting.

Parenting studies conducted primarily among middle-class Anglo American families consistently report that *authoritative parents* who combine warm supportive relationships with firm limits and clear explanations encourage child autonomy and produce the most competent confident children. *Authoritarian parents* who employ strict control and emphasize obedience are characterized as low in warmth and responsiveness and found to produce resentful externalizing children (Baumrind, 1988, 1991). Although this parenting paradigm accurately describes the participants in these studies, it fails to include a parenting style emphasizing strict control and obedience combined with warm and responsive parent–child emotional relationships. This combination of parental strictness and warmth is found to be associated with the most positive child outcomes among a variety of cultural groups, including parents of African American, Chinese, Korean, Puerto Rican, and Iranian heritage (Brody & Flor, 1998; Carlson & Harwood, 2003; Jones & Rao, 1998; Kermani & Brenner, 2000; Yang & Chang, 1999).

Members of these groups tend to emphasize childrearing goals related to family and social interrelatedness as contrasted to the Anglo American emphasis on individual autonomy. This greater emphasis on sociocentric goals may be conceptualized as providing the foundation for more behavior-oriented childrearing and interactive strategies as compared to the language-oriented activities valued in the more individualistic Anglo tradition (Pine, 1992). For example, middle-class mothers in Puerto Rico have been found to use more physical control and more directive utterances in their interactions with their 12-month-old infants than similar middle-class Anglo mothers (Carlson & Harwood, 2003; Harwood et al., 2002). These efforts to control and direct infant behavior are quite consistent with the Puerto Rican mothers' expressed goal of teaching their children to be aware of the needs of others and to interact appropriately in a variety of family and social situations.

In addition, in an extension of this study of low-risk, middle-class Puerto Rican and Anglo mother–infant pairs ($n = 60$), ratings of physical control, emotional expression, and maternal sensitivity during mother–infant interactions in five everyday home settings, videotaped when the infants were 4, 8, and 12 months old, were coded by trained, ethnically matched graduate assistants, blind to the study hypotheses (interrater reliability $r = .91$, range = .86 to .94) (Carlson & Harwood, 2003). Results show evidence of significantly higher use of physical control among the Puerto Rican mothers as compared to the Anglo mothers, $F(1, 57) = 18.13$, $p < .01$, but no significant differences between these groups in ratings of maternal sensitivity or emotional expression. These results provide evidence for caution in generalizing the association of high control with rejection or lack of warmth in any groups other than the middle-class Anglo study participants among whom it was originally noted.

Anglo American mothers demonstrate greater use of language-oriented activities with their infants, including use of praise, offering of choices, and prompting of infant verbal performance (Bornstein et al., 1996; Harwood et al., 2002; Pine, 1992). These activities are consistent with Anglo mothers' stated goals of teaching their children to be assertive, confident, and happy.

A number of current investigations are finding evidence that parenting strategies are clearly related to long-term socialization goals. Among parents who emphasize obedience, respect, and fulfillment of familial roles, child behaviors are carefully monitored and directed. Parents who hope to encourage participation in traditional culture also closely monitor their children, but tend to follow the child's lead more responsively and gently shape the child's motivations to match traditional values. Parents who strongly value the development of individual agency allow and encourage autonomous activity on the part of the child and reward creativity and the violation of norms (Ipsa, Fine, Thornburg, & Sharp, 2001; Martini, 2001; Pauls, Choudhury, Leppanen, & Benasich, 2001; Rao & Pearson, 2001).

Such studies lend support to the hypothesis that parents use culturally defined socialization goals to direct their daily caregiving interactions in meaningful ways. Parenting styles may thus reflect parents' efforts to encourage the development of culturally valued traits in their children. Investigations of the relationships among parental goals, beliefs, expectations, and practices across a variety of cultures are beginning to enhance our understanding of diverse pathways to developmental competence. Parental behaviors that are dissonant with cultural values (e.g., high control among

Anglos who strongly value individual agency) may be more likely to result in negative child outcomes than parenting strategies that are consonant with the surrounding cultural values (e.g., high control among Puerto Ricans who strongly value respectful, appropriate social behavior). Clearly, therapeutic interventions must reflect an understanding of these varied cultural pathways in order to provide appropriate and effective services to diverse families.

Maria holds her daughter in her lap, refusing to release her when she tries to wriggle away, and persistently directs her attention to a simple finger play game. Maria kisses and tickles her daughter to distract the little girl from her attempts to get down, then continues with the finger play until she eventually wins her daughter's attention and participation. Many Anglo American therapists and teachers would be uncomfortable with Maria's persistence in physically controlling and directing her young daughter's activities; however, others who share or understand Maria's goals, parenting beliefs, and expectations would see this interaction as evidence of Maria's warm, positive, and effective parenting skills. Maria would, no doubt, be confused, and perhaps offended, by well-meaning efforts to teach her to follow her child's lead in play, that is, to allow her daughter to direct their interactions. Such failure to recognize Maria's shared cultural goals, expectations, and practices might precipitate a breakdown of communication between Maria and the clinician, and possibly lead to Maria's withdrawal from participation in services.

CULTURE AND ATTACHMENT

How do we reconcile this diversity in developmental pathways to the universal framework of attachment theory? Attachment theory predicts that sensitive, responsive maternal care will lead to the development of secure attachment relationships and subsequent socioemotional competence (Ainsworth, Blehar, Waters, & Wall, 1978). Attachment research among a variety of cultural groups has shown that sampled populations differ significantly in the patterning of attachment classifications as measured by the Strange Situation. Secure attachments predominate quite consistently across cultures, but differences in insecure patterns are striking. A northern German study (Grossmann, Grossmann, Spangler, Suess, & Unzner, 1985) found that nearly all insecure infants were classified as avoidant, whereas similar studies in Japan and Israel found that nearly all insecure infants were classified as ambivalent (Miyake & Campos, 1985; Sagi et al., 1985; van IJzendoorn & Kroonenberg, 1988). Indeed, more recent research comparing Japanese and American attachment patterns calls into question the cross-cultural validity of the Strange Situation paradigm and suggests an inherent fallacy in any measurement methodology that values individualism over relatedness (Rothbaum et al., 2000). In summarizing the findings of cross-cultural attachment research, van IJzendoorn and Sagi (1999) point out that the database is small and representative of only a few of the major cultural groups in our world. Nonetheless, they find evidence to support "a balance between universal trends and contextual determinants" (p. 730) in attachment theory. Further investigation of these contextual differences requires careful consideration of the cultural meanings assigned to attachment behaviors and caregiving responses.

Recent meta-analytic findings are more compatible with a *sensitivity hypothesis* in which maternal sensitivity is one of several important precursors of secure attachment instead of the single, primary precursor (DeWolf & van IJzendoorn, 1997). These findings support the inclusion of other maternal measures, such as emotional expression, control strategies, and broader contextual influences in investigations of the antecedents of attachment among low-risk samples.

Ainsworth et al.'s (1978) operational definition of *sensitivity* emphasizes following the child's lead in interactions and exerting cooperative control by offering choices. Efforts to physically control the infant's behavior or to shape interactions based upon the mother's wishes are rated as interfering and insensitive and have been found to be associated with insecure–avoidant attachment among Anglo mother–infant pairs (Ainsworth, Bell, & Stayton, 1974; Malatesta, Culver, Tesman, & Shepard, 1989). However, as mentioned above, studies among a variety of cultural groups whose members emphasize interdependence over individual autonomy find evidence that the concept of sensitive maternal care includes the expectation that mothers will structure and guide the infant's environment and behavior to enhance appropriate social behaviors and family relationships (Harwood et al., 1999; Jones & Rao, 1998; Knight, Virdin, & Roosa, 1994; Leyendecker & Lamb, 1999; Yang & Chang, 1999). Persistent physical control and strong limitations placed on infant behavior might be seen in this context not as interfering with the infant's development of autonomy, but as positive evidence of efforts to raise a well-behaved, respectful child (Harwood, 1992).

The research mentioned above among middle-class Anglo and Puerto Rican mother–infant pairs using videotaped home interactions at 4, 8, and 12 months to rate maternal use of physical control, emotional expression, and maternal sensitivity also included standardized laboratory-based Strange Situation procedures at 12 months, coded by expert outside coders. Discriminant function analyses using maternal behavior ratings to predict attachment classifications show evidence of an association between high levels of physical control and secure attachment among the Puerto Rican group, whereas high levels of maternal physical control are associated with avoidant attachment among the Anglo group (Carlson & Harwood, 2003).

Kermani and Brenner (2000) also find that parental directiveness and control may be associated with positive social and learning outcomes among preschool Iranian immigrant children. These authors conclude that sensitivity to the child's level of competence and need for support is a more important predictor of positive outcomes than parental use of directive strategies. This research highlights the need to differentiate between culturally appropriate use of directiveness and control versus parental intrusiveness.

These results call into question the use of a single universal definition of maternal sensitivity, instead providing evidence that sensitive caregiving behaviors may be culturally constructed, incorporating the socialization goals, values, and beliefs of the family and community. Typically, attachment theory has conceptualized persistent active maternal structuring of interactions as interfering and rated such behavior as insensitive (Ainsworth et al., 1974). However, the findings reviewed above suggest that high levels of parental directiveness and control may be associated with positive child outcomes and attachment security among cultural groups who emphasize more sociocentric childrearing goals.

Expanding our definitions of maternal sensitivity to include a variety of culture-specific beliefs and practices does not alter the underlying association between sensitive caregiving and secure attachment. Ainsworth et al. (1974) concluded that the most fundamental characteristic of sensitivity is the mother's ability to establish a harmonious relationship with her infant. It may be that harmonious maternal–infant relationships are best established by caregiving practices designed to produce culturally valued traits in the growing infant. In the case of mothers who emphasize more sociocentric childrearing goals, high levels of directiveness and control in the context of warm affectionate relationships may best serve to encourage obedience, respect, and relatedness in their children. A recent investigation of caregiving and security among Anglo American and Columbian mother–infant pairs offers additional support for both the universal association between sensitivity and secure attachment and the cultural construction of particular caregiving and secure-base behaviors (Posada, Carbonell, & Alzate, 2001).

Conceptualizing caregiving as a behavioral system enables understanding of the need for both universality and specificity in our definitions of optimal caregiving (George & Solomon, 1999). The universal goal of providing protection from perceived threats forms the foundation of optimal caregiving. The nature of perceived threats is *universal* with regard to immediate threats to physical well-being and survival. Attachment theory also attests to the universality of responses to emotional loss or isolation from the attachment figure. Other less tangible threats are culturally constructed and may vary widely from one culture to the next. For example, child behavior patterns that are inconsistent with culturally valued behaviors are threats to the child's developing social competence and acceptance in the larger community.

If the caregiving system is investigated using the same behavioral systems approach as attachment theory, then the role of culture must be seen as central to the caregiver's mental representations and interpretations of relationships and experiences. Although the goal of providing protection from situations the parent views as stressful or dangerous remains universal, perceptions of danger or stress and the means of protection will vary widely as a function of cultural meaning systems, contextual differences, and experiential differences. Evidence of the ways in which caregiver socialization goals and parenting practices differentially influence child developmental outcomes among research participants from diverse cultural groups provides preliminary support for the cultural specificity needed in definitions of optimal caregiving. Clinicians who base judgments only upon their own values and beliefs, while disregarding the central role of culture in childrearing and family life, risk ineffective treatments, communication difficulties, and high attrition rates.

FUTURE DIRECTIONS

Understanding that there are a variety of pathways to developmental competence may encourage the cultivation of true cultural reciprocity between culturally different service providers and the families they serve. The mutual benefits of culturally reciprocal and respectful relationships within our increasingly diverse society are too important to be ignored or oversimplified. Further explorations of the role of culture in early relationship formation, caregiving patterns, and child development will require longitudinal evaluations of child outcomes for each cultural group. Culturally varied precursors of attachment as discussed above require further validation, as do any potential cultural variations in the socioemotional outcomes of attachment security among different groups.

Teaching human service professionals that culturally reciprocal practice requires awareness of how personal experiences, beliefs, and values influence their own understanding of development is a necessary first step in our journey toward more inclusive services for diverse individuals and families. Teaching service providers to make proactive efforts to gain understanding of each parent's goals and expectations, and to share their own perspectives respectfully, is the next step in this journey. This step requires a clear understanding of the fact that knowledge of group history and characteristics is valuable, but not sufficient for the development of cultural reciprocity in practice. Only after these steps have been taken, and mutually respectful, collaborative relationships that openly acknowledge cultural differences have been established, can service providers and family members begin to successfully negotiate therapeutic goals and activities.

If professionals are not prepared to actively seek others' cultural perspectives and share their own, communication will frequently remain unilateral, and the effects of interventions may remain minimal. As minority communities in the United States continue to grow in the coming years, the future of our children depends on our understanding of culture and our willingness to participate in personal and professional cultural exploration. As direct service professionals, we must be willing to engage in an active dialogue with cultural researchers—learning, implementing, and providing feedback to increase our collective effectiveness in including culturally diverse populations in family support and educational programming. As Falicov (1998, p. 266) so aptly states, the ultimate challenge lies in "working toward a cohesive society while understanding, respecting, and protecting cultural differences."

ACKNOWLEDGMENTS

This research was made possible through a grant to Robin L. Harwood from the National Institutes of Health (HD32800). Portions of this study were presented at the 1999 and 2001 Biennial Meetings of the Society for Research in Child Development. We are grateful to Glorisa Canino of the University of Puerto Rico School of Medicine for making available the resources of her laboratory for the collection of the Puerto Rican data. We would also like to express appreciation to Margaret Adams, Eugenio Ayala, Delia Collazo, Jorge Colon, Olguimar Cruz, Xin Feng, Zenaida González, Carmen Irizarry, Helena Mendez, Sylvia Meredith, Amy Miller, Erin Reutenauer, Pamela Schulze, and Stephanie Wilson for their assistance with data collection and coding.

REFERENCES

Ainsworth, M. D. S., Bell, S. M., & Stayton, D. J. (1974). Infant–mother attachment and social development: Socialisation as a product of reciprocal responsiveness to signals. In M. J. M. Richards (Ed.), *The integration of a child into a social world* (pp. 99–135). London: Cambridge University Press.

Ainsworth, M. D. S., Blehar, M. C., Waters, E., & Wall, S. (1978). *Patterns of attachment: A psychological study of the Strange Situation.* Hillsdale, NJ: Erlbaum.

Baumrind, D. (1988). Rearing competent children. In W. Damon (Ed.), *Child development today and tomorrow* (pp. 349–378). San Francisco: Jossey-Bass.

Baumrind, D. (1991). Parenting style and adolescent development. In R. M. Lerner, A. C. Petersen, & J. Brooks-Gunn (Eds.), *The encyclopedia of adolescence* (pp. 746–758). New York: Garland.

Bornstein, M. H., Tamis-LeMonda, C. S., Pascual, L. O., Haynes, O. M., Painter, K. M., Galperin, C. Z., & Pecheux, M. (1996). Ideas about parenting in Argentina, France, and the United States. *International Journal of Behavioral Development, 19,* 347–367.

Brody, G., & Flor, D. L. (1998). Maternal resources, parenting practices, and child competence in rural, single-parent African American families. *Child Development, 69*(3), 803–816.

Carlson, V. J., & Harwood, R. L. (2003). Attachment, culture, and the caregiving system: The cultural patterning of everyday experiences among Anglo and Puerto Rican mother infant pairs. *Infant Mental Health Journal, 24*, 53–73.

Cassidy, J., & Shaver, P. R. (Eds.). (1999). *Handbook of attachment: Theory, research, and clinical applications.* New York: Guilford Press.

Cole, M. (1996). *Cultural psychology: A once and future discipline.* Cambridge, MA: Harvard University Press.

D'Andrade, R. G. (1984). Cultural meaning systems. In R. Shweder & R. LeVine (Eds.), *Culture theory: Essays on mind, self, and emotion* (pp. 88–117). New York: Cambridge University Press.

DeWolff, M. S., & van IJzendoorn, M. H. (1997). Sensitivity and attachment: A meta-analysis on parental antecedents of infant attachment. *Child Development, 68*, 571–591.

Dunn, J. (1988). *The beginnings of social understanding.* Cambridge, MA: Harvard University Press.

Falicov, C. J. (1998). *Latino families in therapy: A guide to multicultural practice.* New York: Guilford Press.

Garcia Coll, C., & Magnuson, K. (1999). Cultural influences on child development: Are we ready for a paradigm shift? In A. S. Masten (Ed.), *Cultural processes in child development* (Vol. 29, pp. 1–24). Mahwah, NJ: Erlbaum.

George, C., & Solomon, J. (1999). Attachment and caregiving: The caregiving behavioral system. In J. Cassidy & P. R. Shaver (Eds.), *Handbook of attachment: Theory, research, and clinical applications* (pp. 649–670). New York: Guilford Press.

Grossmann, K., Grossmann, K. E., Spangler, G., Suess, G., & Unzner, L. (1985). Maternal sensitivity and newborns' orientation responses as related to quality of attachment in northern Germany. *Monographs of the Society for Research in Child Development, 50*(1–2, Serial No. 209), 233–256.

Handwerker, W. P. (in press). The construct validity of cultures: Culture theory, cultural diversity, and a method for ethnography. *American Anthropologist.*

Harwood, R. L. (1992). The influence of culturally derived values on Anglo and Puerto Rican mothers' perceptions of attachment behavior. *Child Development, 63*, 822–839.

Harwood, R. L., Handwerker, W. P., Schöoelmerich, A., & Leyendecker, B. (2001). Ethnic category labels, parental beliefs, and the contextualized individual: An exploration of the individualism/sociocentrism debate. *Parenting: Science and Practice, 1*(3), 217–236.

Harwood, R. L., Miller, A. M., Carlson, V. J., & Leyendecker, B. (2002). Childrearing beliefs and practices during feeding among middle-class Puerto Rican and Anglo mother–infant pairs. In J. M. Contreras, K. A. Kerns, & A. M. Neal-Barnett (Eds.), *Latino children and families in the United States* (pp. 133–154). Westport, CT: Praeger.

Harwood, R. L., Miller, J. G., & Irizarry, N. L. (1995). *Culture and attachment: Perceptions of the child in context.* New York: Guilford Press.

Harwood, R. L., Schöoelmerich, A., Schulze, P. A., & Gonzalez, Z. (1999). Cultural differences in maternal beliefs and behaviors: A study of middle-class Anglo and Puerto Rican mother–infant pairs in four everyday situations. *Child Development, 70*(4), 1005–1016.

Ispa, J., Fine, M., Thornburg, K., & Sharp, E. (2001, April). *Maternal childrearing goals: Consistency and correlates.* Poster presented at the biennial meeting of the Society for Research in Child Development, Minneapolis, MN.

Jones, E., & Rao, M. (1998, July). *The differential impact of parental beliefs and practices on Chinese and English preschoolers' social competence.* Paper presented at the 15th biennial meetings of the International Society for the Study of Behavioural Development, Bern, Switzerland.

Kalyanpur, M., & Harry, B. (1997). A posture of reciprocity: A practical approach to collaboration between professionals and parents of culturally diverse backgrounds. *Journal of Child and Family Studies, 6,* 485–509.

Kermani, H., & Brenner, M. E. (2000). Maternal scaffolding in the child's zone of proximal development across tasks: Cross-cultural perspectives. *Journal of Research in Childhood Education, 15,* 30–52.

Knight, G. P., Virdin, L. M., & Roosa, M. (1994). Socialization and family correlates of mental health outcomes among Hispanic and Anglo American children: Consideration of cross-ethnic scalar equivalence. *Child Development, 65,* 212–224.

Leyendecker, B., & Lamb, M. E. (1999). Latino families. In M. E. Lamb (Ed.), *Parenting and child development in "nontraditional" families* (pp. 247–262). Mahwah, NJ: Erlbaum.

Malatesta, C. Z., Culver, C., Tesman, J. R., & Shepard, B. S. (1989). The development of emotion expression during the first two years of life. *Monographs of the Society for Research in Child Development, 54*(1–2, Serial No. 219), 55–82.

Martini, M. (2001, April). *Parents' goals and methods of shaping infant intentionality in four cultural groups.* Poster presented at the biennial meeting of the Society for Research in Child Development, Minneapolis, MN.

Miyake, K. S. C., & Campos, J. J. (1985). Infant temperament, mother's mode of interaction, and attachment in Japan: An interim report. *Monographs of the Society for Research in Child Development, 50*(1–2, Serial No. 209), 276–297.

Pauls, C. D., Choudhury, N., Leppanen, P. H. T., & Benasich, A. A. (2001, April). *The relationship among maternal knowledge and beliefs about infant development, infant temperament, and mother–infant interaction.* Poster presented at the biennial meeting of the Society for Research in Child Development, Minneapolis, MN.

Pine, J. M. (1992). Maternal style at the early one-word stage: Re-evaluating the stereotype of the directive mother. *First Language, 12,* 169–186.

Posada, G., Carbonell, O. A., & Alzate, G. (2001, April). *Maternal caregiving and infant security in two cultures.* Poster presented at the biennial meeting of the Society for Research in Child Development, Minneapolis, MN.

Posada, G., Gao, Y., Wu, F., Posada, R., Tascon, M., Schoelmerich, A., Sagi, A., Kondo-Ikemura, K., Haaland, W., & Synnevaag, B. (1995). The secure-base phenomenon across cultures: Children's behavior, mothers' preferences, and experts' concepts. *Monographs of the Society for Research in Child Development, 60*(2–3, Serial No. 244), 27–48.

Rao, N., & Pearson, E. (2001, April). *Links between socialization goals and childrearing practices in Chinese and Indian mothers.* Poster presented at the biennial meeting of the Society for Research in Child Development, Minneapolis, MN.

Rothbaum, F., Weisz, J., Pott, M., Miyake, K., & Morelli, G. (2000). Attachment and culture: Security in the United States and Japan. *American Psychologist, 55,* 1093–1104.

Sagi, A., Lamb, M. E., Lewkowicz, K. S., Shoham, R., Dvir, R., & Estes, D. (1985). Security of infant–mother, –father, and –metapelet attachments among kibbutz-reared Israeli children. *Monographs of the Society for Research in Child Development, 50*(1–2, Serial No. 209), 257–275.

van IJzendoorn, M. H., & Kroonenberg, P. M. (1988). Cross-cultural patterns of attachment: A meta-analysis of the Strange Situation. *Child Development, 59,* 147–156.

van IJzendoorn, M. H., & Sagi, A. (1999). Cross-cultural patterns of attachment: Universal and contextual dimensions. In J. Cassidy & P. R. Shaver (Eds.), *Handbook of attachment: Theory, research, and clinical applications* (pp. 713–734). New York: Guilford Press.

Yang, Y. S., & Chang, M. J. (1999, April). *The relationships of mothers' parenting and children's characteristics to Korean preschool children's attachment and social competence.* Paper presented at the biennial meeting of the Society for Research in Child Development, Albuquerque, NM.

PART II

MODELS OF CLINICAL INTERVENTION

6

Attachment Theory

A Guide for Couple Therapy

SUSAN M. JOHNSON

The application of attachment theory to adult relationships, which did not occur until the late 1980s (Hazan & Shaver, 1987; Johnson, 1986), was a revolutionary event for the modality of couple therapy. For the first time, a theory of close relationships offered the couple therapist a coherent, relevant, widely applicable, and well-researched framework for understanding the complex phenomenon of the adult love relationship. This is a phenomenon that has preoccupied and perplexed human beings throughout history. Couple therapy, as a modality, has generally been missing a comprehensive theory of relatedness to guide intervention. Over the years a number of general ideas have arisen that have guided the practice of couple therapy—for example, that adult love relationships mirror past relationships with parents, and that we even actively re-create the negative elements of these relationships to resolve inner conflicts; that problems in relationships are due to developmental delays that cause partners to enmesh rather than differentiate; or that partners lack skills, either communication skills or the negotiation skills, with which to create good rational quid pro quo contracts with spouses. There have been many problems with these conceptualizations. For example, the concept of enmeshment confuses caring and coercion (Green & Werner, 1996), and quid pro quo contracts are not generally found in happy couples but only in those who are very distressed (Murstein, Cerreto, & McDonald, 1977). In general, then, as a modality, couple therapy has largely been a set of techniques in search of a coherent theory of relatedness to help direct its interventions. As Anderson (2000) noted in her address at the millennium conference of the American Association of Marriage and Family Therapy, we have set out on a vast and troubled ocean in a very small theoretical boat.

The application of attachment theory to adult love relationships is part of, and consonant with, a larger revolution that has seen adult love relationships and problems in such relationships addressed in scientific inquiry. As Berscheid notes (1999, p. 260), science has at last begun to address the "core mysteries of human relationships." Attachment theory, and the associated research on adult attachment relationships, fits very well with the burgeoning recent research on the nature of relationship distress (Gottman, 1994), and on the impact close relationships have on mental and physical health (Kiecolt-Glasser et al., 1993; Anderson, Beach, & Kaslow, 1999). It is also easily integrated with key perspectives in the couple therapy modality, namely, systems theory and the feminist perspective (Johnson, 2002; Johnson & Best, 2002).

There is nothing so practical as a good theory, and attachment theory helps the couple therapist see into and through the complex, multidimensional drama that is a close relationship in crisis. It helps direct the therapist to the defining features of such relationships, set treatment goals that are relevant and meaningful, and map out the best ways to intervene. A map that outlines the nature of the terrain makes the difference between a glorious adventure and getting lost in the woods and reaching a dead end. If we consider a typical North American distressed couple who arrive in a therapist's office, what does attachment theory tell us about them and their problems?

THE ATTACHMENT PERSPECTIVE ON DISTRESSED RELATIONSHIPS

First, this theory tells us that most significant relationship problems will be about the security of the bond between the partners, about their struggle to define the relationship as a safe haven and a secure base (Bowlby, 1969; Cassidy & Shaver, 1999). Contact with intimate others is the primary way humans have evolved to deal with anxiety and fear. Proximity to an attachment figure tames fear and offers an antidote to feelings of helplessness and meaninglessness. The key issue in distressed relationships is each partner's accessibility and responsiveness to emotional cues. As a distressed woman remarked to her spouse, "It's not the fights that really matter. I could handle disagreements—if I felt like you were there for me. But I can never find you when I need you. I feel alone in this relationship." The spouse becomes the primary attachment figure for the majority of adults, and as such their main source of security and comfort. The attachment to one's partner may be especially crucial at a time and in a culture where there has been a loss of "social capital" (Twenge, 2000). Many people now live in a "community of two," not in the bosom of their extended family or village, and they have no one else to count on for emotional support beside their spouse. Attachment theory also suggests that a therapist may help couples improve their communication skills or gain insight into their past and present relationships, but may be less than effective if he or she does not specifically address the need for comfort and the promotion of the safe emotional engagement and responsiveness that is the basis of a secure bond. This perspective parallels the recent empirical research that stresses the pivotal importance of soothing and supportive responses in defining close relationships and the absolute requirement for safe emotional engagement (Gottman, 1994: Gottman, Coan, Carrere, & Swanson, 1998; Pasch & Bradbury, 1998).

Second, isolation, separation, or disconnection from an attachment figure is inherently traumatizing. Distressed partners who are emotionally disconnected tend to become immersed in fear and insecurity, and to adopt the stances of fight, flight, or freeze that characterize responses to traumatic stress. The more distressed and hopeless the relationship, the more automatic, rigid, and self-reinforcing the emotional responses and the interactional dance between partners will be.

Third, consonant with the current collaborative, nonpathologizing trend in couple and family therapy (Anderson, 1997), attachment theory depathologizes dependency needs (Bowlby, 1988). Bowlby suggests there is no such thing as overdependency or true independence; there is only effective or ineffective dependence (Weinfield, Sroufe, Egeland, & Carlson, 1999). The more effectively dependent a person can be, the more confidently separate and autonomous he or she can be. In general, Western societies have denigrated dependency needs in adults and exalted the image of the separate, self-sufficient individual. Feminist authors remind us that women are often pathologized for their focus on closeness to others (Vatcher & Bogo, 2001). Bowlby also emphasizes that no attachment strategy is dysfunctional in itself. A strategy such as extreme avoidance can be functional in that it can maximize the stability and safety of a specific attachment relationship by minimizing the demands made on an attachment figure. It is when such strategies become rigid and globally applied in new contexts that problems arise. This perspective helps the therapist take a validating, respectful, egalitarian stance toward his or her clients.

Fourth, from an attachment perspective, the patterns of distress in couple relationships are quite finite and predictable and reflect the process of separation distress. Most often, one partner will pursue for emotional connection, but often in an angry critical manner, while the other will placate or withdraw to "keep the peace" or to protect him- or herself from criticism. Each partner's steps then call forth and maintain the others' in a reciprocally determining feedback loop. Gottman (1994) found in his research on relationship distress that negative cycles such as critical complaining and defensive distance predicted the continued deterioration of a relationship. Bowlby (1969) painted a picture of separation distress as naturally proceeding through angry protest, clinging and seeking, depression and despair, and, finally, detachment from the relationship. Occasionally, couples will come for therapy when the pursuing spouse has given up and is beginning to withdraw as a prelude to detachment. This perspective helps the therapist to see the pattern of interactions in a distressed relationship and also to "see beyond" it to the desperation and longing underlying coercive demands and protests and the anxieties and hopelessness underlying stonewalling and withdrawal.

Fifth, depression and anxiety naturally accompany relationship distress (Whisman, 1999), with its attendant loss of security and connection and debilitating sense of isolation, and such distress is likely to maintain these emotional problems. Such distress will also feed into and maintain stress that arises from other sources, for example, posttraumatic stress from violent assault or the echoes of childhood sexual abuse (Johnson & Williams-Keeler, 1998). The resilience fostered by the safe haven and secure base offered in a secure attachment relationship is not to be found. The couple therapist often deals with psychological disorders such as depression as well as with relationship distress per se. Attachment theory suggests specific links between relationship distress and mental disorders, which most clients describe in terms of loss, aloneness, and a sense of helplessness. It thus offers the therapist a clear perspective from which to intervene. It also supports the view of couple therapy as a modality that directly addresses and has an impact on individual functioning and growth.

Sixth, attachment theory directs the therapist's attention to the regulation, processing, and integration of the key emotional responses within a couple relationship (Johnson, 1996). Many models of couple therapy have marginalized emotion, seeing it as a tag-on to cognition or as part of the problem. *Emotion*, which comes from the Latin word meaning "to move," has often been viewed as an intrapersonal, nonsystemic variable. In fact, it is perfectly consistent with systems theory to view emotion and emotional expression as a key link between self and system and as a leading element, an organizer, of the interactional cycles that systems theory has highlighted for couple therapists. Attachment theory emphasizes the importance of emotion as a prime motivator for and organizer of attachment responses. Emotional responses also assign meaning to relationship cues, which are often by nature quite ambiguous, and are a prime means of communicating with others. As Bowlby states (1991, p. 294), "The principal function of emotion is one of communication—namely, the communication to the self and the other of the current motivational state of the individual." Research into the nature of relationship distress also echoes the importance of emotional signals. Facial expressions of emotion are powerful predictors of divorce (Gottman, 1994). Attachment theory suggests that we should pay exquisite attention to the emotions clients bring to couple therapy, which mostly involve anger, sadness and longing, shame, and fear. The therapist can help partners regulate reactive emotions that fuel negative cycles such as attack/defend, and access and articulate marginalized emotions that can be used to move partners into new forms of emotional engagement. For example, expressing desperation pulls a partner closer and cues his or her compassion.

Seventh, the need for secure emotional connection with a few key others is considered to be hard-wired by evolution, and there are a finite number of ways to deal with the loss of such a connection. Thus, there are only a few engagement styles or strategies that the therapist has to take account of. These involve, first, hyperactivating the attachment system and so becoming preoccupied with the relationship, monitoring it constantly, and becoming coercive and aggressive; second, attempting to deactivate the attachment system by "numbing out" and "shutting down" to care less and protect the self; and, third, trying both of the above in sequence. The last strategy is used particularly by trauma survivors who have been violated in close relationships and who, simultaneously, both desperately need and seek, and also desperately fear and avoid, closeness (Johnson, 2002). The considerable research on these engagement strategies helps the couple therapist understand, validate, and begin to deconstruct them in the therapy session (Johnson & Whiffen, 1999: Johnson & Best, 2002).

Eighth, as in other systemic perspectives, attachment focuses on how the self is defined in the context of recurring interpersonal interactions. Bowlby stressed how models of self and models of other, particularly concerning the lovableness of self and the trustworthiness of others, arise from and then guide interactions with others. These models tend to become stable, not simply because they are in place and influence ongoing information processing, but because they tend to be continually confirmed in interactions with significant others. Working models guide people's responses to others and so set up interactions that then pull for confirming feedback (Shaver & Hazan, 1993). The attachment perspective helps the therapist grasp and deal with typical shifts in levels of interaction from explicit content issues (e.g., "You never help with chores.") to more implicit relationship definition/attachment issues (e.g., "Don't speak to me in that tone of voice—like I am nothing to you.") and implicit identity issues (e.g., "You are impossible, you are just too hard to live with."). The therapist can also actively use new positive interactions to challenge negative views of self and other and to promote the construction of a more positive sense of self. Those who feel securely attached to their partners tend to have a more elaborated, articulated, coherent, and positive sense of self (Mikulincer,

1995). The more safely connected I am to those I love, the more I can be myself. Attachment theory helps the therapist conceptualize and therefore address the links between self and system.

Ninth, and finally, attachment theory tells us what the defining moments in a relationship are likely to be, both in terms of the wounds and specific injuries (Johnson, Makinen, & Millikin, 2001) that define the bond as insecure and in terms of the key shifts and change events in therapy that can redefine the relationship as secure and satisfying. Change events in emotionally focused couple therapy (EFT; Johnson, 1996) are associated with specific bonding events called "softenings." In a softening, a newly vulnerable spouse reaches out to a now accessible and engaged partner and asks for his or her attachment needs to be met (Johnson & Talitman, 1997). These pivotal moments appear to offer an antidote to the cycle of negative interactions that have imprisoned the couple for so long. Once such change events are defined and the interventions that lead to them specified (Bradley, 2001), the whole endeavor of therapy is expedited. Pivotal moments where the relationship is defined as unsafe and insecure are also able to be identified. This is crucial in that, if unaddressed, such moments will tend to block change and create impasses in the therapy process. These events, which may be considered relationship traumas, will be discussed in more detail later in this chapter. Attachment theory deepens our understanding of everyday relationship events that have generally been considered to be crucial to relationship satisfaction, such as sexuality. Adult attachment is considered to be reciprocal. It is also representational, in the sense that to know that one is held in the mind of the other, or to hold the other in mind, is often comforting and a source of support. Adult attachment is also sexual (Hazan & Zeifman, 1994). For many partners sexual encounters may be the only time they are held, reassured, and able to connect with their softer feelings and dependency needs.

THE ATTACHMENT PERSPECTIVE ON A POSITIVE RELATIONSHIP

The research on secure attachment offers the couple therapist a clear empirically validated model of healthy connectedness, and thus a specific picture of what couples should, in the best case scenario, be able to do at the end of therapy. The picture of secure attachment that emerges from the research on childhood shows securely attached children being able to regulate their distress on separation from an attachment figure, to send clear assertive signals as to their needs when reunited, to trust and accept comfort and reassurance, and then, confident about their connection with their loved one, to turn to tasks and the exploration of the environment. This picture seems to be equally relevant and applicable to adult partners. More specifically, in terms of affect regulation, securely attached partners should be better able to contain their reactive, negative emotions and to access and articulate their marginalized or numbed-out emotions. So if a secure attachment can be established, the "aggressive blamer" can modify his or her anger and express other emotions such as sadness and longing, and the "stonewalling spouse" can touch and share the helplessness and uncertainty that cues this stance. Securely attached people in general are more able to access and acknowledge their distress in an open congruent way that elicits responsiveness.

As relationships become safer and more secure in the therapy process, partners are able to find exits from negative cycles. Secure attachment is associated with greater self-disclosure (Mikulincer & Nachshon, 1991). Secure partners have greater access to their underlying emotions and can choose to share these emotions and so change the "music" of their relationship "dance." They can also reflect on the process of interaction, and so metacommunicate about the dance. Research suggests that, indeed, secure bonds are characterized by this ability to metacommunicate and so change the direction of an interaction (Kobak & Cole, 1991). In terms of processing information, secure partners are confident enough to engage in cognitive exploration and remain cognitively flexible, even under stress (Mikulincer, 1997). They are more open to new evidence and deal with ambiguity better. In essence, a secure style facilitates the ability to learn from new experience and update models of self and other as necessary. This research parallels the results of the first outcome study on EFT (Johnson & Greenberg, 1985), where partners who were no longer dangling their feet over the cliff of attachment insecurity could, by the end of therapy, tolerate differences, negotiate, and problem solve. In this study, distressed partners who received EFT and increased the security of their bond were as good at problem solving in final sessions as those who had received specific training in this skill as part of the study. Secure partners are also able to reflect on their experience and create integrated coherent narratives about their attachment relationships (Main, Kaplan, & Cassidy, 1985). Insecurity acts to constrict and narrow how cognitions and emotions are processed and dealt with, and so the ability to create such narratives.

The communication of secure partners tends to be more open and direct than that of insecure partners. They tend to disclose more and be more attuned to the communication of others. They are confident enough to assert themselves but tend to offer more empathic support and use rejection less (Feeney, Noller, & Callan, 1994). It is in watershed events when one partner is distressed and the other either provides or fails to provide closeness and comfort that the quality of communication matters most (Simpson & Rholes, 1994). Then the ability to disclose and confide in a direct way about needs and fears and to tune in to the other's experience is crucial if partners are to define or redefine the relationship as a safe haven and a secure base.

COUPLE THERAPY BASED ON ATTACHMENT
AS A THEORY OF RELATEDNESS

A model of intervention based on this theory, such as EFT (Johnson, 1996), should then be characterized by the following:

- A focus on and validation of attachment needs and fears and the promotion of safe emotional engagement, comfort, and support.
- A privileging of emotional responses and communication and direct addressing of attachment vulnerabilities and fears so as to foster emotional attunement and responsiveness.
- The creation of a respectful collaborative alliance, so that the therapy session itself may be a safe haven and a secure base.
- An explicit shaping of responsiveness and accessibility. Withdrawn partners will be reengaged and blaming partners will be supported to soften so that bonding events can occur that offer an antidote to negative cycles and insecurity.
- A focus on how the self is defined and can be redefined in emotional communication with attachment figures.
- An explicit shaping of pivotal attachment responses that redefine a relationship and an addressing of injuries that block relationship repair.

THE EFFECTIVENESS OF INTERVENTIONS
BASED ON ATTACHMENT THEORY

A relevant, coherent, and well-developed theory should give rise to specific interventions that prove to be effective in clinical practice. Attachment theory forms the theoretical basis of EFT, and indeed the literature supports the effectiveness of this intervention (Johnson, Hunsley, Greenberg, & Schindler, 1999). This approach has been found to be more effective than skill-building cognitive-behavioral approaches (Johnson & Greenberg, 1985), and, at present, obtains the best results of any couple intervention in the literature. Studies on EFT have found that 70–75% of couples recover from relationship distress after 10–12 sessions and that 90% rate themselves as significantly improved. The effectiveness of EFT is also apparently not as heavily influenced by initial distress levels as other approaches. Specifically, initial distress was found to account for only 4% of the variance in satisfaction at follow-up compared to an estimated 46% in the behavioral approaches (Whisman & Jacobson, 1990).

In terms of evidence as to the value of the theory, there are two other interesting points that emerge from the outcome research on EFT. First, as in psychotherapy research in general, the quality of the therapeutic alliance appears to predict outcome in EFT. However, it appears to be the task-relevance aspect of this alliance that is the most powerful predictor of outcome, rather than the bond with the therapist or a sense of shared goals. This suggests that couples found the focus on attachment relevant and compelling. Second, EFT does not seem to have the same problem with relapse as other approaches. There is evidence that results are stable, even in very stressed, high-risk relationships where couples would be expected to relapse (Clothier, Manion, Gordon-Walker, & Johnson, 2002), and that there is a trend to continuing improvement after therapy ends (Johnson et al., 1999). If interventions reach to the heart of the matter, they are more likely to create lasting change.

THE CREATION OF SECURE ATTACHMENT: THE EFT MODEL IN PRACTICE

EFT follows the principles outlined above for interventions based on attachment theory. The process of change in EFT occurs in three stages (Johnson, 1996). These stages involve:

1. The deescalation of negative cycles, such as attack–withdraw, that maintain attachment insecurity and block safe emotional engagement and responsiveness. The naming of these cycles and discussion of their impact helps the couple to see these cycles, rather than each other, as the enemy.
2. The shaping of new cycles of responsiveness and accessibility, where initially withdrawn partners take a more involved and active stance and state their needs and fears. Critical, pursuing partners can then begin to ask for their needs to be met in ways that foster compassion and contact. Powerful bonding events can then occur that offer a new emotional experience of connection.
3. The consolidation of gains and the integration of the process of change into the couple's model of the relationship and each partner's sense of self.

A snapshot of an EFT session would capture the therapist constantly involved in two tasks. First, the therapist will be reflecting present patterns in the process of interaction and exploring and expanding the processing of attachment-oriented emotions. The therapist will also explore the cognitive images of self and other that are cued by such emotions. Second, the therapist will be setting interactional tasks, either to enact (and so clarify) present interactional positions or to begin to shape new, more attuned, and more engaged interactions. So, the therapist might ask partners to explore their experience, as in, "What just happened there, as you, Celia, asked him to explain and then [turning to the other spouse] you, Michael, began to give reasons but suddenly looked at Celia's face and threw up your hands and became silent? Was that one of those times you spoke about when the ground opens up at your feet?" The therapist will then help this partner express the emotional reality behind the throwing up of the hands to his spouse, as in, "I see in your face that I will never do it right—I have failed before I begin. So I despair and shut down and then we are stuck." The therapist then helps the other spouse process this message.

In general terms, anxiety and insecurity tend to constrain the way both inner experience and interactional responses are constructed, shaped, and given meaning. The EFT therapist then deconstructs such experience or response, taking the sudden silence of the client Michael above and noting the hopelessness inherent in his response, the sense of self as a failure implied by it, the underlying attachment fears, and the part this response plays in the couple's pattern of interacting. This moment is then reconstructed and expanded and used to prime new interactions. As the therapist helps this spouse tell his wife about his hopelessness and despair, a new level of emotional engagement is initiated and begins to have an impact on how Celia views her husband. Change occurs by the construction of new emotional experience that changes the nature of the attachment bond between spouses.

CORE INTERVENTIONS

The following sections describe the interventions used by the EFT therapist. Some interventions may be used more than others at various stages in therapy.

Reflecting Emotional Experience

To address and reformulate key emotions, the therapist tracks and attunes to each client's relational experience and reflects the essential elements in this experience. For example: "Could you help me to understand? I think you're saying that you become so what you call 'tight' in these situations that you want to hold onto everything, keep everything under control? And then you get very curt with your husband when he begins to 'rock the boat' and talk about what is missing in the relationship. Is that right?"

Main functions: Focusing the therapy process; building and maintaining the alliance; clarifying emotional responses associated with underlying attachment issues and interactional positions.

Validation

Validation is the most basic intervention in EFT. It invites people to engage with their experience and frames their experience as legitimate and acceptable. For example: "It's so hard for you to even hear what he is saying? You just cannot believe that he might want to be close to you—when you feel so small, so needy. You don't feel entitled to be held and comforted right now, is that it?"

Main functions: Legitimizing responses, especially attachment needs and fears; supporting clients to continue to explore how they construct their experience and their interactions; strengthening the alliance.

Evocative Responding

Evocative responding expands by open questions the stimulus, bodily response, associated desires and meanings, or action tendencies implicit in emotions. For example: "What's happening right now, as you say that?" "What's that like for you?" "So when this happens some part of you wants to reach out, but another part of you is screaming out that it is too dangerous?"

Main functions: Expanding elements of experience to facilitate the reorganization of that experience; formulating unclear or marginalized elements of experience; encouraging exploration and emotional engagement.

Heightening

Using repetition, images, metaphors, or enactments, the therapist heightens and elucidates the nature of the clients' experience and how they construct that experience. For example: "So could you say that again directly please, 'I do turn away, I do shut you out,' " or, "This is so difficult for you, you feel lost, like there is no ground under your feet," or, "Can you turn and tell her, 'It's too hard to tell you about my longing?' "

Main functions: Highlighting key experiences that organize responses to the partner and new formulations of experience that will reorganize the interaction.

Empathic Conjecture or Interpretation

In this intervention, the therapist goes one step further in formulating the clients' experience than the clients themselves have done. For example: "You try to protect that raw, sensitive part of you by keeping a 'barrier' between you and the world, but then it gets a little lonely behind there, is that it?"

Main functions: Clarifying and formulating new meanings, especially regarding interactional positions and strategies of engagement that prevent emotional engagement with the partner and definitions of self. These conjectures are always explicitly open to correction and modification by the client.

Tracking, Reflecting, and Replaying Interactions

As the title of this intervention suggests, the therapist holds a mirror up to specific interactions and patterns so that they can be seen more clearly. For example: "Can I stop you for a moment? What just happened here? You smiled at him when he said he loved you, but then you turned your head and said 'Is that right' and began to recount that time he let you down and you decided to be 'separate and strong.' "

Main functions: Slows down and clarifies steps in the interactional dance; replays key interactional sequences so they can be restructured.

Reframing in the Context of the Cycle and Attachment Processes

In this intervention the therapist places specific experience in the context of the interactional patterns and each partner's attachment needs and fears. For example: "You go still and tight because you feel like you're right on the edge of losing her, yes?" "You go still because she matters so much to you, not because you don't care?"

Main functions: Shifts the meaning of specific responses and fosters more positive perceptions of the partner.

Restructuring and Shaping Interactions

The therapist supports the clients to enact present positions and so clarify those positions, as well as enacting new behaviors based upon new emotional responses. The therapist also choreographs specific change events, such as softenings. For example: (1) "Can you tell him, 'I won't, I won't . . . I'm never going to put myself in your hands again?' " (2) "You have just spoken about being sad. Could you tell him right now about that sadness?" (3) "Can you ask him for what you need right now?"

Main functions: Clarifies and expands negative interaction patterns, creates new kinds of dialogue and new interactional steps/positions, leading to positive cycles of accessibility and responsiveness.

These interventions are discussed in more detail elsewhere, together with markers or cues as to when specific interventions are used, and descriptions of the process partners engage in as a result of each intervention (Johnson, 1996, 1999; Johnson & Denton, 2002).

A GOOD MAP LEADS TO NEW DISCOVERIES
AND TERRITORIES: NEW DIRECTIONS IN EFT

Recent developments in EFT illustrate how an attachment perspective can help the therapist treat complex forms of relationship insecurity and distress, such as those found in the relationships of trauma survivors (Johnson, 2002) and address specific kinds of impasses in therapy, such as the recently formulated *attachment injury* (Johnson et al., 2001).

The delineation of attachment injuries illustrates how a relationship theory can clarify impasses in the change process and expedite effective intervention. Attachment theorists have pointed out that incidents in which one partner responds or fails to respond at times of urgent need seem to disproportionately influence the quality of an attachment relationship (Simpson & Rholes, 1994). Such incidents either shatter or confirm each partner's assumptions about attachment relationships and the dependability of the other. Negative attachment-related events, particularly abandonments and betrayals, often then cause seemingly irreparable damage to close relationships. Many partners enter therapy not only in general distress, but also with the goal of bringing closure to such events and so restoring lost intimacy and trust. During the therapy process, these events, even if they are long past, often reemerge in an alive and intensely emotional manner, much like a traumatic flashback, and overwhelm the injured partner, creating an impasse and hindering the process of change. These incidents, usually occurring in the context of life transitions, loss, physical danger, or uncertainty, when attachment needs are most salient and compelling, can be considered relationship traumas. Attachment theory offers an explanation of why certain painful events, such as specific abandonments, become pivotal in a relationship, as well as an understanding of what the key features of such events will be, how they will impact a particular couple's relationship, and how such events can be optimally resolved. Indeed these injuries *must* be resolved if a couple are to repair their bond and create lasting change in their relationship. The resolution of such an injury is presented as part of the case illustration below.

EFT has also been used for many years in a hospital clinic to improve the relationships of clients with relationship distress that is exacerbated by complex posttraumatic stress disorder (Herman, 1992). This disorder, where others are experienced simultaneously as the source of and the only respite from terror, is usually the result of abuse by attachment figures in childhood. It often leads to the adoption of a fearful–avoidant engagement strategy in adult relationships (Shaver & Clarke, 1994). This strategy is characterized by extreme neediness and extreme fear of closeness and exposure. Attachment theory also helps link specific qualities in a primary relationship to individual problems such as depression and posttraumatic stress disorder. If couple therapists can help traumatized partners create a more secure bond, they can also create a potent healing environment where such trauma can be addressed and trust in self and others restored (Johnson, 2002). The map provided by attachment theory has proved invaluable in adapting EFT to these relationships. If the treatment of trauma is essentially about the taming of fear, attachment theory offers the couple therapist the possibility of helping the couple create the "primary protection against feelings of helplessness and meaninglessness" (McFarlane & van der Kolk, 1996, p. 24), a secure connection with a loved one.

CASE PRESENTATION: NO-MAN'S-LAND

Louise and Jim had been married for 14 years. She was a professional artist and he was a successful lawyer. They had met in their early 20s and had had a long-distance relationship for 5 years before they finally married. They had no children and were comfortable with this choice. They came in with a long story of alienation from each other and recounted their previous experience in couple therapy which had ended 9 months earlier and had been negative. In particular, it had contained one session that Louise had experienced as "catastrophic" and which she refused to talk about.

The way they described their everyday interactions was that they were both distant and withdrawn. However, they stated that up until 2 years ago they fought quite regularly. These fights would be about how Louise was pursuing Jim for closeness, while he remained reserved and, in her terms, "cold." In the last 2 years, after a family crisis where her mother had a heart attack and died, Louise had "shut down" and stopped pursuing and began to avoid any kind of physical contact with Jim. Louise said, "We are distant friends. It's a case of going through the motions. Like a no-man's-land. I think maybe we shouldn't be married at all." Louise also spoke of long-term problems with anxiety attacks and bouts of depression and had had individual therapy at various times in her life. She felt that the problem had been that she had grown up alone; she had been "close to no one—except Jim—at first—maybe." Jim also spoke of having no model for "whatever she means by closeness" and coming from a very "reserved" family. He had understood for years that Louise had been disappointed by the relationship and had "hunkered down and just avoided confrontation." He spoke of missing sexual contact and being confused about what his wife wanted from him. He asked, "I do need space sometimes. Do I have to give myself up to stop her from leaving me?" When pressed, Jim agreed that he too was lonely. He added, " I think we're stuck. She talks about divorce. We chill out so much—where are the feelings for each other?"

What were the key moments/episodes in Louise and Jim's journey toward secure attachment? After a few sessions, I began to understand that the "catastrophic" past therapy session had involved an attachment injury for Louise. She stated that the therapist and Jim had agreed in that session that she was too needy, immature, and "dependent," and that she had to learn to give Jim the space he needed. She said that "something had snapped," and she had "switched off." She was not now willing to take risks and to pursue Jim, as in the past. Jim expressed anger at this point, and said he was fed up with walking on eggshells and trying to meet Louise's expectations. Louise then commented that the only emotion she ever saw from him was anger. This couple was easy to work with, except for the fact that Louise needed time and reassurance to feel safe in the alliance with me after her previous experience. Jim seemed to have generally used avoidant, "cool your jets" strategies, while Louise described herself as lonely and preoccupied and as using an "upping the ante" strategy, before she had moved to a more fearful–avoidant stance.

Deescalation of this couple's negative cycle of defensive withdrawal was a relatively easy process. We began to talk about the cycle they were caught in, and both were able to state that they did not want to lose the marriage. Using an attachment perspective and fostering the exploration of underlying feelings, Louise was able to begin to express her anger at Jim's inaccessibility and how he had labeled her the "big, bad, needy one" and discounted her distress. Jim, while at first very intellectual and reserved, began to be able to talk about how he did have feelings, even though his natural style was to be "detached." In fact, with the therapist's help, he began to name his sense of being "flooded and exhausted" from the effort of being "so careful" in the relationship. They began to be more open and sympathetic with each other in the sessions, and both agreed that secure emotional connectedness was a "foreign country" for them, neither being able to remember such a bond in their childhood. They began to share more and to speak of each other as friends, as well as to express some hope for their relationship.

In the second stage of therapy, it seemed imperative to encourage Jim to emotionally engage and become more responsive, and then to try to foster Louise's trust and heal her attachment injury. I began to reflect and heighten Jim's feelings and prompt him to confide in his spouse. He began to access feelings of helplessness and frustration at "not knowing what to do—how to give her what she wants." With support, he was able, even though Louise often sat silent and tight-mouthed, to express his pain and fear of disappointing and so losing his wife.

THERAPIST: What is happening right now, Jim? Your voice sounds very calm, but you are talking slower and more and more "carefully," and you are rubbing your hands together all the time.

JIM: Am I? Well, maybe I'm learning, but I can't talk on an emotional level all the time you know. I can't be made over instantly into what I am not. I am who I am.

THERAPIST: And you are worried that this may not be acceptable to Louise? (*He nods and his eyes fill with tears.*) Can you tell her about that? (*He shakes his head.*) That would be too hard? To tell her how—well—overwhelming it is—this fear of losing her and how it paralyzes you and makes it even harder to try to open up—is that OK? (*He nods in assent.*) Can you tell her, it's so hard to let you see my fear and confusion?

He does this and she responds relatively sympathetically. After this session and the kind of process encapsulated above, Jim began to emerge from his shell and to talk about his sense of rejection. He was able to talk about how Louise could help him by validating his attempts at sharing and being more tolerant of his "fumblings to be personal." He stated that he too wanted the connection they had glimpsed in the beginning of their relationship. As he became more engaged, Louise began to hold her mouth in a tight-closed line and to speak of being "bored."

The task now was to support Jim to stay engaged and to bring Louise, step by step, into a softening where she would risk emotional engagement with Jim. Louise would swing between cool distance, angry remarks, and brief allusions to fear and sadness. After a week where Jim had been very "busy," she remarked, "If you won't carry the relationship, I'm dropping it." I asked her to tell him, "I won't expose myself again and reach for you. My hurt, my aloneness, weren't important to you." He was able to tell her that it was the sense that he was being tested and was failing that terrified him. We framed his dilemma as one where she was *so important* to him that, ironically, he would "freeze up" and be unable to respond. Louise replied, "If you really wanted me I wouldn't have had to fight so hard to get here." We focused on her anger and her determination not to be hurt again. She did admit, however, that they now were able to cuddle and perhaps "things were shifting." We then moved more intensely into Louise's hurt in the relationship and how hard it was now to risk with Jim after being "shut out" all those years. He validated her struggles and her hurt, told her that he found her coolness "scary," and poignantly asked her not to give up on him and the relationship. But just as I thought she was going to reach for him, she then stepped back and became immersed in the trauma of the previous catastrophic therapy session. She became alternately shaky and then distant. I encouraged her to focus on this experience and after saying there was no point and what was happening now was "too little, too late," she began to speak of her sense of isolation and violation in that past session. The attachment injury frame helped me to clarify her experience into a sense of abandonment (Jim had joined with the previous therapist in discounting her) helplessness (she saw that her pain did not matter to him), and despair (she said, "It was the final blow").

The process then evolved in the steps we have identified as typical of attachment injury resolution, leading into a softening and a bonding event. We can summarize these as:

• Louise accesses and articulates the injury and it's attachment significance: "I didn't matter. You shut me out. You both talked about me like I was a mental case, a nonperson. After all my struggles." I helped her articulate and express her grief and then her determination to protect herself and her ensuing stance of "never again."

• With the support of the therapist, Jim was able to acknowledge her hurt and to admit that he had let her down and shut her out. He elaborated on how terrified he had been in that session and how he had responded to the therapist's suggestion that Louise had to " mature" and change with relief, since it assuaged his own fears of failure. He explained his stance in the incident and I framed it in terms of his fears of losing her, rather than in terms of his callousness or indifference.

• Louise, supported by my validation and structuring of the experience, was then able to articulate the depth of her grief and her sense of isolation. As the only person she had ever felt connected to had turned away from her, her "desperation" had been overwhelming and she had given up on the hope of comfort and closeness. As she put it, "I wanted to die. I couldn't tell you but I was suicidal for days." She wept as she spoke of the sense that she was "disintegrating" as her need for closeness had been disqualified by Jim, as it had in her family relationships.

• Jim moved his chair close and intensely expressed his remorse and regret. He acknowledged again that he had let her down and had not understood her need. He wept with her.

• I asked Louise if she could let Jim comfort her. She refused to do this. We explored this "refusal to be taken in by hope." Jim helped by telling her that he was "desperate" for her forgiveness. Gradually, with my reflecting the process and heightening Jim's messages, she began to hear his remorse and his message that she was important to him. She was then able to tell him how afraid she felt to let the longing for him come up again. I supported her to state this directly and fully to Jim.

• Jim comforted Louise. She began to talk about "trying to find a way back to him" and they begin to piece together a narrative of how they had lost each other and now perhaps had found each other again. They both were able to speak of needing reassurance and comfort. Louise articulated that it was crucial that Jim had acknowledged that she had the right to feel angry and hurt about the session where the injury occurred and the lack of intimacy in the relationship.

Once this injury was resolved, Louise was able to take small steps toward Jim and the trust between them began to grow. She was able to ask for her needs to be met in specific ways that he did not find overwhelming, and he was able to respond to her vulnerability as in a classic EFT softening event. In this event she was able to fully experience and disclose her fear of depending on Jim again and he was able to reassure and comfort her. The couple were then able to move into the consolidation phase of therapy, where the relationship becomes defined as a safe haven and a secure base. The differences between them were now less significant. Louise said, "My needs are really not that huge. If he shows me he needs me too." And Jim said, "I do want to be close—but I have to feel safe enough to learn how to do it." Louise was able to state, "I think I am finding feelings—I forgot I had them—it's tentatively love." We talked of ways that they could reassure each other and keep connected on a daily basis and of how they had worked to restore and renew their relationship. They were also able to formulate, with the therapist's help, a coherent narrative of how their relationship had become distressed and how they had repaired it. As a last comment, Jim remarked, "We have both been so lonely, but now no-man's-land seems to be turning into a field of daisies." He smiled.

CONCLUSIONS

Attachment theory, as it has been developed and related to adult relationships, is a transactional systemic theory that offers the expanding field of couple therapy a much-needed comprehensive theory of adult love and connectedness (Johnson & Best, 2002). It offers the therapist an answer to key questions, such as what to focus on and what elements to target for change in the complex drama of relationship distress. It guides the therapist to the heart of the matter and offers a compelling and empirically supported model of relationship health and dysfunction. It informs the therapist as to the pivotal processes and watershed events that define the nature of a close relationship. All of this is essential to the task that now faces couple therapy as a modality (Johnson & Lebow, 2000). This task is to articulate efficient and effective interventions that can help couples construct stable, long-term, satisfying bonds, interventions that can also address key individual symptoms by changing the nature of an individual's most immediate context. As Gurman (2001) suggests, primary relationships have great healing power, and for change to endure it must be supported in a person's natural environment. This theory has great breadth, but it is also specific enough that it can focus on the agreed priority for most clinicians (Beutler, Williams, & Wakefield, 1993), namely, that of delineating the therapist and client behaviors leading to important moments of change. It is an essential part of the coming of age of couple therapy as a modality and indeed makes couple therapy a glorious adventure.

REFERENCES

Anderson, C. (2000). *The ones we left behind: Family therapy and the treatment of mental illness.* Plenary address, American Association of Marital and Family Therapy, millennium conference, Nashville, TN.

Anderson, H. (1997). *Conversation, language and possibilities.* New York: Basic Books.

Anderson, P., Beach, S. R. H., & Kaslow, N. J. (1999). Marital discord and depression: The potential of attachment theory to guide clinical intervention. In T. Joiner & J. C. Coyne (Eds.), *The interactional nature of depression* (pp. 271–297). Washington, DC: American Psychological Association.

Bowlby, J. (1969). *Attachment and loss: Vol. I. Attachment.* New York: Basic Books.

Bowlby, J. (1988). *A secure base.* New York: Basic Books.

Bowlby, J. (1991). Postscript. In C. M. Parkes, J. Stevenson, R. Hinde, & P. Morris (Eds.), *Attachment across the life cycle* (pp. 293–297). London: Routledge.

Berscheid, E. (1999). The greening of relationship science. *American Psychologist, 54,* 260–266.

Beutler, L., Williams, R., & Wakefield, P. (1993). Obstacles to disseminating applied psychological science. *Applied and Preventative Psychology, 2,* 53–58.

Bradley, B. (2001). *Toward a mini-theory of EFT: Therapist behaviors facilitating a softening.* Unpublished doctoral dissertation, Fuller Theological Seminary, Los Angeles.

Cassidy, J., & Shaver, P. R. (Eds.). (1999). *Handbook of attachment: Theory, research, and clinical applications.* New York: Guilford Press.

Clothier, P., Manion, I., Gordon-Walker, J., & Johnson, S. M. (2002). Emotionally focused interventions for couples with chronically ill children: A two-year follow-up. *Journal of Marital and Family Therapy, 28,* 391–398.

Feeney, J. A., Noller, P., & Callan, V. J. (1994). Attachment style, communication and satisfaction in the early years of marriage. In K. Bartholomew & D. Perlman (Eds.), *Attachment processes in adulthood* (pp. 269–308). London: Jessica Kingsley.

Gottman, J. M. (1994). *What predicts divorce?* Hillsdale, NJ: Erlbaum.

Gottman, J. M., Coan, J., Carrere, S., & Swanson, C. (1998). Predicting marital happiness and stability from newlywed interactions. *Journal of Marriage and the Family, 60,* 5–22.

Green, R., & Werner, P. (1996). Intrusiveness and closeness-care giving: Rethinking the concept of family enmeshment. *Family Process, 35,* 115–153.

Gurman, A. (2001). Brief therapy and couple and family therapy: An essential redundancy. *Clinical Psychology: Science and Practice, 8,* 51–65.

Hazan, C., & Shaver, P. (1987). Romantic love conceptualized as an attachment process. *Journal of Personality and Social Psychology, 52,* 511–524.

Hazan, C., & Zeifman, D. (1994). Sex and the psychological tether. In K. Bartholomew & D. Perlman (Eds.), *Attachment processes in adulthood* (pp. 151–180). London: Jessica Kingsley.

Herman, J. L. (1992). *Trauma and recovery.* New York: Basic Books.

Johnson, S. M. (1986). Bonds or bargains?: Relationship paradigms and their significance for marital therapy. *Journal of Marital and Family Therapy, 12,* 259–267.

Johnson, S. M. (1996). *The practice of emotionally focused marital therapy: Creating connection*. New York: Brunner/Mazel.

Johnson, S. M. (1999). Emotionally focused therapy: Straight to the heart. In J. M. Donovan (Ed.), *Short-term couple therapy* (pp. 11–42). New York: Guilford Press.

Johnson, S. M. (2002). *Emotionally focused couple therapy with trauma survivors: Strengthening attachment bonds*. New York: Guilford Press.

Johnson, S. M., & Best, M. (2002). A systemic approach to restructuring attachment: The EFT model of couple therapy. In P. Erdman & T. Caffery (Eds.), *Attachment and family systems: Conceptual, empirical, and therapeutic relatedness* (pp. 165–192). New York: Springer.

Johnson, S. M., & Denton, W. (2002). Emotionally focused couple therapy: Creating secure connections. In A. S. Gurman & N. S. Jacobson (Ed.), *Clinical handbook of couple therapy* (3rd ed., pp. 221–250). New York: Guilford Press.

Johnson, S. M., & Greenberg, L. S. (1985). The differential effects of experiential and problem solving interventions in resolving marital conflicts. *Journal of Consulting and Clinical Psychology, 53*, 175–184.

Johnson, S. M., Hunsley, J., Greenberg, L., & Schlindler, D. (1999). Emotionally focused couples therapy: Status and challenges. *Clinical Psychology: Science and Practice, 6*, 67–79.

Johnson, S. M., & Lebow, J. (2000). The coming of age of couples therapy: A decade review. *Journal of Marital and Family Therapy, 26*, 23–38.

Johnson, S. M., Makinen, J., & Millikin, J. (2001). Attachment injuries in couple relationships: A new perspective on impasses in couples therapy. *Journal of Marital and Family Therapy, 27*, 145–155.

Johnson, S. M., & Talitman, E. (1997). Predictors of success in emotionally focused marital therapy. *Journal of Marital and Family Therapy, 23*, 135–152.

Johnson, S., & Whiffen, V. (1999). Made to measure: Adapting emotionally focused couples therapy to couples' attachment styles. *Clinical Psychology: Science and Practice, 6*, 366–381.

Johnson, S. M., & Williams-Keeler, L. (1998). Creating healing relationships for couples dealing with trauma: The use of emotionally focused couples therapy. *Journal of Marital and Family Therapy, 24*, 25–40.

Kiecolt-Glaser, J. K., Malarkey, W. B., Chee, M., Newton, T., Cacioppo, J., Mao, H. Y., & Glaser, J. (1993). Negative behavior during marital conflict is associated with immunological down-regulation. *Psychosomatic Medicine, 55*, 395–409.

Kobak, R., & Cole, H. (1999). Attachment and meta-monitoring: Implications for adolescent autonomy and psychopathology. In D. Cicchetti & S. Toth (Eds.), *Disorders and dysfunctions of the self* (pp. 267–297). Rochester, NY: University of Rochester Press.

Main, M., Kaplan, N., & Cassidy, J. (1985). Security in infancy, childhood and adulthood: A move to the level of representation. In I. Bretherton & E. Waters (Eds.), Growing points of attachment theory and research. *Monographs of the Society for Research in Child Development, 50*(1–2, Serial No. 209), 66–106.

McFarlane, A. C., & van der Kolk, B. (1996). Trauma and its challenge to society. In B. van der Kolk, A. C. McFarlane, & L. Weisaeth (Eds.), *Traumatic stress* (pp. 24–46). New York: Guilford Press.

Mikulincer, M. (1995). Attachment style and the mental representation of the self. *Journal of Personality and Social Psychology, 69*, 1203–1215.

Mikulincer, M. (1997). Adult attachment style and information processing: Individual differences in curiosity and cognitive closure. *Journal of Personality and Social Psychology, 72*, 1217–1230.

Mikulincer, M., & Nachshon, O. (1991). Attachment styles and patterns of self-disclosure. *Journal of Personality and Social Psychology, 61*, 321–332.

Murstein, B., Cerreto, M., & MacDonald, M. (1977). A theory and investigation of the effect of exchange-orientation on marriage and friendship. *Journal of Marriage and the Family, 39*, 543–548.

Pasch, L. A., & Bradbury, T. N. (1998). Social support, conflict and the development of marital dysfunction. *Journal of Consulting and Clinical Psychology, 66*, 219–230.

Shaver, P., & Clarke, C. L. (1994). The psychodynamics of adult romantic attachment. In J. Masling & R. Borstein (Eds.), *Empirical perspectives on object relations theory* (pp. 105–156). Washington, DC: American Psychological Association.

Shaver, P., & Hazan, C. (1993). Adult romantic attachment: Theory and evidence. In D. Perlman & W. Jones (Eds.), *Advances in personal relationships* (Vol. 4, pp. 29–70). London: Jessica Kingsley.

Simpson, J. A., & Rholes, W. S. (1994). Stress and secure base relationships in adulthood. In K. Bartholomew & D. Perlman (Eds.), *Attachment processes in adulthood* (pp. 181–204). London: Jessica Kingsley.

Twenge, J. M. (2000). The age of anxiety: The birth cohort change in anxiety and neuroticism, 1952–1993. *Journal of Personality and Social Psychology, 79*, 1007–1021.

Vatcher, C. A., & Bogo, M. (2001). The feminist/emotionally focused therapy practice model: An integrated approach for couple therapy. *Journal of Marital and Family Therapy, 21*, 69–84.

Weinfield, N. S., Sroufe, A. L., Egeland, B., & Carlson, E. A. (1999). The nature of individual differences in infant–caregiver attachment. In J. Cassidy & P. R. Shaver (Eds.), *Handbook of attachment: Theory, research, and clinical applications* (pp. 68–88). New York: Guilford Press.

Whisman, M. A. (1999). Marital dissatisfaction and psychiatric disorders: Results from the National Comorbidity Survey. *Journal of Abnormal Psychology, 108*, 701–706.

Whisman, M. A., & Jacobson, N. S. (1990). Power, marital satisfaction, and response to marital therapy. *Journal of Family Psychology, 4*, 202–212.

7

Attachment Processes in Couple Therapy
Informing Behavioral Models

JOANNE DAVILA

As has been noted in numerous places in this volume, attachment theory has become a prominent theory for understanding functioning in adult romantic relationships. Since the publication of Hazan and Shaver's (1987) seminal paper describing the application of attachment theory to adult romantic relationships, research demonstrating how attachment security affects relationships has burgeoned. However, relatively little of that research has been disseminated to practitioners working with couples or applied systematically to interventions for distressed couples (see Johnson, Hunsley, Greenberg, & Schindler, 1999; Johnson & Whiffen, 1999; Johnson, Chapter 6, this volume, for notable exceptions). The goal of this chapter is to discuss why attachment processes can be an important focus in couple treatment and to describe the role of attachment processes in romantic relationships, with an eye toward highlighting those processes that practitioners may want to be alert to in the couples they treat.

As many readers of this book will know, there is an empirically supported couple treatment, emotionally focused couple therapy (EFT; Greenberg & Johnson, 1988; Johnson, Chapter 6, this volume), that uses an attachment framework to understand and treat relationship dysfunction. However, no other couple treatment, for which empirical support exists, has integrated an attachment focus, and this is particularly true for behaviorally based treatments (e.g., behavioral couple therapy [BCT; Jacobson & Holtzworth-Munroe, 1986]). Therefore, this chapter was written with more behaviorally oriented practitioners in mind and will pay particular attention to what an attachment perspective has to offer them (see also Lawrence, Eldridge, & Christensen, 1998). Before getting to these issues, however, a brief discussion of the history of the emergence of the behavioral and attachment perspectives is provided.

EMERGENCE OF THE BEHAVIORAL
AND ATTACHMENT PERSPECTIVES

In the 1960s, academic psychology was moving away from intrapsychic explanations for behavior (e.g., psychodynamic explanations) to explanations that focused on environmental causes and consequences (e.g., behaviorism). In line with this shift, by the 1970s academic clinical psychologists interested in couple functioning and treatment began to focus on aspects of the interactions between partners rather than on partners' individual qualities. Early research on marital functioning and outcome had focused on spouses' individual differences and had suggested that spouses' personality styles were associated with the quality and outcome of their marriage (e.g., Barry, 1970; Terman & Buttenwieser, 1935; Zaleski & Galkowska, 1978). However, in the 1970s a number of prominent marital researchers (e.g., Gottman, 1979) strongly suggested that individual spousal personality styles were not important in the study of marriage. Rather, *interpersonal variables*, that is, variables that captured the observable behaviors exchanged by couple members, could tell us all that we needed to know about marriage. This was a very valid claim in that marriage, and relationships more broadly, are by definition interpersonal endeavors. Hence, this point of view suggested that something unique emerges out of the interaction between two people, and it is this that should be the focus of attention rather than either spouse's individual qualities.

Although this interpersonal perspective made an extremely important point, it resulted in a number of generations of researchers and practitioners who largely ignored individual difference variables. During this time, research progressed in a fairly atheoretical way and focused largely on describing marital interactions, particularly conflict behaviors, and their effect on marital satisfaction and stability. Indeed, evidence that negative behaviors exchanged by spouses were damaging to the marriage began to accumulate (e.g., Gottman, Markman, & Notarius, 1977; Margolin, 1981; Margolin & Wampold, 1981), and support grew for a behavioral, or social-learning, model of marital dysfunction. Based on principles of reinforcement, this perspective conceptualized marital distress as a function of the ratio of rewarding versus punishing behaviors exchanged by spouses.

Behavioral couple therapy grew out of this social-learning perspective. BCT was designed to teach couples more effective communication and problem-solving behaviors, so as to increase their rewarding interactions and decrease their punishing ones. Reasons for, or the meaning of ineffective behaviors, whether those reasons resided within spouses (i.e., individual differences) or within relational processes (e.g., fears of intimacy, rejection, etc.), were not examined. Treatment was largely skills-based. Subsequent empirical research conducted on BCT supported its efficacy (see Hahlweg & Markman, 1988; Dunn & Schwebel, 1995), allowing BCT to become a prominent intervention for couple problems. Hence, the dominant model of relationships and intervention, at least among many academic clinical psychologists, became a behavioral one.

As the behavioral model became dominant among many academic clinical psychology relationship researchers, attachment models of interpersonal functioning were becoming prominent in very different circles. Attachment theory had been designed as a model of the development of personality, psychopathology, and interpersonal functioning with implications for functioning across the lifespan. Bowlby described the theory's application to normative and nonnormative development and promoted its application to psychotherapy with adults (Bowlby, 1969, 1973, 1980, 1988). However, attachment theory became recognized, largely by developmental psychologists, primarily (if not exclusively) as a way to understand child development. Consequently, the implications of attachment theory for adult functioning took a back seat to those for child functioning for many years.

When researchers finally began examining the implications of attachment theory for adult interpersonal functioning, it was social psychologists that did so while they were attempting to understand adult love. Hence, it was primarily social psychologists, not clinical psychologists, who continued to theorize about and investigate the role of attachment security in interpersonal functioning. As such, attachment theory remained outside the purview of those people most likely to study couple dysfunction and to develop interventions, despite the fact that there was clear evidence that adult insecurity was associated with relationship distress (e.g., Collins & Read, 1990; Davila, Karney, & Bradbury, 1999; Hazan & Shaver, 1987; Kobak & Hazan, 1991; Senchak & Leonard, 1992; Shaver & Hazan, 1993). Hence, behavioral and attachment models of relationships developed largely in isolation from one another. At present, however, the limitations of the behavioral model and treatment are being recognized. It is the contention put forth in this chapter that attachment theory has much to offer in offsetting those limitations.

UTILITY OF AN ATTACHMENT PERSPECTIVE
IN COUPLE THERAPY

There are at least three ways in which attachment theory can inform behaviorally oriented models of relationships and couple therapy. An attachment perspective can shed light on why problems emerge in relationships, on why people behave the way they do in relationships, and on who is at most risk for relationship problems.

Why Do Problems Emerge in Relationships?

Behavioral models have not focused on reasons why problems emerge in relationships. As noted earlier, the focus is on remediation of the maladaptive processes by which couples negotiate problems. This has been a generally successful approach, but, as research has indicated, not all couples respond to it (see Christensen & Heavey, 1999). Christensen, Jacobson, and Babcock (1995) have suggested that the reason that BCT has not been more successful is because it focuses on derivative problems rather than on more major controlling problems that are responsible for relationship distress. They argue that many of the specific problems that couples present in therapy are derivative of more important underlying issues. For example, if a couple is arguing about negotiating household responsibilities, it may not really be household chores that are at issue, but something that they represent. Even if couples learn skills to manage the derivative problems (e.g., the couple begins to communicate about chores and develops an equitable system for accomplishing them), the underlying issues may still exist and undermine couples' use of, or success with, the new skills. Hence, Christensen et al. (1995) suggest that a complete functional analysis be conducted, with a focus not only on specific, observable behaviors, but also on affect and on themes that emerge in couples' descriptions of their situation. It is in this pursuit that an attachment perspective may be particularly useful. Although it is always important to be mindful of each couple's idiosyncratic issues and not apply the same theme indiscriminately, attachment theory can provide a guide to common themes that may underlie relationship distress.

What are the themes that attachment theory would suggest underlie relationship distress? At the broadest level, attachment theory suggests that the goal of all attachment relationships is felt security. Hence, relationship distress may be a manifestation of a failure to feel secure in the relationship or a failure to feel that attachment needs are being met. Attachment needs in adult relationships are much the same as those in parent–child relationships. They include things such as wanting to know that the partner is loving, available, consistent, and supportive. Therefore, felt security has a number of components. It refers to a sense of trust and certainty with regard to the availability and responsiveness of the attachment figure, and it refers to a sense of self-worth in regard to the attachment figure—a sense that one will not be rejected or abandoned. As such, specific attachment-relevant themes typically relate to fears of being unloved or rejected by the partner, a desire for greater closeness or intimacy with the partner, and fears that the partner is not trustworthy or available to provide support when needed.

In order to be sure that attachment needs are being met, adults will monitor their romantic partner's availability and ability to meet their needs, just as children do with their parents (e.g., Hazan & Shaver, 1994; Waters, 1997). Hence, during the course of a relationship, an individual will regularly monitor his or her partner's behavior. Should he or she perceive evidence of the partner's unavailability, lack of support, lack of love, or rejection, this will lead to distress and the development of relationship problems.

Kobak, Ruckdeschel, and Hazan (1994) described this process nicely. They suggested that symptoms of marital distress are actually distorted attachment signals. When the attachment relationship is viewed as threatened (e.g., when a spouse begins to view his or her partner as unavailable), normal negative emotions that signal the threat may get distorted and expressed in a manner that contributes to marital difficulties. For instance, a woman who experiences her partner as distant may become upset and anxious and subsequently become more clingy or demanding of the partner's time. She may perceive everything the partner does as indicative of a lack of intimacy or a rejection. This may lead to arguments and/or increased negative affect, which she is unable to regulate in an adaptive fashion. This couple may then present to treatment with complaints that the wife is too dependent and demanding and that the husband is too disengaged (similar to the common demand–withdraw communication pattern that frequently characterizes distressed marriages; see, e.g., Christensen & Heavey, 1990). The surface problem in this case may be one of communication difficulties. The underlying problem, however, is the threat to attachment security.

In some cases, the threat may be so intense as to be experienced as an attachment injury. Johnson, Maikinen, and Millikin (2001) define an *attachment injury* as an abandonment or betrayal of trust that maintains relationship distress because the injured spouse continues to view the partner as unreliable. Hence, the recurrent attachment fears may date back to a critical event from which the injured spouse never recovered. As Johnson et al. (2001) note, attachment injuries may be responsible for impasses that block relationship repair.

A large body of literature supports the notion that when felt security is compromised people experience and engage in various types of relationship-damaging (or at least distress-inducing) activities at the cognitive, affective, and behavioral levels. For example, individuals who feel insecure in relation to their partners have more negative expectations about their partners, make less benign attributions for their partners' behavior, and generally view their partners more negatively (e.g., Cobb, Davila, & Bradbury, 2001; Collins, 1996; Murray, Holmes, & Griffin, 1996). People who feel insecure report more negative affect about their relationship and have difficulty regulating their emotions (e.g., Davila, Bradbury, & Fincham, 1998; Feeney, 1999). Furthermore, people who feel insecure behave in more negative ways with their partners. They display more negative communication behaviors, are worse at providing support to their partners, and are worse at eliciting and taking in support from their partners (e.g., Feeney, Noller, & Callan, 1994; Kobak & Hazan, 1991; Simpson, Rholes, & Nelligan, 1992). Thus, felt security underlies a host of factors that are related to success in relationships or the lack thereof. When consistent patterns of these thoughts, feelings, and behaviors are present in relationships, it may be useful to explore whether there are underlying attachment fears or injuries. Addressing the attachment fears (i.e., targeting the controlling problem) in addition to how they are manifested and how partners can behave differently may help partners to better meet one another's needs and remain satisfied.

Why Do People Behave the Way They Do in Relationships?

Unlike the prior section, which focused on the origin of relationship problems, this section addresses specific behavior patterns in relationships. Before doing so, however, it is important to note that attachment theory is consistent with the idea that behavior patterns may represent an individual's chronic interpersonal style or a pattern of relating that emerges in specific relationships or, most likely, an interaction of the two. Attachment theory is often perceived as speaking only to persistent individual differences in functioning, but that is not the case. An attachment model of relationships accounts for attachment processes that reside within individuals and for those that emerge in close relationships. That is, attachment theory describes how individual characteristics may drive relationship functioning and also how relationship-specific attachment processes may drive functioning. Hence, attachment theory is not simply about individual differences and how they affect interpersonal functioning. It is also about interpersonal processes and behavior in relationships. This discussion of behavior emphasizes both processes.

First, most people do have characteristic interpersonal patterns that they may enact by default. Attachment theory would thus help us know what interpersonal responses to expect from people with different attachment styles (see also Johnson & Whiffen, 1999, for a discussion of this issue). Adult romantic attachment styles can be described as falling into three categories, secure, preoccupied, and avoidant, much like the original parent–child attachment styles (Hazan & Shaver, 1987), or four categories, which distinguish among two types of avoidance, fearful avoidance and dismissing avoidance (see Bartholomew, 1990). The four categories will be described here, as they allow for greater behavioral distinction. Moreover, most adult attachment researchers agree that adult attachment security can be characterized according to placement along two dimensions: avoidance of intimacy and anxiety about abandonment (e.g., Brennan, Clark, &

Shaver, 1998; Shaver & Hazan, 1993). These two dimensions underlie the styles described by the four-category model.

Secure people are characterized by low levels of avoidance of intimacy and low levels of anxiety about abandonment. In relationships, they are comfortable being close with partners and they engage in self-disclosure. They are likely to turn to partners in times of need, but can also manage stress and their emotions independently. They are available for their partners, can provide necessary support, and respond flexibly to relationship events. They view themselves and their partners positively and feel worthy of love. Hence, they are likely to be open communicators and good problem solvers. They are likely to make relatively benign attributions about partners, and they will be able to manage their experience and expression of affect with partners.

Preoccupied people are also characterized by low levels of avoidance of intimacy, but they differ from secure people because they exhibit high levels of anxiety about abandonment. They question whether they are worthy of love and are extremely worried about being rejected, but they are also extremely needy of and dependent on relationships. Hence, in relationships, they want to be extremely close, both physically and emotionally. They are extremely sensitive and expressive, and often seek reassurance about their partners' love and availability and their own self-worth. They provide a great deal of caregiving, sometimes to the point of excess, and they have the potential to be dominating. Hence, although they may be open communicators, they may be too much so (or not clear communicators), and their ability for adaptive problem solving may become clouded by intense emotion. Although they idealize partners, they may also be demanding and never feel that their needs are fully met.

Dismissing people are characterized by high levels of avoidance of intimacy and low levels of anxiety about abandonment. Unlike preoccupied people, dismissing people have a relatively low need for relationships, do not care much about what others think of them, and are content being self-sufficient, often compulsively so. Hence, in relationships, they show low levels of self-disclosure, emotional closeness, and physical affection. They do not turn to partners in times of stress and often do not see the need to provide support or care to their partners. Although they may do so in tangible ways, they rarely do so in emotional ways. They tend to be poor communicators and problem solvers, preferring instead to manage things on their own or not at all. They are emotionally distant and defended in relationships, are likely to make negative attributions about partners (given their general distrust of people), and can be critical and judgmental.

Finally, *fearful people* are characterized by high levels of avoidance of intimacy and high levels of anxiety about abandonment. Like preoccupied people, fearful people question whether they are worthy of love, are extremely worried about being rejected, and want close relationships. However, unlike preoccupied people, they manage their fears by avoiding intimacy in relationships. Fearful people will get into close relationships, but it often takes them a very long time. Once in relationships, they may have difficulty being emotionally and physically close, may inhibit self-disclosure, and may hold in emotions. They may not turn to partners when upset or in need of support, and they may fail to perceive or believe that partners care about them. They are likely to be very sensitive and vulnerable, and they tend to behave in a passive manner. Hence, they are not good communicators and problem solvers, often sacrificing their own needs.

In sum, each attachment style is marked by characteristic ways of functioning that allow for the prediction of how people will behave in relationships, particularly under times of stress when attachment needs are most evident. Hence, awareness of people's attachment styles can help practitioners to understand, conceptualize, and predict relationship behavior and its causes. However, what I have just described are the *prototypical* ways of functioning, and it is important to note that the large majority of people do not conform to these prototypes perfectly. In fact, most people possess aspects of more than one of the styles. Therefore, it is important to recognize that people may have more than one set of behavioral patterns in their repertoire.

In addition, some of these behavioral patterns may function as both strengths and weaknesses in differing circumstances. For example, the capacity for intense emotional closeness (a preoccupied strategy) may be adaptive when it conveys to partners that they are desired and valued, but maladaptive when it conveys intrusiveness or becomes coercive. As another example, the capacity for dismissing needs and tolerating distance (a dismissing strategy) may be adaptive when it helps someone stay connected to a temporarily distant or busy spouse, but maladaptive when it conveys a lack of interest in or care for the partner. So it is also important to recognize that people who engage in insecure behavioral strategies are not necessarily living maladaptive lives or relationships.

Finally, attachment patterns are malleable. They can change (Davila, Burge, & Hammen, 1997; Davila et al., 1999; Davila & Cobb, in press; Baldwin & Fehr, 1995; Baldwin, Keelan, Fehr, Enns, & Koh-Rangarajoo, 1996). Moreover, people can have different levels of security in different relationships (e.g., Baldwin et al., 1996; Bridges, Connell, & Belsky, 1988; Cook, 2000; LaGuardia, Ryan, Couchman, & Deci, 2000; Lamb, 1977; Main & Weston, 1981). These findings attest not only to the fact that attachment security is both a property of individuals and a property of relationships, but that people have the potential to become more secure in their relationships. Hence, therapy directed at increasing relationship security is not an unreasonable notion.

The prior discussion focused mainly on individual differences and how they may affect relational processes. Now let us turn to relational processes themselves. As noted earlier, attachment is very much about interpersonal behavior. Indeed, inherent in the theory is the notion that interactional behavior is powerful and formative, and that it directs the ongoing course of relationships. Hence, an attachment perspective is similar to a behavioral or social-learning perspective in that they both are interested in the interpersonal behavior in which partners engage with one another. However, the two theories have generally focused on different behaviors.

Attachment theory particularly draws attention to a set of behaviors that have not traditionally been the focus of behavioral models, but that have been shown to play an important role in relationship satisfaction and stability: social support behaviors (e.g., Pasch & Bradbury, 1998). Traditionally, behavioral models have focused on conflict, and the goal of treatment was its successful management. Attachment theory, as it is applied to adult relationships, instead puts a much greater emphasis on social support.

As noted earlier, security is maintained in relationships when partners perceive one another to be available when needed. Such issues of availability are directly linked to social support in relationships. According to attachment theorists, one of the most important sets of roles played by relationship partners is that of careseeker and caregiver (e.g., Bowlby, 1982; Waters, 1997). As *careseekers*, partners must signal their distress appropriately, convey their needs, connect with their partners, and feel soothed by their partners' attempts at comfort. As *caregivers*, partners must be sensitive to partners' signals, be physically and psychologically available, and be accepting of their partners' needs. As noted earlier, individuals regularly monitor interactions with their partners for evidence of whether partners are sensitive, available, accepting, and responsive. People then base their feelings about and behavior toward their partners on this information. Good careseeking and good caregiving will foster security in relationships for a number of reasons. Good caregiving by partners will provide people with evidence of the availability of their partners. Good careseeking will allow people greater opportunity to get their needs met by their partners. Good careseeking may also reinforce security and further good caregiving behavior because caregivers will feel appreciated and valued by their partners. Hence, from an attachment perspective, the core of adaptive adult couple functioning lies in the ability of partners to seek and provide support and the quality of their supportive interactions, rather than solely in their ability to manage conflict. The goal of successful relationships would thus be to meet one another's needs before conflict arises rather than simply to manage the conflict once it arises. Hence, strategies directed at helping couples become better caregivers and careseekers may be an important component of prevention and intervention programs (see also Cobb & Bradbury, Chapter 13, this volume).

Social support is a relational process that exists in all relationships and must be negotiated regardless of spouses' individual characteristics. Of course, individual levels of security will bear upon peoples' capacity for caregiving and careseeking, but even people who are dispositionally secure may experience attachment fears in relationships, difficulty seeking support, and difficulty providing support, depending on the circumstances. Hence, it is important to note that it is not only the insecure who must face the challenges of getting their attachment needs met and the challenges of meeting the needs of their partners. Secure people do as well.

In this section I have attempted to do two things. First, to point out how maladaptive relationship behaviors may be understood from the perspective of individual attachment patterns. Second, to describe a set of relationship behaviors that attachment theory would suggest are at the heart of adaptive couple functioning. In doing so, I have attempted to make clear that attachment theory can speak both to the stable individual differences that people bring to relationships and to the interpersonal challenges that all couples face during the course of their relationships. Hence, attachment theory can help us to understand the types of maladaptive relationship behavior that may be most central to relationship distress and the reasons people engage in certain behaviors.

Who Is at Most Risk for Relationship Problems?

In many ways, the question of who is at risk for relationship problems is no different than either of the questions addressed previously. And at this point it should be clear and not surprising that people who are more insecure, or who become trapped in patterns of interactions in particular relationships that erode felt security, are at greater risk for relationship problems. However, the more pertinent questions may be, Who is in most need of intervention or preventative efforts and what do they need? These are questions that have rarely been addressed. Most treatments and prevention efforts were not designed with specific types of couples in mind. In fact, the most common behaviorally oriented marital distress prevention and intervention programs, such as the Prevention and Relationship Enhancement Program (PREP; see Floyd, Markman, Kelly, Blumberg, & Stanley, 1995) and behavioral or cognitive-behavioral marital therapy (e.g., Baucom, Epstein, & Rankin, 1995; Jacobson & Holtzworth-Munroe, 1986) were not designed to address any unique risk factors. The failure of programs to take specific risk factors into account might even be responsible for the somewhat weak, although promising, effects shown to date in the prevention literature (see Bradbury, Cohan, & Karney, 1998) and the disappointing long-term results in the behavioral treatment literature (see Christensen & Heavey, 1999).

Therefore, an important goal for the future is to identify various types of at-risk couples who may be most in need of intervention. Attachment theory may help us to do this. As I have stressed throughout this chapter, there may be both individual difference (e.g., a partner who is dispositionally insecure) and relational risk factors (e.g., a couple who fails to support one another adequately) that deserve attention. An individual difference-based attachment perspective on risk has been the focus of recent work that I have conducted with my colleague Thomas Bradbury. We have hypothesized that attachment insecurity binds spouses together in a chronically unhappy marriage (Davila & Bradbury, 2001). Specifically, we have suggested that insecurity decreases the likelihood that spouses will be happy in their marriage, while at the same time increasing the likelihood that unhappy spouses will stay married (see Kirkpatrick & Davis, 1994, for a similar argument pertaining to dating relationships). Therefore, insecure spouses may be particularly at risk for chronically unhappy relationships.

We focused on a particular type of insecurity—concerns about abandonment and love-worthiness—that are at the core of a preoccupied attachment style. People who have such concerns tend to be characterized by a dependent manner of relating, low self-worth, and an excessive desire to gain others' approval (e.g., Bartholomew, 1990). They tend to be excessively focused on relationships and attachment-related information, high in proximity seeking, and constantly monitoring their attachment figure. They are frequently unhappy in their relationships, but they experience high levels of distress when relationships end and they do not like to be without relationships. Therefore, it follows that people with these characteristics are likely to attempt to maintain relationships at all costs, even if it means remaining in an unsatisfying one. Hence, people who are concerned about abandonment are likely to remain in relationships that are chronically unsatisfying. This is exactly what our research has shown.

We followed 172 newlywed couples over the first 4 years of marriage and found that concerns about abandonment were highest among those spouses who were married, but chronically unhappy, compared to those who were happily married and those who divorced. Importantly, this association was not explained by other factors that might account for staying in an unhappy marriage (e.g., holding attitudes against divorce, the presence of a child), or by broader dysfunctional personality traits that might subsume concerns about abandonment (e.g., neuroticism, low self-esteem). Although the study was correlational in nature, the findings suggest that spouses' insecurity (and the relational patterns that sustain it) may make them unhappy in their marriage and at the same time keep them in their marriage. Hence, the stability of such marriages may be based in insecurity rather than in satisfaction. If that is the case, then spouses who are concerned about abandonment are particularly at risk for relationship dysfunction and may need specific interventions or premarital preparation programs designed to increase security.

Our research had two additional implications for how we might approach the prevention and treatment of marital distress. First, different types of insecurity may have different effects on marital functioning and course. Specifically, only people who were concerned about abandonment remained in chronically unhappy marriages. People who reported a different type of insecurity, the avoidance of intimacy, did not. This suggests that we should not treat all types of insecurity in a similar manner. To target the risk for staying in unhappy marriages, intervention strategies should focus specifically on alleviating abandonment concerns.

Interestingly, a recent study found that compared to secure and preoccupied spouses (the latter of whom are frequently concerned about abandonment), dismissing spouses, who typically avoid intimacy, divorce more frequently (Ceglian & Gardner, 1999). This is not surprising, given that divorcing may be a good way to avoid intimacy for people who want to do so. Therefore, people who avoid intimacy may be at a different type of risk and may need different prevention and intervention strategies to manage their particular type of attachment insecurity.

A second issue involved in staying in an unhappy marriage is that doing so may have negative *individual* consequences as well as negative *marital* consequences. We found that compared to happily married spouses and divorced spouses, spouses who were married but unhappy showed the highest levels of depressive symptoms both early in their marriage and over the course of their marriage. The importance of this finding is compounded by research indicating that insecurity and depression are associated within and across partners in relationships. For example, Whiffen, Kallos-Lilly, and MacDonald (2001) found that depressed wives were more insecure than their nondepressed counterparts. Moreover, the husbands of chronically depressed wives were particularly insecure, and their insecurity predicted the maintenance of their wives' depressive symptoms. Hence, an ongoing cycle of chronic insecurity, depression, and relationship distress may characterize the relationships of some couples, and we may need to pay particular attention to such couples at both the prevention and the intervention levels. Given that behavioral marital treatments have already demonstrated some efficacy in relieving both depressive symptoms and marital distress (e.g., Jacobson, Dobson, Fruzzetti, Schmaling, & Salusky, 1991; O'Leary & Beach, 1990), there may be utility in exploring the incorporation of interventions designed to address relationship insecurity as well. A number of researchers and clinicians have now begun to do so (Anderson, Beach, & Kaslow, 1999; Whiffen & Johnson, 1998).

ATTACHMENT-BASED STRATEGIES FOR PREVENTING AND INTERVENING IN MARITAL DISTRESS

In this last section, a number of suggestions for incorporating an attachment-based perspective into behavioral treatment are discussed. These suggestions draw directly in many cases on other treatments, including EFT (Greenberg & Johnson, 1988; Johnson, Chapter 6, this volume) and integrative behavioral couple therapy (Christensen et al., 1995) and on the writings of other attachment scholars (Kobak et al., 1994; Johnson et al., 1999, 2001). These suggestions are not intended as a new form of therapy, nor are they intended to address the complexities involved in developing or integrating attachment-based treatment strategies into behavioral treatments. Rather, it is hoped that they provide a framework from which to begin considering attachment-based models.

Suggestion 1: Conduct an Assessment of Attachment Security

A first step in incorporating an attachment-based focus would be to assess spouses' levels and patterns of security. Assessment is an important aspect of behavioral programs and an attachment assessment early on could provide practitioners with important information about the types of problems to which couples may be vulnerable (e.g., couples with a preoccupied partner may face problems with trusting and relying on their partner), the types of behaviors spouses may exhibit (e.g., spouses who are fearful may tend to be submissive or withdraw in the face of conflict), and who will be most at risk for particular types of problems (e.g., among distressed couples, those with a preoccupied partner may remain chronically unhappy, whereas those with a dismissing partner may be at risk for divorce). Hence, assessment would be the first step in being able to focus treatment more specifically around the couples' unique attachment issues.

Although the assessment of attachment security and patterns has faced its share of controversy in the research literature, there are a number of ways that practitioners could gain insight into spouses' patterns. First, attachment security can be assessed quickly, easily, and inexpensively via self-report. There are a number of self-report measures that would be appropriate, including Bartholomew's Relationship Questionnaire or Relationship Styles Questionnaire (Bartholomew & Horowitz, 1991), Collins and Read's Adult Attachment Scale (Collins & Read, 1990), and Brennan's Experiences in Close Relationships Scale (Brennan et al., 1998). Such screening may be very cost-effective if it can help identify those spouses at greatest risk for marital distress. Of course, self-report measures are limited in that they are vulnerable to reporting biases. For example, some people may lack sufficient insight into their own relational patterns to report accurately or some people may intentionally misrepresent themselves. However, as brief screening instruments these measures may suffice.

More extensive attachment-relevant information may be gathered through interview procedures that focus on couple attachment, such as the Current Relationship Interview (Crowell & Owens, 1996) or the romantic relationship section of the Peer Attachment Interview (Bartholomew & Horowitz, 1991). Unfortunately, these interview procedures typically require extensive training in administration and coding, as they were developed as research instruments. However, for interested practitioners, these interviews may yield the most extensive and rich information about attachment patterns. Clues about attachment patterns within couples may also be gleaned from observing couples interact (either formally or informally). Practitioners should be attuned to indicators of abandonment fears and signs of intimacy avoidance. The former may be evident in intense affect and in behaviors that are demanding, dependent, or submissive. The latter may be evident in displays of, for example, withdrawal, minimizing behavior, contempt, intellectualization, and restricted emotionality.

Suggestion 2: Conceptualize the Controlling Problem as Attachment Based

Once an assessment is made regarding the ways in which insecurity is manifested in a particular couple and in their interaction style, interventions can be developed and applied within the couple's particular attachment context. At the simplest level, the function of couples' behavior in maintaining or exacerbating insecurity, and hence dissatisfaction, would be conveyed to couples and behavioral interventions would be taught from the perspective of how they would change the experience of security at cognitive, emotional, and behavioral levels. Doing so is consistent with Christensen et al.'s (1995) goal of identifying controlling, rather than derivative, problems. Hence, the couple would continually be provided with an idiographic attachment-relevant explanation for the function and goal of behavior change across multiple problem areas.

Suggestion 3: Emphasize Support Skills in Addition to Conflict Resolution Skills

The traditional focus in behavioral treatments is on helping couples communicate and problem solve more effectively in order to facilitate conflict resolution. As noted earlier, an attachment perspective would shift this focus away from conflict resolution toward support seeking and provision. Hence, integrating an attachment perspective into behavioral treatment would require an explicit focus on helping couples to become more effective support seekers and providers. This could be done in a number of ways. Just as education is provided regarding conflict resolution and problem solving, couples could be educated about the function of support, both in general and from an attachment perspective, and could be taught ways to appropriately seek and provide support. Many of the techniques that couples are taught to facilitate problem solving could easily be adapted to the context of support. For example, the use of receptive and expressive communication strategies (e.g., Jacobson & Holtzworth-Munroe, 1986) would be helpful for discussions that couples have during which they are attempting to seek or provide support.

Couples could also be taught skills specific to support interactions. For example, it would be particularly useful to help couples increase their positive behaviors such as empathy and validation, and to decrease their negative behaviors such as criticism and ignoring. It would also be important to help partners identify their needs for support, the circumstances under which they would feel safe seeking support from the partner, and what they would like to get from their partner. Once each partners' support needs and goals are identified and linked to their attachment concerns, therapists could help couples determine ways to support one another that would disconfirm attachment fears and foster feelings of security.

Suggestion 4: Reduce Abandonment Fears and Increase Comfort with Intimacy

Because research suggests that abandonment fears may be associated with chronic marital distress and that discomfort with intimacy may be associated with divorce, interventions designed to specifically target these issues may be useful. Consistent with other theorists (Christensen et al., 1995; Greenberg & Johnson, 1988; Kobak et al., 1994; Johnson, Chapter 6, this volume; Johnson et al., 1999, 2001), these issues may be best addressed from a more emotional or experiential standpoint, in which couples can actually experience in-session interactions that disconfirm fears and increase intimacy. Although skills training in, for example, receptive and expressive communication may facilitate communication about abandonment and intimacy, it may not necessarily produce naturally the kinds of interactions that will feel genuinely secure. Therefore, in session, therapists may need to facilitate partners' awareness of each other's underlying attachment concerns by helping partners to develop insight into these concerns and then to express them. Therapists may need to facilitate partners' development of empathy for each other's concerns by, for example, encouraging the expression of soft emotions and disclosures and discouraging blaming. As partners become more able to see their own and their partners' concerns, more able to express these concerns, and more able to empathize with one another's concerns, they are likely to naturally feel more comfortable with intimacy and less likely to be fearful of abandonment because the self-disclosures and the ensuing partner responses will validate such experiences. Once couples begin to have these experiences in session, it may be appropriate to then help them consider how they can foster the same security-building experiences in other domains.

CONCLUSIONS

The goal of this chapter was to discuss why attachment processes can be an important focus in couple treatment with a particular emphasis on how attachment theory can inform traditional behavioral models and interventions. It was suggested that an attachment perspective can shed light on why problems emerge in relationships, on why people behave the way they do in relationships, and on who is at most risk for relationship problems—all questions that have not been addressed sufficiently in behavioral treatments. In answer to these questions, it was suggested that relationship problems can be conceptualized as breaches in felt security and in partners' inability to get their attachment needs met. It was suggested that the seeking and provision of support through careseeking and caregiving behaviors was the central set of relationship behaviors to be negotiated by couples and the central way in which attachment needs are enacted and met. Finally, it was suggested that spouses who do not feel secure, particularly those who have concerns about abandonment and their own love-worthiness, are most likely to be unhappy in their relationship and yet to stay in their relationship. Thus attachment insecurity can bind partners together in a chronically unhappy relationship. Hence, couples with insecure partners are at risk for chronic relationship distress and should be targeted for both prevention and treatment efforts. It is hoped that the processes outlined here have demonstrated the utility of attachment theory for understanding relationship processes and will spur the application of an attachment perspective on relationships to current behavioral models of relationships and couple intervention.

REFERENCES

Anderson, P., Beach, S. R. H., & Kaslow, N. J. (1999). Marital discord and depression: The potential of attachment theory to guide integrative clinical intervention. In T. E. Joiner & J. C. Coyne (Eds.), *The interactional nature of depression: Advances in interpersonal approaches* (pp. 271–297). Washington, DC: American Psychological Association.

Baldwin, M. W., & Fehr, B. (1995). On the instability of attachment style ratings. *Personal Relationships, 2,* 247–261.

Baldwin, M. W., Keelan, J. P. R., Fehr, B., Enns, V., & Koh-Rangarajoo, E. (1996). Social-cognitive conceptualization of attachment working models: Availability and accessibility effect. *Journal of Personality and Social Psychology, 71,* 94–109.

Barry, W. A. (1970). Marriage research and conflict: An integrative review. *Psychological Bulletin, 73,* 41–54.

Bartholomew, K. (1990). Avoidance of intimacy: An attachment perspective. *Journal of Social and Personal Relationships, 7,* 147–178.

Bartholomew, K., & Horowitz, L. M. (1991). Attachment styles among young adults:

A test of a four-category model. *Journal of Personality and Social Psychology, 61*, 226–244.

Baucom, D. H., Epstein, N., & Rankin, L. A. (1995). Cognitive aspects of cognitive-behavioral marital therapy. In N. S. Jacobson & A. S. Gurman (Eds.), *Clinical handbook of couple therapy* (pp. 65–90). New York: Guilford Press.

Bowlby, J. (1969). *Attachment and loss: Vol. I. Attachment.* New York: Basic Books.

Bowlby, J. (1973). *Attachment and loss: Vol. II. Separation: Anxiety and anger.* New York: Basic Books.

Bowlby, J. (1980). *Attachment and loss: Vol. III. Loss.* New York: Basic Books.

Bowlby, J. (1988). *A secure base.* New York: Basic Books.

Bradbury, T. N., Cohan, C. L., & Karney, B. R. (1998). Optimizing longitudinal research for understanding and preventing marital dysfunction. In T. N. Bradbury (Ed.), *The development course of marital dysfunction* (pp. 279–311). New York: Cambridge University Press.

Brennan, K. A., Clark, C. L., & Shaver, P. R. (1998). Self-report measurement of adult attachment: An integrative overview. In J. A. Simpson & W. S. Rholes (Eds.), *Attachment theory and close relationships* (pp. 46–76). New York: Guilford Press.

Bridges, L., Connell, J. P., & Belsky, J. (1988). Similarities and differences in infant–mother and infant–father interaction in the Strange Situation. *Developmental Psychology, 24*, 92–100.

Ceglian, C. P., & Gardner, S. (1999). Attachment style: A risk for multiple marriages? *Journal of Divorce and Remarriage, 31*, 125–139.

Christensen, A., & Heavey, C. L. (1990). Gender and social structure in the demand/withdraw pattern of marital conflict. *Journal of Personality and Social Psychology, 59*, 73–81.

Christensen, A., & Heavey, C. L. (1999). Interventions for couples. *Annual Review of Psychology, 50*, 165–190.

Christensen, A., Jacobson, N. S., & Babcock, J. C. (1995). Integrative behavioral couple therapy. In N. S. Jacobson & A. S. Gurman (Eds.), *Clinical handbook of couple therapy* (pp. 31–64). New York: Guilford Press.

Cobb, R., Davila, J., & Bradbury, T. (2001). Attachment security and marital satisfaction: The role of positive perceptions and social support. *Personality and Social Psychology Bulletin, 27*, 1131–1144.

Collins, N. L. (1996). Working models of attachment: Implications for explanation, emotion, and behavior. *Journal of Personality and Social Psychology, 71*, 810–832.

Collins, N. L., & Read, S. J. (1990). Adult attachment, working models and relationship quality in dating couples. *Journal of Personality and Social Psychology, 58*, 644–663.

Cook, W. L. (2000). Understanding attachment security in family context. *Journal of Personality and Social Psychology, 78*, 285–294.

Crowell, J. A., & Owens, G. (1996). *Current Relationship Interview and scoring system.* Unpublished manuscript, Department of Psychology, State University of New York at Stony Brook.

Davila, J., & Bradbury, T. N. (2001). Attachment insecurity and the distinction between unhappy spouses who do and do not divorce. *Journal of Family Psychology, 15*, 373–393.

Davila, J., Bradbury, T. N., & Fincham, F. D. (1998). Negative affectivity as a mediator of the association between attachment and marital satisfaction. *Personal Relationships, 5,* 467–484.

Davila, J., Burge, D., & Hammen, C. (1997). Why does attachment style change? *Journal of Personality and Social Psychology, 73,* 826–838.

Davila, J., & Cobb, R. (in press). Predicting change in self-reported and interviewer-assessed adult attachment: Tests of the individual difference and life stress models of attachment change. *Personality and Social Psychology Bulletin.*

Davila, J., Karney, B. R., & Bradbury, T. N. (1999). Attachment change processes in the early years of marriage. *Journal of Personality and Social Psychology, 76,* 783–802.

Dunn, R. L., & Schwebel, A. I. (1995). Meta-analytic review of marital therapy outcome research. *Journal of Family Psychology, 9,* 58–68.

Feeney, J. A. (1999). Adult attachment, emotional control, and marital satisfaction. *Personal Relationships, 6,* 169–185.

Feeney, J. A., Noller, P., & Callan, V. J. (1994). Attachment style, communication, and satisfaction in the early years of marriage. *Advances in Personal Relationships, 5,* 269–308.

Floyd, F. J., Markman, H. J., Kelly, S., Blumberg, S. L., & Stanley, S. (1995). Preventive intervention and relationship enhancement. In N. S. Jacobson & A. S. Gurman (Eds.), *Clinical handbook of couple therapy* (pp. 212–226). New York: Guilford Press.

Gottman, J. M. (1979). *Marital interaction: Experimental investigations.* New York: Academic Press.

Gottman, J. M., Markman, H. J., & Notarius, C. (1977). The topography of marital conflict: A sequential analysis of verbal and nonverbal behavior. *Journal of Marriage and the Family, 39,* 461–477.

Greenberg, L. S., & Johnson, S. M. (1988). *Emotionally focused therapy for couples.* New York: Guilford Press.

Hahlweg, K., & Markman, H. J. (1988). Effectiveness of behavioral marital therapy: Empirical status of behavioral techniques in preventing and alleviating marital distress. *Journal of Consulting and Clinical Psychology, 56,* 440–447.

Hazan, C., & Shaver, P. R. (1987). Romantic love conceptualized as an attachment process. *Journal of Personality and Social Psychology, 52,* 511–534.

Hazan, C., & Shaver, P. R. (1994). Attachment as an organizational framework for research on close relationships. *Psychological Inquiry, 5,* 1–22.

Jacobson, N. S., Dobson, K., Fruzzetti, A. E., Schmaling, K. B., & Salusky, S. (1991). Marital therapy as a treatment for depression. *Journal of Consulting and Clinical Psychology, 59,* 547–557.

Jacobson, N. S., & Holtzworth-Munroe, A. (1986). Marital therapy: A social learning-cognitive perspective. In N. S. Jacobson & A. S. Gurman (Eds.), *Clinical handbook of marital therapy* (pp. 29–70). New York: Guilford Press.

Johnson, S. M., Hunsley, J., Greenberg, L., & Schindler, D. (1999). Emotionally focused couples therapy: Status and challenges. *Clinical Psychology: Science and Practice, 6,* 67–79.

Johnson, S. M., Makinen, J. A., & Millikin, J. W. (2001). Attachment injuries in couple relationships: A new perspective on impasses in couples therapy. *Journal of Marital and Family Therapy, 27,* 145–155.

Johnson, S. M., & Whiffen, V. E. (1999). Made to measure: Adapting emotionally focused couple therapy to partners' attachment styles. *Clinical Psychology: Science and Practice, 6,* 366–381.

Kirkpatrick, L. A., & Davis, K. E. (1994). Attachment style, gender, and relationship stability: A longitudinal analysis. *Journal of Personality and Social Psychology, 66,* 502–512.

Kobak, R. R., & Hazan, C. (1991). Attachment in marriage: Effects of security and accuracy of working models. *Journal of Personality and Social Psychology, 60,* 861–869.

Kobak, R. R., Ruckdeschel, K., & Hazan, C. (1994). From symptom to signal: An attachment view of emotion in marital therapy. In S. Johnson & L. Greenberg (Eds.), *The heart of the matter: Perspective on emotion in marital therapy* (pp. 46–71). New York: Brunner/Mazel.

LaGuardia, J. G., Ryan, R. M., Couchman, C. E., & Deci, E. L. (2000). Within-person variation in security of attachment: A self-determination theory perspective on attachment, need fulfillment, and well-being. *Journal of Personality and Social Psychology, 79,* 367–384.

Lamb, M. E. (1977). Father–infant and mother–infant interaction in the first year of life. *Child Development, 48,* 167–181.

Lawrence, E., Eldridge, K. A., & Christensen, A. (1998). The enhancement of traditional behavioral couples therapy: Consideration of individual factors and dyadic development. *Clinical Psychology Review, 18,* 745–764.

Main, M., & Weston, D. R. (1981). The quality of toddler's relationship to mother and father: Related to conflict behavior and the readiness to establish new relationships. *Child Development, 52,* 932–940.

Margolin, G. (1981). Behavior exchange in happy and unhappy marriages: A family cycle perspective. *Behavior Therapy, 12,* 329–343.

Margolin, G., & Wampold, B. E. (1981). Sequential analysis of conflict and accord in distressed and nondistressed marital partners. *Journal of Consulting and Clinical Psychology, 49,* 554–567.

Murray, S. L., Holmes, J. G., & Griffin, D. W. (1996). The self-fulfilling nature of positive illusions in romantic relationships: Love is not blind, but prescient. *Journal of Personality and Social Psychology, 71,* 1155–1180.

O'Leary, K. D., & Beach, S. R. H. (1990). Marital therapy: A viable treatment for depression and marital discord. *American Journal of Psychology, 147,* 183–186.

Pasch, L. A., & Bradbury, T. N. (1998). Social support, conflict, and the development of marital dysfunction. *Journal of Consulting and Clinical Psychology, 66,* 219–230.

Senchak, M., & Leonard, K. E. (1992). Attachment styles and marital adjustment among newlywed couples. *Journal of Social and Personal Relationships, 9,* 51–64.

Shaver, P. R., & Hazan, C. (1993). Adult romantic attachment: Theory and evidence. *Advances in Personal Relationships, 4,* 29–70.

Simpson, J., Rholes, W., & Nelligan, J. (1992). Support seeking and support giving within couples in an anxiety provoking situation: The role of attachment styles. *Journal of Personality and Social Psychology, 62,* 434–446.

Terman, L. M., & Buttenweiser, P. (1935). Personality factors in marital compatibility. *Journal of Social Psychology, 6,* 143–171.

Waters, E. (1997, April). *The secure base concept in Bowlby's theory and current re-*

search. Paper presented at the annual meeting of the Society for Research in Child Development, Washington, DC.

Whiffen, V. E., & Johnson, S. M. (1998). An attachment theory framework for the treatment of childbearing depression. *Clinical Psychology: Science and Practice, 5*, 478–493.

Whiffen, V. E., Kallos-Lilly, V., & MacDonald, B. J. (2001). Depression and attachment in couples. *Cognitive Therapy and Research, 25*, 421–434.

Zaleski, Z., & Galkowska, M. (1978). Neuroticism and marital satisfaction. *Behaviour Research and Therapy, 16*, 285–286.

8

Caring for the Caregiver

An Attachment Approach to Assessment and Treatment of Child Problems

ROGER KOBAK
TONI MANDELBAUM

The family therapy literature has been guided by several general themes. First and foremost, family therapists have emphasized viewing individual problems in the context of family relationships. As a result, therapists face the challenge of persuading parents and children that individual problems can be most effectively treated in the context of family relationships. A variety of techniques have been developed to address this challenge. A second general theme in family therapy has centered on identifying mechanisms through which family relationships help to shape individual dysfunction or pathology. Theory has played an important role in differentiating between the various schools of family therapy. For instance, structural theory emphasizes the interrelated subsystems of the family and the maintenance of appropriate boundaries and hierarchical structure. Bowen's (1978) approach focuses on the individual's ability to differentiate from the family by establishing increased cognitive control over the emotional processes that dominate dysfunctional family relationships. The strategic approach stresses techniques for introducing novel perspectives to unbalance "stuck" or rigid family relationships and symptomatic behavior (Madanes,1981). In spite of a common focus and diversity of approaches, family therapists have often relied more on theory than on an empirical understanding of parent–child and marital relationships.

Attachment theory and research can provide an empirical understanding of how parent–child and intimate adult relationships contribute to individual adaptation and psychopathology (Bowlby, 1988). Attachment relationships are a double-edged sword. On the one hand, well functioning parent–child and adult attachments provide individuals with a critical resource for coping with stress and for employing flexible problem solving (Shaver & Mikulincer, 2002). On the other hand, attachment relationships can also become a major source of dysfunctional anxiety, anger, and distorted communication (Bowlby, 1973; Johnson, 2002; Kobak, 1999). Our basic assumption is that the negative emotions that accompany insecure attachments are a major source of the distress that motivates families to seek treatment. As such, an attachment approach can provide a valuable guide to therapists in assessing and understanding family distress. Further, an understanding of secure attachment bonds provides the therapist with a guide for managing distress and restoring family members' confidence in each other.

Despite the potential contribution of an attachment approach to family and couple therapy, previous attachment research has been limited in several critical respects. First, attachment researchers have shed more light on the child's than on the parent's motivation for maintaining the parent–child relationship (George & Solomon, 1999). In this chapter, we discuss the importance of the parent's caregiving system for assessing family dysfunction and motivating change in *parent–child relationships*. A second limitation follows from the first. Caring for children occurs in the context of the parent's relationships with other adults. Cooperative sharing of caregiving responsibilities, or what we term the *caregiving alliance*, can either support or undermine the caregiver's capacity to care for children. Finally, parents' own *adult attachment relationships* can provide a secure base for meeting the challenges of raising children or can be the source of much anxiety and distress. Each of these relational systems, the parent–child, the caregiving alliance, and the adult attachment relationship can enhance or impede caring for children. Security and cooperation in one system can enhance functioning in the others. Alternatively, distress in one subsystem can "leak" into the others and may divert attention from the source of the difficulty. For instance, feelings of anxiety, anger, and distress that accompany an insecure adult attachment relationship may be misdirected toward the child or may absorb the caregiver's attention in ways that reduce the child's security and generate symptoms in the child. The failure to encapsulate stress generated from adult relationships increases the likelihood of burdening children with problems they are unable to manage. These "boundary violations" often result in failed problem solving that further increase the caregiver's sense of frustration and helplessness.

Treatment and assessment of family relationships are closely linked. The goal of assessment is to clearly identify the sources of relationship distress and how distress may undermine effective caregiving. As the therapist uses assessment information to establish a therapeutic focus, the caregiver may gain new perspectives on his or her self and the family relationships. Increased awareness creates new opportunities for more effective communication and stress management. By accurately identifying and effectively encapsulating family distress, the parent can become more available to his or her children and reassure them of his or her ability to provide protection and security. In the first section of this chapter, we develop an attachment model of the family system and use this model to guide therapeutic assessment and treatment planning. In the second section, we consider techniques for establishing and maintaining a focus for family treatment.

AN ATTACHMENT MODEL OF FAMILY RELATIONSHIPS

Attachment theory views family relationships in an evolutionary context that considers the individual's core motivational systems and their biological function (Cassidy, 1999). From this perspective, the child's attachment to a caregiver serves the function of protection, providing the child with a safe haven in times of distress and a secure base from which to learn about and explore the world. The child's basic security is derived from his or her confident expectation that the caregiver will be available and responsive if called upon for help (Ainsworth, 1990; Bowlby, 1973). When the parent's availability is threatened or jeopardized, the child experiences strong feelings of anxiety, anger, or sadness that in normal circumstances will communicate the importance of the relationship to adult caregivers (Bowlby, 1973). By early childhood, the child's growing capacity for verbal communication and perspective taking transform the infant attachment relationship into a cooperative partnership with the parent (Kobak & Duemmler, 1994). This give-and-take often occurs through conversations in which points of view are openly expressed, understood, and negotiated. Parents' availability remains of fundamental importance, although now availability is expressed through the parent's efforts in establishing and maintaining a sense of cooperation and partnership with the child.

The parents' side of the relationship is motivated by a caregiving system whose biological function is to provide protection and support for the developing child (George & Solomon, 1999). The caregiving system engages the parent in ongoing monitoring of the child's needs and accounts for the parent's investment in the child's success in growing up and ultimately reproducing and caring for the next generation. Successful maintenance of a caregiving relationship can account for a very strong sense of generativity and pride for the parent. Alternatively, if the child experiences difficulties in adjustment, the parent is likely to experience guilt and a sense of failure. The caregiving system promotes a sensitivity to the child's signals that complements the child's need to experience the parent as available and responsive. At the most basic level, parental sensitivity depends on the ability to attend to child signals (Crowell & Feldman, 1988). However, competing demands that physically or emotionally separate the parent from the child may substantially reduce parental availability. A long list of problems, including depression, employment difficulties, and substance abuse, may interfere with parents' abilities to attend to their child. These types of problems are likely to be further exacerbated by stressful family interactions.

The child's confidence in his or her caregiver's availability is readily observable in the quality of parent–child communication (Bretherton, 1990). Open and cooperative communication is a hallmark of a secure attachment relationship. When the child has confidence in the parent, feelings are communicated directly, both the child's and the parent's ability to empathize and take each other's perspective is enhanced, and differences in point of view are open to negotiation (Kobak & Duemmler, 1994). Negative emotions arising from conflicts or frustration thus serve an important signal function in allowing partners to better understand each other and maintain confidence in their relationship (Kobak, Hazan, & Ruckdeschel, 1994). As a result, negative emotions are likely to be short-lived and positive emotions can play an increased role in the relationship.

Caregiving is substantially more complex than the workings of the child's attachment system. Not only must the caregiver continually adapt to the child's growing capacities for maintaining a partnership, but he or she must manage caregiving in the context of other adult relationships. These adult relationships can be either an invaluable source of support or a major source of anger, anxiety, and distress. When parents establish a *caregiving alliance* in the interest of protecting and educating their children, parenting becomes a shared responsibility and each caregiver has a partner with whom to manage the day-to-day stresses of raising children. Perhaps most important, the caregiving alliance can provide parents with a context for "reflective dialogue" about caring for the child. Reflective dialogue provides the parent with a place to understand disruptions in the caregiver–child relationship, examine feelings, empathize with the child, and repair breaches in caregiving availability (Marvin, Cooper, Hoffman, & Powell, 2002). *Adult attachment relationships* may also provide for caregivers' own attachment needs. In successful adult attachments, the adults form a partnership in which they reciprocally act as attachment figures to one another. These relationships are most commonly formed with spouses. However, a variety of other individuals, including a relative, a close friend, or in some cases religious institutions, may serve as attachment figures and the development of an attachment relationship may provide an invaluable source of support for coping with distress.

Attachment Distress, Boundary Violations, and Symptom Formation

An understanding of the motivational systems that foster the development and maintenance of family relationships provides a guide to the emotional dynamics that structure parent–child and intimate adult relationships. The core assumption of our attachment model is that child symptoms and parent–child distress are more likely to emerge at times when the child perceives threats to the caregiver's availability. Perceived threats are accompanied by strong feelings of fear and anger and are often expressed in distorted or symptomatic forms. A caregiver's response may further distort the child's concerns by dismissing or exaggerating the child's problems. When the child's strategies for maintaining the relationship break down, the parent and child often interact in ways that further fuel the child's anxiety and the parent's sense of frustration and failure.

Distress in the parent–child dyad normally motivates the caregiver to seek support from other adults. If support is available, distress can be contained and the child problem can be addressed. However, if the caregiver feels abandoned by his or her caregiving partner, the child problem quickly becomes compounded with the caregiver's own feelings of anxiety and anger. The caregiving alliance can rapidly be reduced to mutual criticism and competition over the children. In such instances, basic caregiving boundaries that normally protect the child are violated and the child is exposed to adult distress that further erodes his or her confidence in the parents' availability. Child symptoms may also be produced by distress that originates in the caregiving alliance or in the adult attachment relationship. The family therapy literature has provided extensive examples of times when distress originating in the adult relationships is poorly managed and undermines the parent–child relationship. The initial challenge for therapists is moving from the presenting problems or symptoms to the relationship processes that produce or maintain them.

ASSESSMENT: A FRAMEWORK FOR REFRAMING CHILD SYMPTOMS

The first step in assessment is determining whether attachment insecurity has either perpetuated or contributed to the child's symptoms. Some child difficulties, including learning disabilities and attention-deficit/hyperactivity disorder, may often create stress in the parent–child relationship, but these difficulties can usually be overcome with psychoeducational support for the parent about the child's difficulties. In other cases, the child's problems are closely linked to perceived threats to the parent's availability and high levels of distress in family relationships. In assessing the child's symptoms, the therapist must systematically move from an initial focus on negative child behavior to the quality of the caregiver–child dyad. After understanding the child's problems in the context of the parent–child relationship, the therapist moves to considering the caregiver's adult relationships and how these may be reducing his or her capacity for empathizing with and attending to the child's needs. Two aspects of the caregiver's adult relationship are of particular concern. First, what is the quality of the caregiving alliance or support available to the caregiver for parenting? Second, what is the quality of the caregiver's adult attachment relationships? A thorough assessment should increase the therapist's empathy with the caregiver and result in a formulation that establishes treatment priorities that support the caregiver, thereby increasing the caregiver's availability to his or her child.

Assessing the Problem Child–Primary Caregiver Dyad

After obtaining a clear understanding of the child's presenting problems, the focus of assessment moves to evaluating the quality of the relationship between the child and his or her primary caregiver. In most families, the primary caregiver is the person who has the most involvement with the child and is often most distressed about the child's difficulties. The process of evaluating parent–child attachment involves careful consideration of both the caregiver's availability and the child's confidence in the caregiver's availability. Observations of caregiver–child communication provide the therapist with information for assessing attachment quality. On the one hand, markers of attachment security include the caregiver's ongoing capacity to empathize with and understand the child's goals, directly communicate appropriate parental goals and concerns, and flexibly negotiate conflicts (Kobak & Duemmler, 1994). On the other hand, insecure attachment is often evident in severe restrictions of the caregiver's capacity for empathy or reflective function (Fonagy & Target, 1997). When feelings of anxiety and anger take precedence, the parent's view of the child shifts from one of a cooperative partner to that of a hostile antagonist. The caregiver's frustration with the child further reduces mental freedom for exploring alternative views, perspective taking, and problem solving (Bugental, 1992). As a result, the parent will often adhere to a view of the child as negativistic, uncooperative, or hostile and have difficulty perceiving the underlying sources of the child's fear, rage, or sadness. The caregiver's diminished capacity for empathizing with the child substantially reduces his or her capacity for soothing the child and restoring a sense of cooperative partnership (Kobak & Esposito, in press).

Close observation of parent–child interaction provides the therapist with important information on caregiving difficulties. First, it is important to assess the degree to which the parent is able to attend to and read the child's signals. Assessing the caregiver's understanding of the child can be difficult when the child is strongly disengaged or noncommunicative. However, the therapist can often play a useful role in supporting child communications and then monitoring caregiver response. It is important to observe how the caregiver responds to the child's communications. Many times child disengagement results from a history of parents' ignoring, misunderstanding, or outright rejecting the child's initiatives and signals.

A second aspect of parent–child communication involves parents' ability to clearly communicate their own thoughts and feelings (Baumrind, 1967; Kobak & Duemmler, 1994). An important part of parental communication is establishing clear and developmentally appropriate expectations for the child's behavior. The appropriateness and emotional tone of parental communications can set a context for establishing cooperative and growing maturity on the part of the child. Alternatively, parents can communicate in ways that reduce the child's sense of wanting to cooperate and could actively anger the child and increase the likelihood of noncompliance. A related aspect of caregiving communication involves determining what should *not* be communicated to the child. Generally, the parent's own distress needs to be contained or minimally communicated to a child, which in turn helps the child to better understand and cooperate with the parent.

Finally, successful communication requires a capacity for negotiation and problem-solving flexibility. This type of flexibility requires a freedom to explore different perspectives on the problem and to develop creative ideas about how to reconcile different agendas. Generally such problem solving occurs in an emotionally secure climate where both the parent's and the child's goals are directly communicated and mutually understood. This type of problem solving is dependent on the caregiver being capable of clear communication of his or her own expectations and empathy with the child's needs. The absence of direct communication and empathy in distressed relationships usually eliminates the negotiation and problem solving that make cooperation possible. Perhaps the most important feature of successful caregiving is the parent's ability to identify and correct the child's perception of the parent as being unavailable, unresponsive, or rejecting. This capacity requires empathy with the child and an ability to acknowledge failures in a way that restores the child's confidence in the parent's availability (Diamond & Stern, Chapter 10, this volume).

In distressed parent–child relationships, the parent's difficulties in communicating with and engaging his or her child often put pressure on the therapist to take over caregiving from the parent. This pressure often is produced by the parent's own sense of failure, frustration, and uncertainty about how to help the child. If the therapist does not take over from the parent, the parent will often resort to alternative means of managing anxiety by focusing on the child's problem behavior or diverting discussion to other topics. As a result, in assessing the problem child–primary caregiver dyad, it is important for the therapist to find elements of caregiving competence that provide a basis for encouraging the parent to remain engaged with the child.

While parent–child communication provides the initial focus for assessment, the therapist needs to link the child's symptoms to perceived threats to the caregiver's availability. Difficulties in parent–child communication foster the child's perceptions of the parent as unavailable. These perceptions, in turn, increase the child's anxiety, anger, and defensive behavior, and usually contribute to the child's presenting problems (Bowlby, 1973; Miccuci, 1998). By identifying the child's attachment-related fears, the therapist can see beyond the child's defensive, disengaged, or hostile behavior to core insecurities that are maintaining the child's symptoms and poor communication with the caregiver. Perceived threats to caregiver's availability fall into several major categories: relationship disruptions, caregiver helplessness, and parental anger or rejection.

Unanticipated or unplanned separations can create relationship disruptions that shake the child's confidence in the caregiver's availability (Kobak, Little, Race, & Acosta, 2001). The timing of the child's problems and their association with disruptions in the family relationships are critical factors for the therapist to consider. The impact of these disruptions on the child's confidence largely depends on the circumstances surrounding the event. Separations accompanying divorce can be particularly disturbing to children insofar as the separation is often accompanied by anger and conflict. Disruptions can also occur as a result of illness or sudden emergencies that are not anticipated by either the child or the caregiver. Loss of the caregiver represents an extreme form of disruption, but how this impacts on the child' expectations will depend on the circumstances surrounding the loss and the availability of alternative caregivers (Bowlby, 1980). There are many less obvious disruptions in attachment relationships. Stressful life events may occupy the parent's attention and be perceived by the child as a major disruption in the relationship. Job loss, work difficulties, reactions to loss of parents, or conflict with relatives are all potential sources of stress to parents that may have the effect of disrupting the relationship with the child.

Caregiver helplessness represents a major threat to the child's confidence in the caregiver's availability (Lyons-Ruth & Jacobvitz, 1999; Main & Hesse, 1990). If the child perceives the parent as being depressed or overwhelmed by his or her own difficulties, he or she is likely not only to experience reduced attention from the parent, but also may actively try to protect the parent. Not all forms of caregiver distress necessarily result in "parentification," or role reversal with the child. Parents can inform children of stresses in other parts of their lives and prevent the children from assuming blame or responsibility for these problems. Such an understanding can promote accommodation and help the child to maintain confidence in the caregiver's availability. In contrast, if the child senses distress in the caregiver that is not clearly identified, he or she may become burdened and more anxious about the caregiver's well-being.

A final possible threat to a caregiver's availability comes from parental anger and rejection. If the parent is chronically irritable or prone to angry outbursts, the child can usually adapt by learning to avoid the parent or reduce contacts that are likely to trigger anger. Although the child's expectation of rejection may result from accumulated episodes of hostile behavior, specific episodes of ruptures in the relationship may become prototypical symbols of caregiver rejection and abandonment. These ruptures can result from poorly managed stresses in the life of the parent or from unresolved issues dating from the parent's own childhood experiences, such as child sexual abuse. However, anger that is expressed in frightening or critical ways can do much to undermine the child's sense of being loved and can sensitize the child to the notion that the parent may reject him or her. Rejection and abandonment at a time of intense need may also create impasses in therapeutic efforts to restore the child's confidence in the parent or in parents' trust for each other (Johnson, Makinen, & Millikin, 2001).

Assessing Caregiving Context: The Role of Other Adults in the Family

Once the therapist has linked the child's symptoms to attachment insecurity and perceived threats to the caregiver's availability, the next step involves understanding the sources of stress and support in the caregiver's life. The role of secondary caregivers can vary enormously within family systems and can create many types of caregiving arrangements (Howes, 1999). In families with an effective caregiving alliance, it may be difficult to make a distinction between primary and secondary caregivers. In other families, secondary caregivers may be completely absent. The secondary caregiver's role in the family forms an important part of the attachment assessment (Cowan, Powell, & Cowan, 1997). In some families, as the relationship between the child and the primary caregiver becomes distressed, the secondary caregiver's availability can be an important source of support for the child. When this occurs, it is likely to reduce the severity of family distress and provides an important avenue for treating the family. A secondary caregiver who is responsive to both the child and the primary caregiver can serve as a source of support and keep distress contained to the primary attachment relationship. In contrast, a disengaged secondary caregiver may greatly increase anxiety in both the child and the primary caregiver. Lack of availability at a time of high stress can readily be perceived as emotional abandonment. The quality of the attachment bond between caregivers can have an enormous impact on the overall emotional climate of the family. A secure bond can provide both primary and secondary caregivers with a secure base for parenting children, managing day-to-day stresses, and pursuing other important goals.

The presence of a cooperative *caregiving alliance* provides an initial indicator of the security of the adult attachment. There are several markers of a cooperative caregiving alliance. First and foremost is the willingness of the secondary adult to participate in joint sessions. Participation indicates a sense of shared responsibility and involvement. When both caregivers are present, the therapist can directly observe the way in which caregivers work together to support each other in relation to the child. Communications about the child can differ dramatically depending on the quality of the caregiving alliance. In a well-functioning alliance, caregivers can help each other to better understand the child as well as generate new and constructive perspectives on the child. Caregivers can often provide useful feedback about parenting or model alternative ways of responding to the child's signals. The key to the caregiving alliance is a shared sense of responsibility and respect for partners as caregivers to the child.

The absence of a caregiving alliance can be noted in several ways. Some caregivers have difficulty discussing the child without lapsing into mutual criticism or blame. In these relationships, caregivers often undermine each other's sense of competence as a parent, and view each other as antagonists rather than allies in the task of caring for the child. In other families, the absence of a cooperative caregiving alliance is marked by too much agreement about the child. In these relationships, conversations focus on the child as the problem. Although caregivers may derive a sense of partnership from this approach to the child, such conversations may fail to generate an understanding of the child or suggest ways to engage the child more positively. Instead, they result in an implicit decision to reject and blame the child for shortcomings in the parent–child relationship. Rather than enhance parental availability, this type of caregiving alliance reduces availability and tends to perpetuate child problems.

Problems in maintaining a caregiving alliance are often, but not always, rooted in an insecure *adult attachment* relationship. Where partners lose confidence in each other's availability and responsiveness, the threat of abandonment and loss evokes the most basic attachment emotions of fear and anger. Coping with such feelings tends to take precedence over other issues in the adult's life, and reduces the caregiver's availability to the child. As a result, problems in the caregiving alliance should usually be followed up by assessment of the quality of the adult attachment relationship. High levels of adult attachment distress can be readily identified. Distressed individuals are often quick to report their anger or anxiety about their partner and his or her lack of commitment to maintaining the relationship. If both partners are present, the therapist can often readily observe negative interaction cycles that are well documented in distressed marriages (Johnson,

1996). These may take the form of mutual accusations, pursuit-and-with-drawal patterns, or mutual avoidance, and may impact the child's relation-ship with his or her caregivers in several ways. First, difficulties in main-taining positive communication between adults will make it more difficult for the adults to remain engaged in a cooperative manner about childcare issues. Many times, marital distress will result in the primary caregiver be-coming more involved with the child and the secondary caregiver becoming less involved. This leads to a common pattern in distressed families in which the mother is characterized as overinvolved while the father is char-acterized as disengaged or absent (Luepnitz, 1988).

Formulation: Stress Management and Caregiver Availability

The goal of this assessment phase is to link the child's symptoms to the ma-jor sources of distress and support in the family system. A diagram of the assessment issues is presented in Figure 8.1.

    If the child's problems are linked to perceived threats to the caregiver's availability, the next step is to arrive at a balanced understanding of the sources of stress and support in the primary caregiver's adult relationships

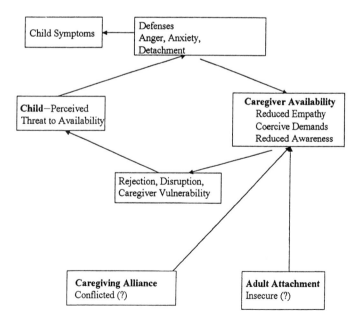

FIGURE 8.1. A diagram of the child's assessment issues.

and how those stresses and lack of support are interfering with the caregiver's capacity to be available to and supportive of the child. In many respects, the primary caregiver is the focal point for an attachment-based formulation of the child's problems. By understanding the caregiver's difficulties, assessment can point to ways that the therapist can enter the family system to support the caregiver and ultimately increase the caregiver's availability to the child.

Assessment information can be organized into two major categories of factors that facilitate or hinder caregiving. The first category includes those aspects of family relationships that support the caregiver's capacity to be available and responsive to the child. Such support can come from within the family, in the form of a caregiving alliance, or it can come from outside the family, in the form of close friends who provide a context for discussing child-related issues and provide normative information about how other parents may be dealing with similar issues in raising children. Perhaps most important, support for caregiving can be provided through an adult attachment relationship that gives the caregiver a place to meet his or her own attachment needs and a secure base for facing the changing demands of growing children. Finally, the caregiver's relationship with his or her family of origin can provide an important source of support for caregiving.

Second, what are the stresses and competing demands that reduce the caregivers' availability? The research on stressful life events has identified a number of events such as residential moves, job loss, financial problems, and illness that adults report as stressful. These types of stresses can reduce parental availability in a variety of ways. However, we believe that families become most vulnerable when stresses actually occur within attachment relationships that normally serve as a source of support. *More specifically, when parent–child, caregiving alliance, and adult attachment relationships become distressed and undermine the adult's confidence as a caregiver and partner in an adult attachment relationship, distress can escalate in an exponential fashion and fundamentally jeopardize the caregiver's capacity for remaining available to the child.* Distress occurring within family relationships represents simultaneously a loss of critical support and a major potential threat to security and well-being.

When caregivers experience a "compound fear situation" (Bowlby, 1973), involving the loss of support and perceived rejection from loved ones, their capacity to compartmentalize and manage stress may be severely challenged. The breakdown in stress management can take a variety of forms. The caregiver may at some times feel overwhelmed and helpless and at other times may feel angry (Lyons-Ruth & Jacobvitz, 1999). Anger can be readily displaced from another adult to the child. A caregiver can shift his or her unmet needs for support from another adult to his or her child. These forms of mismanaged stress create basic violations in the boundaries that define the caregiver's relationship with the child, and are readily perceived by the child as threats to the caregiver's availability, including caregiver helplessness, rejection, or abandonment.

CASE ILLUSTRATION:
THE OVERWHELMED AND DEPRESSED CAREGIVER

Cathy, the mother, wanted therapy for Donna, her 16-year-old daughter, whom she felt had been inexplicably noncompliant. She and her husband had found Donna smoking, and they suspected she was drinking with her friends. Cathy vacillated between helpless and hostile stances toward her daughter. She cried as she talked of Donna's childhood and her guilt at resenting having to care for Donna's severe asthma. Guilt shifted to anger as she accused Donna of "paying her back" by acting out. Donna looked away as her mother talked, clearly used to her mother's tears, and just as clearly unmoved by them. It was apparent that there was more to the story than just Donna's acting out. The initial session generated a number of questions. First, although there was clearly substantial anger and poor communication, the link between the daughter's problems and the mother–daughter relationship needed to be explored. Second, although the mother was clearly distressed enough to seek treatment, the sources of her distress needed further evaluation. The therapist tentatively hypothesized that there may be some caregiver helplessness and possibly a history of rejection in the mother–daughter relationship. A family assessment was scheduled to further evaluate support for the mother.

In the first family sessions, Dan (14) and Donna (16) sat between their parents. David (52) and Cathy (48) did not address each other directly, instead looking at their children when talking. The mother and daughter were caught in a cycle of mutual blame and accusation. Donna was quick to say that she "just wanted her mother to lay off" and her mother countered with "How can I trust you?" As Donna tried to reassert her position, Cathy became tearful and accused Donna of trying to punish her. Cathy's own distress undermined her daughter's efforts to assert herself, leading Donna to disengage and dismiss her mother's concerns. The pursue–withdraw pattern of defensive and distorted communication was often repeated at home. Cathy would become overwhelmed and needy, with Donna reacting either with fiery anger or with silent withdrawal.

Donna's disengaged and hostile behavior were symptoms of her frustrations in gaining her mother's attention. Instead of having an available parent, Donna had to adjust to her mother's distress, hostility, and helplessness. Every time Donna had an asthma attack, her mother cried, felt overwhelmed, and would tell Donna that "if your father really loved you, he'd be here now." Donna's father, David, was often physically and emotionally absent. In session, David spoke for minutes on end without monitoring how others were receiving his monologue. Neither child seemed to place much import on what their father had to say. Two years prior to the start of therapy David had left Cathy for 12 months to pursue an affair and had fundamentally shaken his children's confidence in his availability.

The parents' lack of availability to the children was maintained by an ineffective caregiving alliance. Although it was obvious to the therapist that Cathy and David both cared a great deal for their children, they did not seem to understand the impact of their communications. For example, Cathy would tell Donna: "I can't deal with you on my own. Why are you so difficult? Don't you understand what I'm dealing with?" David repeatedly explained that he had returned to his family after a year's hiatus only because he did not want his children to grow up without a father. Yet his attempts to rejoin the family tended to engender more distress. Cathy's tears enraged David, who spoke of feeling unfit as a husband, while David's anger left Cathy tearful and confused. They both were very uncomfortable with one another and uncertain of their role as parents. Their mutual displeasure with their daughter provided their only topic of conversation.

Difficulties in the caregiving alliance led to further assessment of Cathy and David's attachment relationship. The couple's relationship history illustrated a pattern in which David responded to conflict by escaping to bars, while Cathy struggled to care for their children. David's affair turned Cathy's worst fears of abandonment into a reality. She acknowledged that she turned much of her anger and anxiety toward the children. Cathy and David were caught in an anxious/preoccupied, critical/avoidant defensive cycle that left them both exhausted and hopeless. David's affair represented an attachment injury that exacerbated and crystallized the insecurity in their relationship (Johnson et al., 2001). David's return to the marriage did not assuage Cathy's fears of rejection since he repeatedly stated that he had only returned to the marriage for the sake of his children. He refused to tell Cathy that she was important to him and reserved the right to leave again should their issues remain unresolved. Because neither member of the couple was assured of the other's commitment or availability, their energies were expended on anxiously monitoring each other. The stress they were under prevented them from focusing on their children's needs. Fears of rejection and abandonment crippled the caregiving alliance.

Case Formulation: Stress Management and Caregiver Availability

At the time Cathy sought treatment for Donna's problems, the family was experiencing considerable distress. In spite of a history of insecure attachment and asthma-related worries, the mother–daughter relationship had been relatively stable. Only as Donna moved toward more adolescent autonomy did their relationship become less tenable. Cathy's difficulty in managing this transition was further increased by distress in her marriage. She had very little positive support and her own anxiety and anger at David's abandonment further increased her distress and reduced her ability to listen to or communicate effectively with her children. David, newly sober, also had little support and often voiced feelings of loneliness and isolation. He was unable to socialize with his friends, all of whom continued to drink. With little support from each other and strong fears of rejection and abandonment, David and Cathy struggled with managing the feelings that were produced by an insecure attachment relationship. Cathy tended to focus her distress on her relationship with the children and turned to them for solace. This sense that Cathy had become a burden was reflected in Donna's desire to "get my mother off my back."

ESTABLISHING A FOCUS FOR TREATMENT: A SECURE BASE FOR THE CAREGIVER

Our attachment model integrates assessment information into a formulation for establishing treatment goals and a therapeutic contract. At the heart of our model is the assumption that child problems can often be most effectively addressed by caring for the caregiver. *The central notion is that change in families is most likely to occur when the caregiver establishes greater confidence in the availability of another adult.* The feeling of increased security creates the conditions for the caregiver to more accurately monitor his or her self, consider alternative perspectives on his or her child, and engage in new and more positive approaches to the child's problematic behavior. A secure adult relationship also provides the caregiver with an ally or partner who can introduce new information and perspectives on the child that facilitate problem solving and increase cognitive flexibility. Depending on the family structure, this other person can be either an adult partner or the therapist. When the caregiver feels supported, preferably by other significant adults and/or by the therapist, he or she becomes more capable of repairing breaches and perceived threats to his or her availability to the child. While providing the caregiver with a secure relationship is a central ingredient in change, the therapist must also establish a focus for treatment that clearly identifies how treatment can reduce the child's symptoms and family distress. A clearly defined treatment focus can in itself provide therapeutic benefit to family members by labeling and encapsulating the sources of family distress. Depending on the assessment, there are several possible treatment foci, beginning with the parent–child dyad.

In choosing a focus the therapist often begins with the presenting problem, but gradually refocuses treatment to the source of the greatest distress. If the primary source of distress is in the parent–child relationship, refocusing from the child problem to communication in the parent–child relationship may be relatively direct. The therapist would work to support the parent in understanding the child's problems as linked to perceived threats to parental availability. In linking the child's symptoms to perceived threats to parental availability, the therapist actively takes on the child's perspective and points to concerns that may have been suppressed or not openly acknowledged by the child. A reframing approach that focuses on allowing each person in the family to receive equal responsibility enables the therapist to highlight the crucial issues without blaming or accusing any particular family member. Utilizing an unbalancing technique, the therapist can become a voice for the child and can direct the parent's attention to how family circumstances may be impacting the child. Child symptoms are reframed from this perspective as a distorted form of communicating the importance of the parent's availability to the child. Establishing this link provides a way of understanding the symptom and reframing the problem in relational terms.

Refocusing on the parent–child relationship must be done in a way that supports the parent (Diamond, Diamond, & Liddle, 2000). It must also be clearly linked to the presenting problem. In presenting the child's concerns, the therapist can stress the parent's significance to the child, involve the parent in understanding the child's perspective, and open discussion of ways to increase the parent's positive attention to and engagement with the child. In exploring the issues involved in reassuring the child, the therapist and the parent can form a caregiving alliance that provides the caregiver with a secure base for examining his or her parenting and aspects of his or her life situation that have become obstacles to attending to his or her child. A balanced and nonaccusatory formulation of the problem in attachment terms can be presented in a way that would elicit acceptance from both the child and the caregiver.

As the therapist and the caregiver move toward a common understanding of the child's problems, they must next establish a treatment focus. For the most part, the nature of the problem as formulated will guide the therapist and the caregiver toward particular treatment goals. If assessment has identified parental anger as the primary threat to the caregiver availability, the therapist can move toward a focus on communication around issues involving conflict. If the primary threat to caregiver availability results from parental stress, the treatment recommendation can center on enhancing the parent's ability to monitor and communicate with the child about the situation. Loyalty conflict between caregivers can be addressed by conjoint sessions with the child and caregivers that focus on discussion of differences and enhancing mutual support. Finally, caregiver helplessness can be addressed by helping the caregiver to create a secure base with his or her adult partner.

An overarching goal for treatment is providing the caregiver with a secure base for exploring his or her relationship with the child. The notion of a secure base for caregiving centers on the parent's confidence that he or she has an ally who shares his or her interest in protecting and supporting the child's development. In better functioning families, the caregiving alliance provides parents with a secure base for problem solving child-related issues, gaining new perspectives on the child, and testing out ideas. As each caregiver feels more secure, his or her capacity to consider alternative perspectives of him- or herself, acknowledge difficult feelings, and problem solve childcare issues increase. As a result, we see the establishment of a secure relationship with the therapist as a precondition to being able to be open to new experiences in the therapy sessions. A secure base is likely to increase the parent's overall confidence and increase engagement with the child in a competent caregiving role. The relationship with the therapist can provide an important platform for identifying sources of distress that are interfering with the caregiver's capacity to attend to the child and for exploring negative attributions and feelings about the child. For instance, discussions with the therapist allowed Cathy to identify her feelings of abandonment by and anger toward David. From this standpoint she could more readily acknowledge how these feelings were at times displaced on the children and interfered with her ability to accurately interpret Donna's own anger.

The transition from the parent–child dyad to a focus on the caregiving alliance is in many respects a natural one and can lead to a focus on the adult attachment relationship if this is needed. Assignments that test the caregivers' abilities to work together to gain child cooperation can serve to increase the family's awareness of discomfort or conflict between caregivers. The success of the focus on the caregiving alliance will often determine whether the therapist needs to further shift the focus to adult attachment issues. In cases where fear and anger dominate the adult's attachment relationship and undermines efforts to build a caregiving alliance, couple therapy becomes the primary treatment modality. Emotionally focused therapy (EFT) provides the approach of choice for a therapist pursuing an attachment model, and has produced impressive outcomes (Johnson, Hunsley, Greenberg, & Schendler, 1999). However, in cases that begin with the child as the identified patient, it is important that the therapist continue to monitor the impact of the couple work on the parent–child relationship and the children. This can be done by reports from the parents and by occasional sessions directly involving the children.

CASE ILLUSTRATION, CONTINUED: ESTABLISHING A TREATMENT FOCUS

At least three treatment possibilities emerged from the assessment phase. The therapist could focus on the mother–child dyad with the goal of improving communication, reducing the pursue–withdraw cycle that characterized the mother–daughter relationship, and establishing a reparative conversation about the perceived threat to the mother's availability (Diamond & Stern, Chapter 10, this volume). The therapist could work with both parents to establish a more effective caregiving alliance, or he or she could work with the couple around issues of marital distress and attachment insecurity directly through couple therapy. Although both husband and wife were very distressed over their relationship, the links between adult attachment insecurity and the presenting child problem were not apparent to the family. As a result, therapy initially focused on the parent–child relationship. In the early sessions, Donna was able to clearly voice her perceptions of her relationship with her mother. She acknowledged disappointment at not being able to talk with her mother, but was able to convey a sense that she understood that her mother really cared about her in spite of being "really messed up." Cathy was able to acknowledge that she at times burdened Donna with her own distress. Both mother and daughter could see how helping Cathy gain support from David might improve their ability to communicate with each other.

The focus on building a more effective caregiving alliance had several advantages. First, a focus on the caregiving alliance provided direct support to Cathy in a way that could reduce her sense of being overwhelmed and alone in addressing the children's problems. Strengthening this alliance also helped Cathy to more effectively manage caregiving stress and increased her capacity for more positive engagement with her children. In addition, an enhanced caregiving alliance clarified David's caregiving role for his children, allowing him to feel more competent and involved. Increasing both parents' availability then reduced Donna's anxiety about her parents' availability and created conditions that allowed her to become more cooperative and open with her parents. For instance, while admitting that she had experimented with smoking and drinking, Donna acknowledged that her parents' concerns were legitimate and reassured them that she would tell them if she smoked or drank in the future.

The main challenge facing the therapist in this case was to shift attention from the child's symptoms to the need to build more cooperation between the parents. An enactment served to highlight the parents' need to work together. When Donna refused to attend therapy and sat in the car, the therapist supported the parents in insisting that Donna leave the car and join the session. With much support, the parents both went out and asked their daughter to join the session. The ensuing discussion allowed the couple to acknowledge their feelings of helplessness in their caregiving roles and to begin to support each other. To reinforce a focus on the caregiving alliance, the parents were told to set a time to be together during which they were not allowed to discuss anything to do with their children. When they returned the next week, David and Cathy commented on how difficult it was for the two of them to be alone. They were extremely uncomfortable without their children as buffers. Turning to the parents, the therapist suggested that they come in alone for a few sessions to work on feeling more comfortable and less helpless as parents. The focus of the therapy had thus shifted to increasing support and competence in the caregiving alliance.

David and Cathy then began to work on their relationship and demonstrated great commitment in couple therapy. The therapist adopted an EFT approach to restoring security in the marital relationship (Johnson, 1996). This work initially focused on accessing attachment-related fears of abandonment. By helping Cathy and David identify their attachment failures, and engage in direct and open conversation about their concerns, the therapist increased trust and security in the relationship. As a result, David's anger was connected to his fear of not being accepted by Cathy, allowing the therapist to reframe his anger as a sign of Cathy's importance to him. This understanding increased Cathy's empathy and decreased her defensiveness. Most weeks, the couple arrived feeling more confident in the other's availability. David became much more direct in communicating his need to rely on Cathy. Although Cathy was skeptical at first, she gradually came to trust in David's commitment to the relationship. Toward the end of therapy she stated, "It was hard for me to believe when he first said he was ready to commit to the relationship, but now I can really believe him. He not only says he loves me but he shows it." The increased security in their own relationship freed the parents to attend more effectively to their children. Donna's hostile outbursts decreased and Cathy was able to "lay off" Donna, allowing her more freedom to be a teenager. After 6 months, the couple ended treatment, describing their relationship as more secure.

CONCLUSION

Our attachment model provides an overall guide to understanding the attachment dynamics that generate distress in families seeking therapy. For the therapist, the model identifies the interrelated subsystems of the parent–child relationship, caregiving alliance, and adult attachments, and the markers of distress in each of those subsystems. It is often the case that distress in one of the family subsystems creates leakage or boundary violations that undermine confidence and cooperation in other subsystems. Identifying the most distressed subsystem in the family can provide the basis for establishing an effective focus for therapy. Regardless of whether treatment focuses on the parent–child relationship, the caregiving alliance, or the adult attachment relationship, the key to effective treatment centers on increasing support for the caregiver in the family system. By providing a secure base to the caregiver, the therapist can provide the platform from which the caregiver can more effectively identify sources of distress, increase empathy with self and children, and engage in reparative conversations. When the caregiver feels secure, child problems can be managed much more effectively and the child's confidence in the parent's availability can be restored.

REFERENCES

Ainsworth, M. D. S. (1990). Some considerations regarding theory and assessment relevant to attachments beyond infancy. In M. Greenberg, D. Cicchetti, & E. M. Cummings (Eds.), *Attachment in the preschool years: Theory, research, and intervention* (pp. 463–488). Chicago: University of Chicago Press.

Baumrind, D. (1967). Child care practices anteceding three patterns of preschool behavior. *Genetic Psychology Monographs*, 75, 43–88.

Bowen, M. (1978). *Family therapy in clinical practice*. New York: Aronson.

Bowlby, J. (1973). *Attachment and Loss: Vol. II. Separation*. New York: Basic Books.

Bowlby, J. (1980). *Attachment and Loss: Vol. III. Loss*. New York: Basic Books.

Bowlby, J. (1988). *A secure base: Parent–child attachment and healthy human development*. New York: Basic Books.

Bretherton, I. (1990). Open communication and internal working models: Their role in the development of attachment relationships. In R. A. Thompson (Ed.), *Nebraska Symposium on Motivation: Socioemotional development* (pp. 57–113). Lincoln: University of Nebraska Press.

Bugental, D. (1992). Affective and cognitive processes within threat-oriented family systems. In I. E. Sigel, A. V. McGillicuddy-DeLisi, & J. J. Goodnow (Eds.), *Parental belief systems: Psychological consequences for children* (2nd ed., pp. 219–248). Hillsdale, NJ: Erlbaum.

Cassidy, J. (1999). The nature of the child's ties. In J. Cassidy & P. R. Shaver (Eds.), *Handbook of attachment: Theory, research, and clinical applications* (pp. 3–20). New York: Guilford Press.

Cowan, P., Powell, D., & Cowan, C. P. (2000). Parenting interventions: A family systems perspective. In W. Damon, I. E. Sigel, & K. A. Renninger (Eds.), *Handbook of child psychology: Vol. 4. Child psychology in practice* (5th ed., pp. 57–89). New York: Wiley.

Crowell, J. A., & Feldman, S. (1988). Mothers' internal working models of relationships and children's behavioral and developmental status: A study of mother–child interaction. *Child Development*, 59, 1273–1285.

Diamond, G. M., Diamond, G. S., & Liddle, H. A. (2000). The therapist–parent alliance in family-based therapy for adolescents. *Journal of Clinical Psychology*, 56, 1037–1050.

Fonagy, P., & Target, M. (1997). Attachment and reflective function: Their role in self-organization. *Development and Psychopathology*, 9, 679–700.

George, C., & Solomon, J. (1999). Attachment and caregiving: The caregiving behavioral system. In J. Cassidy & P. R. Shaver (Eds.), *Handbook of attachment: Theory, research, and clinical applications* (pp. 649–670). New York: Guilford Press.

Howes, C. (1999). Attachment relationships in the context of multiple caregivers. In J. Cassidy & P. R. Shaver (Eds.), *Handbook of attachment: Theory, research, and clinical applications* (pp. 671–687). New York: Guilford Press.

Johnson, S. (1996). *Creating connection: The practice of emotionally focused marital therapy.* New York: Brunner/Mazel.

Johnson, S. M. (2002). *Emotionally focused couple therapy with trauma survivors: Strengthening attachment bonds.* New York: Guilford Press.

Johnson, S., Hunsley, J., Greenberg, L., & Schindler, D. (1999). Emotionally focused couple therapy: Status and challenges. *Clinical Psychology: Science and Practice, 6,* 67–79.

Johnson, S., Makinen, J., & Millikin, J. (2001). Attachment injuries in couple relationships: A new perspective on impasses in couple therapy. *Journal of Marital and Family Therapy, 27,* 145–155.

Kobak, R. (1999). The emotional dynamics of disruptions in attachment relationships: Implications for theory, research, and clinical intervention. In J. Cassidy & P. Shaver (Eds.), *Handbook of attachment: Theory, research, and clinical applications* (pp. 21–43). New York: Guilford Press.

Kobak, R., & Duemmler, S. (1994). Attachment and conversation: Toward a discourse analysis of adolescent and adult security. In D. Perlman & K. Bartholemew (Eds.), *Advances in personal relationships: Vol. 5. Attachment processes in adulthood* (pp.121–149). London: Jessica Kingsley.

Kobak, R., & Esposito, A. (in press). Levels of processing in parent–child relationships: Implications for clinical assessment and treatment. In L. Atkinson (Ed.), *Attachment and psychopathology* (2nd ed.). New York: Guilford Press.

Kobak, R., Hazan, C., & Ruckdeschel, K. (1994). From symptom to signal: An attachment view of emotion in marital therapy. In S. Johnson & L. Greenberg (Eds.), *Emotions in marital therapy* (pp. 46–71). New York: Brunner/Mazel.

Kobak, R., Little, M., Race, E., & Acosta, M. (2001). Attachment disruptions in seriously emotionally disturbed children: Implications for treatment. *Attachment and Human Development, 3,* 243–258.

Kochansa, G., Aksan, N., & Koenig, A. L. (1995). Mother–child mutually positive affect, the quality of child compliance to requests and prohibitions, and maternal control as correlates of early internalization. *Child Development, 66,* 236–254.

Luepnitz, D. (1988). *The family interpreted: Feminist theory in clinical practice.* New York: Basic Books.

Lyons Ruth, K., & Jacobvitz, D. (1999). Attachment disorganization: Unresolved loss, relational violence, and lapses in behavioral and attentional strategies. In J. Cassidy & P. R. Shaver (Eds.), *Handbook of attachment: Theory, research, and clinical applications* (pp. 520–554). New York: Guilford Press.

Madanes, C. (1981). *Strategic family therapy.* San Francisco: Jossey-Bass.

Main, M., & Hesse, E. (1990). Parents' unresolved traumatic experiences are related to infant disorganized attachment status: Is frightening and/or frightened parental behavior the linking mechanism? In M. T. Greenberg, D. Cicchetti, & E. M. Cummings (Eds.), *Attachment in the preschool years* (pp. 121–160). Chicago: University of Chicago Press.

Marvin, R., Cooper, G., Hoffman, K., & Powell, B. (2002). The Circle of Security Project: Attachment-based intervention with caregiver–pre-school dyads. *Attachment and Human Development, 4,* 107–124.

Micucci, J. A. (1998). *The adolescent in family therapy: Breaking the cycle of conflict and control.* New York: Guilford Press.

Shaver, P., & Mikulincer, M. (2002). Attachment-related psychodynamics. *Attachment and Human Development, 4,* 133–161.

9

Creating and Repairing Attachments in Biological, Foster, and Adoptive Families

TERRY M. LEVY
MICHAEL ORLANS

Children's early development depends, to a large extent, on the health and emotional well-being of their parents or other primary caregivers. This caregiving relationship is a major environmental influence that affects every aspect of the children's learning and development—mind, brain, emotions, relationships, and morality (Shonkoff & Phillips, 2000). A significant number of children are exposed to traumatic and damaging environmental influences (e.g., abuse, neglect, violence, parental substance abuse, and severe psychological problems) that can produce serious and lasting social, emotional, and regulatory impairments. Many of these children are placed in foster homes and/or become members of adoptive families. It then becomes the task of these caregivers to provide the commitment, consistency, and emotional connection necessary to help these children recover from prior damage and develop the capacity for positive growth and development.

Research and clinical experience have shown two major findings. First, many children with backgrounds of abuse, neglect, and compromised attachment do improve dramatically when fostered by or adopted into healthy and loving families, highlighting the importance of sensitive and stable parenting. Second, a substantial number of these children continue to experience severe psychosocial impairments even after they are living long term in much better environments, and do not form secure attachments with foster and/or adoptive parents (Chisholm, 1998; O'Conner, Bredenkamp, Rutter, & English and Romanian Adoptees Study Team, 1999). These children and families need specialized interventions to promote positive change.

There are two major goals of this chapter. First, we describe the essential elements and ingredients that go into the development of secure attachment in parent–child relationships and family systems. Next, we describe the components and processes that are inherent in repairing compromised attachment in foster and adoptive families, including *corrective attachment parenting* and *corrective attachment therapy* (Levy & Orlans, 1998; Levy, 2000).

THE NATURE AND FUNCTIONS OF ATTACHMENT

Human relationships are the building blocks of healthy development, and attachment forms the core of these relationships. Attachment is a deep-seated and abiding biological, psychological, and social connection established between a child and caregiver(s) in the first several years of life (Ainsworth, 1973; Bowlby, 1969; Levy & Orlans, 1998). The genesis and development of attachment resides in the interaction of both nature (biology) and nurture (experience). The inborn attachment system motivates the infant to seek closeness and communication with parents or surrogate caregivers. The attachment figures instinctively protect, nurture, and guide the development of their young, and provide cues that promote secure attachment (e.g., through smiles, eye contact, positive affect, touch, holding, and rocking). Specific attachment behaviors are learned, the culmination of ongoing reciprocal interactions between child and caregiver. Children learn to trust dependable and safe caregivers, who provide love, limits, need fulfillment, and encouragement to explore. This process of interacting and connecting is a "mutual regulatory system," with the caregiver and the child influencing one another over time (Tronick & Weinberg, 1997). Further, attachment is influenced by the broad emotional network of family and community systems, including father, siblings, marital subsystem, extended kin, and external social systems (Donley, 1993).

Secure attachment serves many crucial functions for the developing child:

- Affords a safe haven for the vulnerable infant via proximity to a consistently available caregiver.
- Directly affects the structure, function, and growth of the developing brain: "Human connections create neuronal connections" (Siegel, 1999, p. 85).
- Allows the child to explore the environment with a tolerable level of

anxiety (providing a "secure base"), facilitating healthy cognitive, emotional, and social development.

- Teaches basic trust, intimacy, and reciprocity, which serves as a template for meaningful relationships throughout the lifespan.
- Promotes physiological and emotional self-regulation, a cornerstone of early childhood development.
- Results in the formation of a positive sense of self, including feelings of competency, self-worth, and positive core beliefs (an "internal working model" of self).
- Fosters the internalization of prosocial morality and values, including compassion, empathy, and the development of a conscience.
- Serves as a protective factor that increases resourcefulness and resilience, thereby minimizing the negative effects of stress and loss throughout life.

Attachment patterns affect people throughout their lifespans. Research has documented the importance of secure attachment in the adult years; adults who feel nurtured, supported, and loved are more likely to be happier and healthier, have a lower risk of developing a serious illness, and recover from disease more rapidly than those lacking satisfying attachments. In a 35-year study, adults who reported the lack of a warm and close relationship with their mothers when growing up were over twice as likely to be diagnosed with serious diseases, such as coronary artery disease and alcoholism (Russek & Schwartz, 1997). Large-scale community studies found that adults who lacked close emotional connections had five times the risk of premature death from all causes, compared to those with close family ties and supportive social networks (Berkman, 1995; Reynolds & Kaplan, 1990).

CREATING SECURE ATTACHMENTS

Studies have demonstrated that secure attachment in the early years is highly correlated with positive psychological outcomes: high self-esteem; independence and autonomy; trust, intimacy, and affection; resilience; self-regulation; enduring relationships; prosocial coping skills and morality; positive core beliefs; empathy and compassion; and academic success. Disrupted and anxious attachment has been found to be associated with aggression, impulsivity, conduct disorders, relationship deficits, negative self-images, and antisocial attitudes and behaviors (Egeland, Pianta, & O'Brien, 1993; Erickson, Sroufe, & Egeland, 1985; Renken, Egeland, Marvinney, Mangelsdoft, & Sroufe. 1989; Sroufe, Egeland, & Kreutzer, 1990).

The following is a list of the key factors that create secure attachments in children, parent–child relationships, and family systems. This discussion is based on theoretical, empirical, and clinical contributions from the fields of attachment, family systems, child development, clinical psychology, neurobiology, and parenting skills approaches.

Sensitivity to Child's Signals and Cues

The caregiver is able to accurately perceive the child's needs and signals, and responds appropriately. Parents are attuned to the rhythms, cues, and state of mind of their infant, including smiles, glances, gestures, and cries. The child begins to develop trust, positive core beliefs, and the ability for self-regulation and interactive problem solving (Figure 9.1). As development unfolds, parents continue to tune into the child's needs and respond in age-appropriate ways (e.g., setting limits, encouraging autonomy and exploration). Sensitive parents have the ability to reflect on the emotional and mental states of their children, as well as their own, in a realistic and coherent way (this constitutes the "reflective function" associated with secure attachment; see Fonagy, Target, & Steele, 1997). They are also tuned into the unique qualities and individual differences of each child.

Affective Attunement and Reciprocity

The emotions expressed by both child and parent are in synch and contingent on one another. For example, parents and infants experience emo-

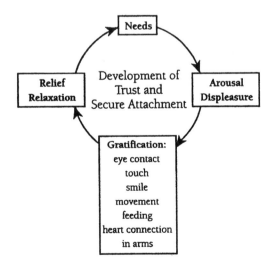

FIGURE 9.1. First-year attachment cycle. From Levy and Orlans (1998). Copyright 1998, Child Welfare League of America. Reprinted by special permission of the Child Welfare League of America, Washington, DC.

tional synchrony and communication via gaze, gestures, voice, and facial expressions. These ongoing reciprocal exchanges form the basis for learning important cognitive and social skills, including the child's sense of mastery ("I can get others to respond"), morality ("I am treated with empathy and care, and will treat others the same"), self-identity ("I am worthwhile and lovable"), cognitive development ("There are consequences to my actions"), and self-regulation ("I am learning self-control by experiencing consistent external control"). It is not necessary to be in synch at all times. Securely attached parents and children have moderate levels of synchrony and positive emotional interactions, as well as moments of stress and negativity. Attunement and empathic sensitivity occurring only 30% of the time can result in secure attachment (Tronick & Cohen, 1989). Parents and children must learn to effectively handle times when they are "not on the same page." Children can deal with parental imperfections as long as they are balanced by sufficient love and understanding (Biringen, 2000; Biringen & Robinson, 1991; Stern, 1985; Tronick & Weinberg, 1997).

Nurturing, Compassionate, and Loving Care

Nurturing and loving care fosters the capacity for trust, empathy, and a positive sense of self. Empathic parents rear empathic children. Children with secure attachments during infancy, compared to those with insecure–anxious attachments, were found to be more caring and compassionate toward peers and had the best friendships by ages 3, 4, and 5 (Sroufe, 1983; Troy & Sroufe, 1987; Waters, Wippman, & Sroufe, 1979). Nurturing and loving parents can set limits and express displeasure and anger in a controlled and nonthreatening manner, but are generally patient and understanding. These parents are able to regulate their emotions and impulses, therefore being healthy role models and safe disciplinarians. Children internalize parental values and respect parental rules and limits when they are offered with love and nurturance; they have a desire and willingness to please their parents. Children develop beliefs and expectations about themselves and relationships based on the quality of care they receive ("internal working models of self and other"; see Bowlby, 1969, 1988; Zeanah & Zeanah, 1989). Loving and nurturing care results in positive core beliefs ("I am wanted, worthwhile, competent, and lovable; my caregivers are trustworthy, caring, and responsive").

Clear and Consistent Structure

Providing appropriate rules and expectations engenders feelings of safety and security in children. Effective leadership provides healthy role models, sends a message that parents are in charge, and enhances the child's respect. Developmentally appropriate rules and roles engender a sense of order and predictability, and create a foundation for social and emotional learning. Family rules that include the four R's (respect, responsibility, resourcefulness, reciprocity) lead to secure attachment. Respect involves showing deference and high regard for others, and expecting the same for oneself. By demonstrating respectful attitudes and behaviors toward parents and others children learn self-respect. Responsibility entails holding children accountable for their choices and actions. For example, chores help children learn responsibility, cooperation, and a sense of accomplishment. Resourcefulness involves learning to utilize and have confidence in one's own inner strengths and abilities in order to cope with challenges. Reciprocity is at the basis of all these qualities; parents and children learn a healthy "give-and-take."

Parents' Attachment History

Parents' attachment histories influence their childrearing practices, marital relationships, and general psychosocial functioning. Parents either copy the behaviors modeled by their own caregivers ("replicative script") or make an effort to raise their children differently ("corrective script") (Byng-Hall, 1995). These reactionary strategies are not effective when parents have significant unresolved psychological wounds, and they become a barrier to creating a framework of love, sensitivity, and security for their children. A parent's state of mind with regard to attachment has a significant influence on the child's attachment. *State of mind* refers to the adult's way of processing emotions, memories, and perceptions of his or her own attachment histories. Adults who value attachment and are able to resolve past attachment wounds and so process their own histories realistically and coherently, typically have children with secure attachments (Dozier, Albus, Stovall, & Bates, 2001; Main, Kaplan, & Cassidy, 1985; van IJzendoorn, 1995). These parents or caregivers can perceive their children accurately and meet their needs appropriately because their own emotional issues do not interfere with their parenting. Parents with painful early emotional experiences can "earn" secure attachment for themselves and facilitate it in their children, however, by self-reflection, communication with significant others, and the formation of secure and loving relationships in their current lives (Hesse, 1999).

Autonomy and Connectedness

Secure attachment encompasses an ongoing balance of closeness and separateness, dependence and independence. Early secure attachment becomes a vehicle for later autonomy and independence. The infant is basically helpless and dependent. Over time, the sensitively attuned parent allows more independent exploration and autonomous action. Parents and children negotiate a way of maintaining connection and creating distance that is mutually acceptable. The balance between connection and autonomy changes in accordance with the developmental needs and capabilities of the child. The ability to achieve this balance is basic to all healthy human relationships. Connectedness involves the ability to experience intimacy and vulnerability, rely on and trust a significant other, and communicate honestly about needs and emotions. Autonomy is the ability to experience oneself as distinct and separate with unique assets and liabilities, manage one's life independently, and enjoy solitude and aloneness (Lewis & Gossett, 1999). Achieving a balance of high connectedness and high autonomy is often characterized as optimal for healthy relationships.

Discipline with Love and Limits

To provide effective discipline one must understand the child's developmental needs. Creating secure attachment involves basic trust and security via consistent need fulfillment. For example, parents who respond quickly to their infants' cries have babies who cry less over time (Solter, 1995). As the first year progresses, the baby actively maintains closeness to the attachment figure, notices his or her absence, wanders off to explore, and soon returns to the safety of that attachment figure. As the child becomes more mobile and independent, consistent limits become increasingly important.

Toddlerhood involves the development of autonomy, self-identity, and self-control (Figure 9.2). The parent must provide limits (e.g., communicate "no") and offer appropriate consequences. The child develops frustration tolerance, adapts to other's needs, handles external boundaries, and experiences mastery over feelings of disappointment. Limits need to be given with understanding and patience, which enables the toddler to internalize and accept the structure provided. Limits given in a punitive manner damage the attachment relationship and the child's self-esteem. When appropriate limits are lacking, children become self-centered, controlling, and learn that authority figures are not to be respected or trusted. The child who is securely attached is able to demonstrate competency in four areas: knowledge, skills, judgment, and self-control. Security of attachment leads to optimal learning and cognitive development, attaining emotional and social skills, and the ability to modulate feelings and impulses.

Family and Community Systems

Although the mother–infant relationship is crucial, it is necessary to understand the context of the whole family, as well as external social influences, when considering attachment security and child development. The family system approach focuses on three major influences on attachment: marital relationship, attachment histories of parents, and extended social network.

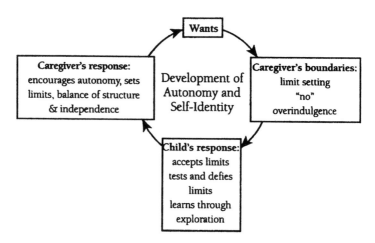

FIGURE 9.2. Second-year attachment cycle. From Levy and Orlans (1998). Copyright 1998, Child Welfare League of America. Reprinted by special permission of the Child Welfare League of America, Washington, DC.

Studies show that the quality of the marital relationship influences children's attachment. For example, depressed caregivers are more likely to have insecurely attached babies, but a supportive spouse or partner reduces the risk of depression (Beach & Nelson, 1990). Mothers who breast-fed their babies reported feeling more confident and competent when their partners were understanding and supportive (Pedersen, Yarrow, Anderson, & Cain, 1978). Women who were insecurely attached as children were more likely to have children with anxious attachment, unless they had an intimate and trustful marital relationship (Lewis & Gossett, 1999).

Patterns of attachment are transmitted over generations. A child attaches not only to the primary caregivers, but also to the entire emotional network. Factors external to primary family relationships include extended kin (e.g., friends, mentors, kinship placement), community support systems (e.g., religious groups, schools, neighborhood programs), and social service agencies (e.g., foster care, protective services, juvenile justice system). Social service programs can support and empower family relationships and attachment. These programs can also "dilute" family relationships through interventions that undermine connections among family members (Colapinto, 1995).

Communicating for Secure Attachment

Physiological and emotional communication between parents (particularly the mother) and fetus begins during pregnancy (Verny & Kelly, 1981). The fetus decodes the emotional state of the mother through a neurohormonal dialogue (Borysenko & Borysenko, 1994). The infant's ability to communicate to the caregiver, and the caregiver's ability to read those signals accurately and respond appropriately, is crucial to the development of the attachment relationship (Brazelton & Cramer, 1990).

Communication continues to serve a primary function in determining attachment relationships as development unfolds. Effective communication involves the content of the message to the child and the way in which that message is expressed (the "metamessage"). Parents who send warm and validating messages are more likely to facilitate secure attachment. Positive attachment communication utilizes the primary cues of secure attachment. For example, eye contact and loving touch facilitates effective listening in a respectful way. "Thinking words" promote positivity and cooperation (e.g., "Please join us for lunch as soon as you clean your room"); "fighting words" invite defiance and hostility (e.g., "You can't eat until you clean your room"). Rather than lecturing and criticizing, a more constructive problem-solving tool is a resource model of communication: "Tell me what happened. What did you think and feel at that time?; How did you respond?; What were the results?; How can you handle the situation differently next time in order to get a better result?" This method of communication guides the child to find his or her own solutions, avoids power struggles, and sends the message "You are smart, capable, and lovable."

Belonging

Secure attachment includes being a part of a relationship network. Doing something helpful for the family teaches reciprocity, cooperation, and caring, and enhances feelings of belonging. Being a part of a social network, and considering the wants and needs of others, was in our evolutionary interest. Feelings of security and connectedness are triggered in the "old brain" and emotional system of the child via family interaction and involvement (Kagan, 1981; MacLean, 1982).

ATTACHMENT AND FOSTER CARE

Twenty-four million infants, toddlers, and preschoolers are currently growing up in the United States (Shonkoff & Phillips, 2000). More and more of these children are being raised in high-risk families (e.g., because of poverty, abuse and neglect, parental substance abuse, domestic violence, and psychological disorders). Seventy-five percent of children entering foster care have a family history of mental illness or drug and alcohol abuse (Chernoff, Combs-Orne, Risley-Curtiss, & Heisler, 1994). Research has shown that up to 80% of high-risk families create severely compromised attachment in their children (Lyons-Ruth, 1996). The foster care system is flooded with these wounded children.

There are more children in foster care now than ever before (over 500,000 in 2000), a 90% increase since 1986. At the same time, the number of foster parents has been declining, due to inadequate salaries; lack of recognition, training, and support; the poor image of the foster care system; the increased needs and problems of foster children; and role confusion (Child Welfare League of America, 1996; Klee, Kronstadt, & Zlotnick, 1997). Foster parents are expected to play a number of roles in the lives of children: help them cope with separation and loss, build self-esteem, and encourage positive relationships and secure attachment (Dougherty, 2001).

All interactions in the foster home milieu have a potential to be therapeutic. Via their actions, reactions, and the creation of a safe and predictable environment, foster parents provide a context in which children can achieve many positive changes. The list that follows offers strategies and solutions that therapists can use to help foster parents facilitate secure attachment.

Understand Internal Working Models

Early experiences with caregivers shape children's beliefs about self, relationships, and life in general. Children with negative core beliefs as a result of aversive attachment relationships perceive parents as untrustworthy and threatening. Therapeutic parenting can change the child's internal working models and subsequent behavior. To impact these negative working models, foster parents can tune into the child's perceptions and interpretations; give praise and approval for specific behaviors, as unconditional positives are incongruent with their negative internal working models and can result in an escalation of negative behavior; and resist personalizing the child's negative behaviors.

Balance of Connection and Control

Therapeutic parenting is a balance of love and limits, that is, connecting with the child while also providing the necessary structure to engender respect and trust. Parenting approaches that exclusively focus on control instigate power struggles and an adversarial climate. A focus on attachment emphasizes that control often means survival to a child with a history of loss and maltreatment. Foster parents can create a healing emotional climate by being proactive rather than reactive. They can model caring, nonjudgmental, and sensitive attitudes and behavior; provide clear and consistent limits and consequences; and give choices rather than commands.

Teach Reciprocity

These children tend to be self-centered and demanding, and they usually lack the ability to give and receive. They avoid needing others and being vulnerable, due to a lack of trust and a self-perception of being unworthy of love and caring. Foster parents can encourage the child to ask for help; promote contributions to the family, as pitching in allows the child to be a part of the family and have a sense of accomplishment; engage in reciprocal interactions via play, rituals, homework, and other cooperative activities; and negotiate conflicts by teaching problem solving, communication, and the acceptance of individual differences.

Meet Individual Needs

Foster parents must attempt to understand the needs, thoughts, and attachment patterns of each child. Caregiver attunement to the developmental needs and signals of the child facilitates secure attachment. Foster parents can know each child's attachment history, patterns, and triggers (e.g., anniversary reactions); look beyond negative behavior into the child's deeper attachment needs and fears; and provide the sensitive need fulfillment absent in the child's early years.

Increase Parents' Self-Awareness

Caregivers bring their own mind-sets and emotional "baggage" into relationships with children. Therapeutic parents must be aware of their histories, sensitivities, and emotional reactions. Solutions are dictated by the way you frame the problem, and one's mind-set is formed by prior relationship experiences. Foster parents can complete a *Life Script*, a self-report tool that generates awareness of one's attachment history; be aware of predictable reactions such as anger, withdrawal, and depression; and take good care of themselves by systematically planning how to reduce stress and meet personal needs.

Learn to Manage Emotions

These children have considerable anger, fear, sadness, and shame due to unresolved loss and maltreatment. They never learned to identify, regulate, and effectively communicate their emotions, which are often masked under a global response of anger and avoidance to reduce vulnerability. Foster parents can help by remaining emotionally neutral in response to negative behaviors and expressing positive emotion in response to positive behavior. They can teach children to identify and talk about emotions in a safe and empathic context, and they can model the healthy management and communication of emotions. They can also promote positive emotions such as joy, fun, love, pleasure, and pride.

Understanding Attachment Styles

As a result of inadequate caregiving, children develop several attachment patterns. The *avoidant* child has learned to avoid closeness, does not seek comfort, and projects an image of self-reliance ("I don't need you or care about you"). The *ambivalent* child is clingy, demanding, and hypervigilant regarding rejection. These children are preoccupied with their parents' moods, fear separation, are not easily soothed, and act infantile and controlling in an effort to connect ("I will force closeness because I know you will leave me"). Children with a *disorganized* attachment pattern have experienced extreme trauma (e.g., violence, severe abuse, multiple losses) and typically have posttraumatic stress disorder. They lack an organized strategy to handle relationships, and can be punitive and dangerous ("I am constantly frightened and will not be close; I hate myself and others"). Foster parents can respond based on the child's attachment pattern:

> *Avoidant*: keep the child close and provide considerable support and comfort.
>
> *Ambivalent:* set limits, encourage autonomy, and be consistent and predictable.
>
> *Disorganized*: utilize support systems to create safety for parent and child (i.e., ongoing therapy, appropriate medication, support of social services). This child may need highly structured placement such as in a residential treatment center.

Increasing the Sense of Belonging

The primary experience of foster children is loss and abandonment. These children lack identification with family, cultural background, and community. Foster parents can encourage participation to feel a part of the family and community; respect their cultural roots and rituals, as well as prior connections (e.g., biological family); and have children placed early and do not move them, in order to allow the time and consistency necessary to feel connected.

ATTACHMENT AND THE ADOPTIVE FAMILY

Adoption affects the lives of over 50 million Americans. Many children, particularly when adopted early, develop secure attachments to their adopted parents and families, and live healthy and productive lives (Schaffer & Lindstrom, 1989). Promoting attachment security involves many of the same ingredients experienced in healthy biological families, including the first-year attachment cycle, positive interaction cycle, and claiming. The first-year attachment cycle is initiated by the child's needs and arousal, and is followed by the parent's response of gratification. The positive interaction cycle is parent-initiated. Parents are proactive: set a positive tone, create clear and consistent structure, and encourage physical and emotional closeness to create a positive reciprocal relationship. Claiming involves a feeling of loyalty and commitment to one another; children must learn to feel a sense of connection and belonging.

In the past, parents did not typically talk to their children about adoption, worrying that it would be damaging, and feeling unsure due to a lack of information and guidance. Parents are now encouraged to discuss adoption with their child, usually between 3 and 4 years of age. This normalizes adoption issues, provides practice in communicating and confiding, and helps the child form a positive self-image.

As children grow older, especially in the latency stage (ages 8 to 12), issues regarding identity and adoption are heightened. Children in this stage will often ask questions (e.g., "Why did my birth mother give me up?", "Do I have brothers and sisters?", "Was it my fault?"). Parents should answer questions in an honest and developmentally sensitive way. This is an opportunity for trust building, a cornerstone of secure attachment. Parents' own insecurities may block open communication ("Why do you ask so many questions?", "Are you unhappy with our family?"). It is important for parents to seek professional guidance if conflicts arise when addressing adoption concerns (American Academy of Pediatrics, 1999; Brodzinsky & Schechter, 1990).

Many children who are adopted have histories of disrupted attachment. The key factors regarding the severity of attachment disorder are age at adoption, number of prior moves, abuse and neglect in the early stages, and prenatal trauma (e.g., fetal alcohol syndrome). These factors seriously hamper the child's ability to form close attachment relationships in the adoptive family. A high number of adopted children with compromised attachment come to the attention of the mental health, social services, and criminal justice systems. These children are five times more likely to be referred for psychological treatment, twice as likely to display psychological symptoms in later life, and are diagnosed with attention-deficit/hyperactivity disorder 10 times more than their nonadopted peers. They comprise only 2% of children under 18 in the United States, but represent over one-third of children placed in residential treatment centers (Jones, 1997).

The majority of the families seen at our corrective attachment therapy program present with children adopted from foreign orphanages or foster care programs (Levy & Orlans, 1998). The children display many challenging symptoms and behaviors. They are oppositional, controlling, and mistrustful. They tend to have negative core beliefs, antisocial attitudes, and antisocial behaviors. The adoptive parents were often intellectually and emotionally unprepared to deal with the child's problems and the subsequent negative impact on their family. Parents were often not given adequate preplacement services, including full disclosure of the child's history and a realistic appraisal of risks. Parents often had unrealistic fantasies about helping a needy child and suffer from their own unresolved losses and family-of-origin issues. After the adoption, negative and destructive relationship patterns created a family climate of tension, hostility, and despair.

A child's adaptation to the adoptive family is dependent on the nature and quality of his or her prior attachments and reactions to separation and loss. A physiological and psychological attachment bond between mother and baby develops during pregnancy, intensifies at birth, and exists forever. Adopted children have a significant loss of this bond, and must resolve their grief regarding this loss in order to form subsequent attachments (Levy & Orlans, 2000b). Young children do not have the cognitive and psychological tools to successfully resolve these losses. Children who experience severe losses typically react in one of two ways. They may provoke the very rejection they fear ("I'll reject you before you leave me"), and become defiant and aggressive. Conversely, they may present as overly compliant and placating ("If I am docile, maybe you will not leave me"), and become withdrawn and dysphoric. Regardless of the reaction, assistance must be provided to help children resolve loss and grief, in order to attach to their adoptive family.

Parents have often experienced losses that can form a barrier to securely attaching to their adoptive child. Those without biological children must resolve the loss associated with infertility. It is also necessary to grieve the loss the of the parent's adoption fantasy: "We will bring this child into our family and receive appreciation and love." Instead, the parents are often recipients of rejection and hostility.

Loyalty conflicts also present a barrier to attachment in the adoptive family. Children who have not resolved prior losses maintain an emotional allegiance to birth or foster parents. Adoptive parents feel confused and threatened by the child's desire to place past caregivers "on a pedestal." A child's negative working model of self and other can also prevent healthy attachment. The child has developed a self-image as unwanted, damaged, and undeserving of love, and perceives the adoptive parents as unsafe and threatening. The negative belief system of the child is then reinforced by any parental anger and emotional distancing.

Parents and siblings commonly experience secondary traumatic stress disorder, the result of chronic stress associated with living with these challenging children. Family burnout from the breakdown of a collective commitment to one another and the refusal to work together cooperatively leaves family members emotionally exhausted and disillusioned (Figley, 1998).

Adopted children with histories of maltreatment and derailed attachment typically reenact their negative relationship patterns learned earlier in life. For example, children will try to provoke rejection or abuse in order to confirm their core beliefs (e.g., "I'm not worth loving"), maintain control, and avoid emotional closeness. The parents often become angry, punitive, and rejecting, and the parent–child interactions become dominated by power struggles. These children believe their survival is contingent upon manipulation and control. Parents, as well as others who influence the children's lives, are often unable to effectively manage these controlling and coercive behaviors.

Triangulation, in which a child forms a coalition with one adult against another, is a common form of manipulation and control. For example, the child may be hostile toward mother and charming with father, or oppositional with parents while compliant with the teacher. It is crucial for all the significant adults in the child's life to form a collaborative alliance so that these manipulative strategies are curtailed.

Marital stress and conflict is extremely high in these families. All couples must deal with the challenges of relating to these children. Couples who have a history of serious conflict prior to adoption often experience a total breakdown in their marital relationships. Parents need guidance in order to learn effective communication and conflict-resolution skills, and to promote closeness, commitment, and a fulfillment of their own emotional needs.

Sibling conflicts are magnified in these families. Adoptive children with compromised attachment are commonly abusive and manipulative toward siblings. They are jealous and resentful of siblings, particularly biological siblings, who have positive and loving relationships with their parents. Siblings commonly feel neglected and resentful toward their parents because of the vast amount of time and resources devoted to the "problem" child. Family life can become extremely restricted. For example, siblings will stop inviting friends to their home and avoid family activities due to persistent conflict.

Parents often feel isolated and alone at a time when they need support and understanding the most. They are often blamed by family members and those in the school and mental health systems for their child's acting-out behaviors. One of the first goals of family treatment is to eliminate the blame directed toward parents and establish a trusting working alliance.

CORRECTIVE ATTACHMENT THERAPY

Corrective attachment therapy (CAT), described in depth in *Attachment, Trauma and Healing* (Levy & Orlans, 1998), is an integration of family systems and attachment-oriented principles. The treatment framework must make available the physical, emotional, and social ingredients of secure attachment. That is, those same ingredients of attachment found in secure parent–child relationships must be available in the therapist–child relationship, which requires the following:

- *Structure.* The therapist provides limits, rules, and boundaries similar to the clear and consistent structure provided by the sensitive and appropriately responsive caregiver. For example, the therapist informs the child of the rules of therapy, and together they establish an explicit contract that defines their responsibilities and goals.
- *Attunement.* The therapist works hard to be "in synch" with the child's needs, emotions, and internal working model, and provides the message: "I know what you need in order to feel safe, and I will offer it." For example, it is understood that the child's hostile and controlling demeanor is a defensive strategy, a reaction to feelings of vulnerability and anxiety regarding unresolved loss.
- *Empathy.* Just as the loving parent cares deeply about his or her child, the therapist conveys a heartfelt level of caring and compassion. The therapist is proactive and empathic, and does not react negatively to hostility and distancing behavior. The message conveyed is: "How sad that those terrible things happened to you; I am sorry you were treated badly; I understand what you feel and how much pain you must be in."
- *Positive affect.* The therapist maintains a positive demeanor, particularly when the child is distancing or acting out. This prevents the reenactment of dysfunctional patterns, such as mutual rejection or escalation of power struggles. The message to the child is: "I will not allow you to control our relationship in unhealthy and destructive ways."
- *Support.* The therapist provides support tailored to the developmental needs and capabilities of the child. Initially, the emphasis is on rules, expectations, and natural consequences. As therapy progresses, the focus shifts to reinforcing the child's independent achievements.
- *Reciprocity.* The securely attached child achieves a "goal-corrected partnership" with caregivers, characterized by a sharing of control, values, and emotions. The therapist guides the child toward a reciprocal relationship based on mutual respect and sensitivity. As the child becomes more securely attached, he or she learns to balance his or her own needs with those of others.
- *Love.* Secure attachment involves the ability to feel a deep and genuine caring for and commitment to another. Children with disrupted attachment are generally incapable of giving and receiving love. Therapy guides the child to a place where love can be experienced. The open expression of loving feelings occurs with parents holding their children "in arms, eye-to-eye, face-to-face." Children, however, will only feel safe in experiencing

love if the parent(s) are available to receive that level of intimacy. Thus, therapy must facilitate the parents' emotional availability to the child.

Treatment Goals and Methodologies

Therapeutic effectiveness is contingent on clear goals and a comprehensive assessment (Tables 9.1 and 9.2; Levy & Orlans, 1998). A basic treatment goal is the formation of a constructive context in which family members invest in the treatment process (i.e., by contracting), promoting a genuine desire to change.

Treatment goals focus on the child, parents, family system, and external social systems. Child-oriented goals involve resolving prior maltreatment and disrupted attachment, modifying the negative working model, and developing prosocial coping skills and values. Goals for parents include addressing family-of-origin and marital issues, providing support, and teaching the concepts and skills of *corrective attachment parenting*. Family system goals focus on promoting secure attachments and enhancing an emotional climate of intimacy and optimism. Social system goals involve establishing a collaborative relationship with school, social service, and other helping agencies.

A number of therapeutic interventions are used and will be described

---

TABLE 9.1. Assessment of the Child

- Presenting problem:
  - Six symptom categories: behavioral, cognitive, affective, social, physical, and moral/spiritual.
  - Environmental factors.
  - Frequency, duration, and severity.
  - Child's interpretation of problems; behavior during assessment.
  - Family systems context.

- Developmental history:
  - Birth parents and family; pre- and perinatal factors.
  - Postnatal experiences and developmental milestones.
  - Attachment history.
  - School history.
  - Relationship history.
  - Sexual history.
  - Strengths and resources.
  - Additional problems and concurrent diagnoses.

- Internal working model:
  - Core beliefs about self, caregivers, and life in general.
  - Assessment methods: sentence completion, first-year attachment cycle, inner child metaphor, drawings, psychodramatic reenactment.

Note. From Levy and Orlans (1998). Copyright 1998, Child Welfare League of America. Reprinted by special permission of the Child Welfare League of America, Washington, DC.

TABLE 9.2. Parent and Family Assessment

- Parents' attachment history:
  - Family background.
  - Additional family-of-origin information.
  - Education and employment history.
  - Assessment methods: autobiography, life script, adult attachment interview, and clinical interview.

- Parents' current functioning:
  - Psychosocial and physical health.
  - Marital and other significant relationships.

- Parenting attitudes and skills:
  - Parenting history.
  - Parenting practices with siblings.
  - Parenting practices with child with attachment disorder.
  - Parental commitment.
  - Out-of-home placements.
  - Parenting philosophies and competencies.

- Family system:
  - Structure, dynamics, and relationship patterns.
  - Support systems.
  - Stressors and stress management.

Note. From Levy and Orlans (1998). Copyright 1998, Child Welfare League of America. Reprinted by special permission of the Child Welfare League of America, Washington, DC.

below. Some of these interventions occur within the context of the *holding nurturing process* (HNP), an "in arms" experience that promotes secure attachment. The HNP is not a method. It is a relationship context within which interventions are employed. The HNP stimulates the part of the brain (limbic system) that regulates attachment, reduces the effects of the alarm reaction caused by trauma, promotes self-regulation, and facilitates corrective emotional and interpersonal experiences.

In the HNP, the child lays prone on a couch in the parent's lap, in a face-to-face position. One parent, usually the mother, provides the primary nurturing role while the other parent sits by her side in a supportive role. When presented in a confident and nonchalant manner, most children do not protest being held "in arms" because of their need for nurturance and structure. If a child is reluctant and/or apprehensive, the therapist explains the purpose of the HNP and answers all questions, often reducing anxiety.

An intervention that focuses on the adoptive parents is the *Life Script* interview. This is a structured interview that provides detailed information about parents' attachment histories. Sample questions include: "Give several adjectives that describe your primary caregivers and yourself from your perspective as a young child; What were the major messages your parents gave you about yourself and how to deal with life?; How did your parents handle conflict, emotion, and discipline?; Who did you turn to for comfort and support when upset, and what happened?" The Life Script is used for adult assessment and as a therapeutic tool during marital and parent–child interventions.

Another intervention is *attachment communication training* (ACT), a vehicle for teaching specific communication skills (e.g., sharing, empathic listening, verbal/nonverbal attunement) and conflict management skills. ACT facilitates safe and constructive communication and problem solving as the husband and wife (or parent–child) sit knee-to-knee. Ground rules specify no blaming, criticizing, or interrupting. Sharing skills (e.g., "I" statements rather than questions; be concise and honest; make eye contact; be aware of own perceptions) and listening skills (e.g., do not censor or rehearse rebuttal; maintain a nonjudgmental and empathic attitude; give feedback that indicates messages are received accurately) are practiced and utilized. Therapists facilitate accurate and sensitive communication, which fosters intimacy and connection. The combination of effective communication and awareness of prior attachment issues (revealed from the Life Script) promotes a positive marital and parental relationship.

Other interventions focus more on the adopted child him- or herself. Children are informed about the *rules* of therapy, which spell out expectations for their behaviors and attitudes. Clear and consistent ground rules promote a feeling of safety and security. Examples of rules include maintain eye contact when communicating; provide quick answers; "I don't know" is not acceptable (guess or ask for help); we will work hard but you must work hardest. The child-generated *problem list* provides insight into the child's interpretation of issues and events. The therapist makes a list of the child's "problems," as reported by the child. Three sets of *contracts* are established (i.e., therapists–child, parents–child, therapists–parents). Contracts define each person's responsibilities, provide structure, and promote motivation and collaboration. Therapeutic rules and the child-generated problem list form the basis of the contract with the child.

Teaching the child about the *first-year attachment cycle* (Figure 9.1) helps the child learn about early attachment experiences. The therapist discusses the four stages with the child (need–arousal–gratification–trust) in the HNP, as it pertains to his or her early life. This provides a normalizing experience ("You adapted to an unhealthy environment to survive"), and a foundation for cognitive-affective revision.

The *inner child metaphor* is a guided imagery and dialogue intervention in which the child revisits early life experiences, using a teddy bear to symbolize the self. While talking to the "younger self," the child expresses emotions and reveals core beliefs, which helps heal attachment traumas and enhance self-identity.

Psychodramatic reenactment involves the child and others in role-playing relationship scenarios from the child's early life. Role plays are done twice, first depicting the real-life negative experiences (e.g., helpless and fearful), and next depicting them in a more positive and hopeful way (e.g., with support and power). This intervention enhances genuine involvement, encourages open expression of perceptions and emotions, and promotes resolution of trauma.

The *magic wand* intervention allows the child to have a conversation with prior attachment figures (e.g., birth parents), who act as if they are healthy and can listen to the child. This experience facilitates "letting go" of anger and pain, and fosters psychological integration so that the child is no longer controlled by negative memories and emotions.

CASE STUDY: ATTACHMENT AND ADOPTION

Kathy was born in Korea. Her birth mother was a young factory worker who grew up in an orphanage and ran away at age 13. Her birth father was physically abusive with the mother, and she left him during the pregnancy. Kathy was placed in an orphanage at birth, as the mother did not believe she could take care of her. She was subsequently placed in a foster home, hospitalized at age 5 months for dysentery and convulsions, then adopted by John and Tina at age 6 months and brought to the United States.

The parents reported that Kathy did not cry or protest as an infant. They thought this was a sign of her "good nature," only to later learn it was a symptom of severely compromised attachment. Kathy had developed an avoidant attachment pattern (i.e., a deactivated attachment system) after learning that her needs would not be met by caregivers and that it was not safe to be vulnerable. She developed into a bright, creative, but very troubled child and teenager. She would lie, steal, and be demanding and abusive to her parents and younger brother (also adopted from Korea). Despite many years of counseling, Kathy was not improving and the parents were desperate. They came to our treatment program when Kathy was 18 years old, after she had flunked out of college and had wrecked several cars.

We focused on the parents' family-of-origin issues and need for parent training during the initial phase of treatment (2-week intensive CAT). Father was raised in a rural farm family where there was minimal communication and emotional attachment with his parents. He learned to avoid emotional sharing and to fear conflict and confrontation. Mother grew up in a large urban Italian family in which there was considerable communication, overt but manageable conflict, and close affectional bonds. She was the oldest of five children, and learned to take charge, protect others, and be "overresponsible." She did all the worrying in the current family, which resulted in chronic anxiety and physical shakiness and quivering.

Kathy was initially manipulative and superficial. She was adept at getting others to work hard, while she played the game of resistance and control. As an attempt to set appropriate boundaries for Kathy, while modeling effective limit setting for the parents, we provided the following messages: "We will work hard to help you, providing you work the hardest; we will not coerce or convince you, therapy is your choice; there are consequences to all choices, and you will be held accountable." A *therapeutic contract* was established with the parents; they agreed to set limits with Kathy, as per our direction, and to work on their marital and personal issues. After several attempts at testing the therapists and parents, Kathy decided to genuinely participate in treatment. For example, when the therapists and her parents collaboratively suggested she *not* come to therapy, Kathy walked 3 miles to our clinic. Interventions that circumvent control battles, such as "prescribing the symptom," are crucial with control-oriented children and young adults. At this point, goals and a therapeutic contract were established based on Kathy's *problem list* (e.g., increase honesty and responsibility; develop a closer relationship with parents; enhance self-esteem).

While discussing the *first-year attachment cycle* in the context of the HNP ("in arms" with therapist, with parents observing on a TV monitor in another room), Kathy began to explore early attachment experiences, including loss of her birth mother and the basis of her negative internal working model. For the first time in her life, she became genuinely emotional, crying about the rejection from her birth mother and various caregivers prior to adoption. She acknowledged and shared how she perceived herself: "I felt like no one wanted me and I didn't deserve love—I still feel that way." The session ended with Kathy "in arms" with her mother, sharing insights and feelings, and one-half hour of nonverbal connecting (eye contact, nurturing, gentle and loving touch, smiles). Mother reported her surprise and delight at the level of closeness.

While in the HNP, the therapist explained the reasons for using the *inner child metaphor* and Kathy agreed to participate. Kathy told "little Kathy" (symbolized by a small stuffed bear) the story of her life, including specific memories, perceptions of events, emotional reactions, and relationship experiences. She shared her pain of feeling "different," her unresolved loss of birth mother and culture, and how she projected anger and blame on her adoptive parents (especially mother). She also spoke of her jealousy and anger toward her brother, who is "easier to love," and her chronic self-doubts and self-contempt. The session concluded with honest communication between Kathy and her parents, and quality connecting time ("in arms" with mother, father in supportive role). The following day, the parents reported that Kathy had been genuinely affectionate and close for the first time.

Kathy was able to acknowledge and share the perceptions and emotions of her younger self in *psychodramatic reenactment*, which became a vehicle for cognitive/affective revision. She expressed hate and pain toward her birth mother for abandoning her and giving her the message: "You are not worth keeping, you are defective and unlovable." She began rehearsing and accepting the alternative positive mind-set: "I was a good and lovable baby; my birth mother had problems; it was not my fault." Again, Kathy and her parents spent considerable time "in arms" sharing and connecting at the end of the session. Kathy told her mother she was sorry for the mean and rejecting way she had treated her in the past, and asked for forgiveness. She was genuinely moved by her father's tears and they cried and laughed together. There was closeness and connection between all family members.

ACT was used for the relationship dyads (husband–wife, mother–daughter, father–daughter) to promote effective communication and problem-solving skills, and enhance emotional attachment via safe and constructive confiding. Marital interaction changed from the prior pattern of Tina speaking and John silent to a pattern of mutual sharing and listening. This not only improved the marital relationship, but also resulted in cooperative coparenting, as opposed to the responsibility resting with the mother. The parent–daughter dialogues enabled mother and Kathy to express their concerns, resentments, and needs. Kathy no longer relied on manipulation and blaming. She was more adult-like in her sharing and listening. The parents were also able to express themselves honestly without prompting a defensive and hostile reaction from their daughter. Kathy accepted more responsibility for her choices and actions, and allowed a genuine emotional closeness with her parents.

Using the *magic wand* intervention, Kathy "talked with" her birth mother and father, who were seen as being able to truly listen to her feelings. Kathy shared her pain and anger with them while in the protective arms of her adoptive parents. She ended the dialogue by expressing "forgiveness" and deciding to let go of the past hurts and disappointments. Mother was able to be supportive without rescuing and father was emotionally available to both wife and daughter. The family dynamics had changed, and attachment among all family members was significantly increased.

Six-month follow-up revealed a number of positive individual and interpersonal changes. Mother was less anxious and more confident, and no longer assumed the role of rescuer and enabler. Father became more emotionally available and involved in the marriage and in the parental role. Marital communication improved, and they both participated as a parental team. Kathy stopped stealing and began taking responsibility for her choices and behaviors. She moved into an apartment, got a full-time job, began paying for her own car insurance and other expenses, and displayed an increased level of caring and compassion on her visits home. She gave her father a birthday card and wrote, "A journey begins with the first step." When she moved to her new apartment she returned home to get something she forgot, her little bear ("Baby Kathy"). She reported that she wanted to take good care of herself on her new journey into adulthood. It appears that Kathy had achieved a more favorable balance of connection and autonomy. Her newfound ability to attach to her parents allowed her to begin exploring individuation in a positive way.

CONCLUSION

In conclusion, it is necessary to understand the importance of attachment as a lifespan issue. Attachment is crucial for healthy child development, meaningful adult relationships, and effective and loving parenting. Foster and adoptive parents must obtain the knowledge, skills, and support necessary to facilitate secure attachment with their children. Training and education of mental health and social service professionals is also crucial. Although awareness of attachment issues has increased over the last decade, many child welfare professionals are still not cognizant of its importance for families and society. Combining child development, family systems, and attachment perspectives are effective for assessment and treatment with challenging clients. Our longitudinal outcome studies demonstrate an 80% reduction of children's severe symptoms, maintained over time, with enduring positive changes in family relationships (Levy & Orlans, 1998).

REFERENCES

Ainsworth, M. D. S. (1973). The development of infant–mother attachment. In B. M Caldwell & H. N. Ricciuti (Eds.), *Review of child development research* (Vol. 3, pp. 1–94). Chicago: University of Chicago Press.

American Academy of Pediatrics. (1999). *Adoption: Guidelines for parents*. Elk Grove Village, IL: Author.

Beach, S. R. H., & Nelson, G. M. (1990). Pursuing research on major psychopathology from a contextual perspective: The example of depression and marital discord. In G. Brody & I. Sigel (Eds.), *Methods of family research: Biographies of research projects: Vol 2. Clinical populations* (pp. 110–132). Hillsdale, NJ: Erlbaum.

Berkman, L. F. (1995). The role of social relations in health promotion. *Psychosomatic Medicine, 57*, 245–254.

Biringen, Z. (2000). Emotional availability: Conceptualization and research findings. *American Journal of Orthopsychiatry, 70*(1), 104–114.

Biringen, Z., & Robinson, J. L. (1991). Emotional availability: A reconceptualization for research. *American Journal of Orthopsychiatry, 61*(2), 258–271.

Borysenko, J., & Borysenko, M. (1994). *The power of the mind to heal*. Carson, CA: Hay House.

Bowlby, J. (1969). *Attachment and Loss: Vol. I. Attachment*. New York: Basic Books.

Bowlby, J. (1988). *A secure base: Parent–child attachment and healthy human development*. New York: Basic Books.

Brazelton, T. B., & Cramer, B. G. (1990). *The earliest relationship*. New York: Addison-Wesley.

Brodzinsky, D. M., & Schechter, M. D. (1990). *The psychology of adoption*. New York: Oxford University Press.

Byng-Hall, J. (1995). Creating a secure family base: Some implications of attachment theory for family therapy. *Family Process, 34*(1), 45–58.

Chernoff, R., Combs-Orne, T., Risley-Curtiss, C., & Heisler, A. (1994). Assessing the health status of children entering foster care. *Pediatrics, 93*, 594–601.

Child Welfare League of America. (1996). *Family foster care survey*. Washington, DC: Author.

Chisholm, K. (1998). A three year follow-up of attachment and indiscriminate friendliness in children adopted from Romanian orphanages. *Child Development, 69*(4), 1092–1106.

Colapinto, J. A. (1995). Dilution of family process in social services: Implications for treatment of neglectful families. *Family Process, 34*(1), 59–74.

Donley, M. G. (1993). Attachment and the emotional unit. *Family Process, 32*(1), 3–20.

Dougherty, S. (2001). *Expanding the role of foster parents in achieving permanency*. Washington, DC: Child Welfare League of America Press.

Dozier, M., Albus, K. E., Stovall, K. C., & Bates, B. C. (2001). Foster infants' attachment quality: The role of foster mother state of mind. *Child Development, 72*(5), 1467–1477.

Egeland, B., Pianta, R., & O'Brien, M. A. (1993). Maternal intrusiveness in infancy and child maladaptation in early school years. *Development and Psychopathology, 5*, 359–370.

Erickson, M., Sroufe, L. A., & Egeland, B. (1985). The relationship between quality of attachment and behavior problems in preschool and a high-risk sample. In I. Bretherton & E. Waters (Eds.), Growing points of attachment theory and research. *Monographs of the Society for Research in Child Development, 50*(1–2, Serial No. 209), 147–166.

Figley, C. (1998). *Burnout in families: The systemic cost of caring*. New York: CRC Press.

Fonagy, P., Target, M., & Steele, M. (1997). Morality, disruptive behavior, borderline personality disorder, crime, and their relationships to security of attachment. In C. Atkinson & K. J. Zucker (Eds.), *Attachment and psychopathology* (pp 223–274). New York: Guilford Press.

Hesse, E. (1999). The Adult Attachment Interview: Historical and current perspectives. In J. Cassidy & P. Shaver (Eds.), *Handbook of attachment: Theory, research, and clinical applications* (pp. 395–433). New York: Guilford Press.

Jones, A. (1997). Issues relevant to therapy with adoptees. *Psychotherapy, 34*(1), 64–68.

Kagan, J. (1981). *The second year: The emergence of self-awareness*. Cambridge, MA: Harvard University Press.

Klee, L., Kronstadt, D., & Zlotnick, C. (1997). Foster care's youngest: A preliminary report. *American Journal of Orthopsychiatry, 67*(2), 290–299.

Levy, T. (Ed.). (2000). *Handbook of attachment interventions*. San Diego: Academic Press.

Levy, T., & Orlans, M. (1998). *Attachment, trauma and healing: Understanding and treating attachment disorder in children and families*. Washington, DC: Child Welfare League of America Press.

Levy, T., & Orlans, M. (2000a). Attachment disorder as an antecedent to violence and antisocial patterns in children. In T. Levy (Ed.), *Handbook of attachment interventions* (pp. 1–26). San Diego: Academic Press.

Levy, T., & Orlans, M. (2000b). Attachment disorder and the adoptive family. In T. Levy (Ed.), *Handbook of attachment interventions* (pp. 243–259). San Diego: Academic Press.

Lewis, J. M., & Gossett, J. J. (1999). *Disarming the past: How an intimate relationship can heal old wounds.* Phoenix, AZ: Zeig, Tucker, & Co.

Lyons-Ruth, K. (1996). Attachment relationships among children with aggressive behavior problems: The role of disorganized early attachment patterns. *Journal of Consulting and Clinical Psychology, 64*(1), 64–73.

MacLean, P. D. (1982). The co-evolution of the brain and the family. *L. S. B. Leakey Foundation News, 1,* 14–15.

Main, M., Kaplan, N., & Cassidy, J. (1985). Security in infancy, childhood and adulthood: A move to the level of representation. In I. Bretherton & E. Waters (Eds.), Growing points of attachment theory and research. *Monographs of the Society for Research in Child Development, 50*(1–2, Serial No. 209), 66–104.

O'Connor, T. G., Bredenkamp, D., Rutter, M., & The English and Romanian Adoptees (ERA) Study Team. (1999). Attachment disturbances and disorders in children exposed to early severe deprivation. *Infant Mental Health Journal, 20*(1), 10–29.

Pedersen, F., Yarrow, L., Anderson, B., & Cain, R. (1978). Conceptualization of father influences in the infancy period. In M. Lewis & L. A. Rosenblum (Eds.), *The social network of the developing infant* (pp. 203–221). New York: Plenum Press.

Renken, B., Egeland, B., Marvinney, D., Mangelsdoft, S., & Sroufe, L. A. (1989). Early childhood antecedents of aggression and passive-withdrawal in early elementary school. *Journal of Personality, 57,* 257–281.

Reynolds, P., & Kaplan, G. A. (1990). Social connections and risk for cancer: Prospective evidence from the Alameda County Study. *Behavioral Medicine, 16*(3), 101–110.

Russek, L. G., & Schwartz, G. E. (1997). Feelings of parental caring predict health status in midlife: A 35-year follow-up of the Harvard Mastery of Stress Study. *Journal of Behavioral Medicine, 20,* 1–13.

Schaffer, J. S., & Lindstrom, C. (1989). *How to raise an adopted child.* New York: Crown.

Shonkoff, J. P., & Phillips, D. A. (Eds.). (2000). *From neurons to neighborhoods: The science of early childhood development.* Washington, DC: National Academy Press.

Siegel, D. J. (1999). *The developing mind: How relationships and the brain interact to shape who we are.* New York: Guilford Press.

Solter, A. (1995). Why do babies cry? *Pre and Perinatal Psychology Journal, 10*(1), 21–43.

Sroufe, L. A. (1983). Infant–caregiver attachment patterns of adaptation in preschool: The roots of maladaptation and competence. In M. Perlmutter (Ed.), *Minnesota Symposium in child psychology* (Vol. 16, pp. 41–81). Hillsdale, NJ: Erlbaum.

Sroufe, L. A., Egeland, B., & Kreutzer, T. (1990). The fate of early experience following developmental change. *Child Development, 61,* 1363–1373.

Stern, D. N. (1985). *The interpersonal world of the infant: A view from psychoanalysis and developmental psychology.* New York: Basic Books.

Tronick, E. Z., & Cohen, J. F. (1989). Infant–mother face-to-face interaction: Age and gender differences in coordination. *Child Development, 60,* 85–92.

Tronick, E. Z., & Weinberg, M. K. (1997). Depressed mothers and infants: Failure to form dyadic states of consciousness. In L. Murray & P. Cooper (Eds.), *Postpartum depression and child development* (pp. 54–84). New York: Guilford Press.

Troy, M., & Sroufe, L. A. (1987). Victimization among preschoolers: The role of attachment relationship history. *Journal of the American Academy of Child and Adolescent Psychiatry, 26,* 166–172.

van IJzendoorn, M. H. (1995). Adult attachment representations, parental responsiveness, and infant attachment: A meta-analysis on the predictive validity of the Adult Attachment Interview. *Psychological Bulletin, 117,* 387–403.

Verny T., & Kelly, J. (1981). *The secret life of the unborn child.* New York: Delta.

Waters, E., Wippman, J., & Sroufe, L. A. (1979). Attachment, positive affect, and competence in the peer group: Two studies in construct validation. *Child Development, 50,* 821–829.

Zeanah, C. H., & Zeanah, P. D. (1989). Intergenerational transmission of maltreatment: Insights from attachment theory and research. *Psychiatry, 52,* 177–196.

10

Attachment-Based Family Therapy for Depressed Adolescents
Repairing Attachment Failures

GUY S. DIAMOND
RICHARD S. STERN

Attachment-based family therapy (ABFT) for depressed adolescents focuses on repairing the relational fabric between adolescents and their parents by facilitating conversations about past family traumas or ongoing interactional conflicts that have damaged trust. The model is characterized by five distinct, yet interrelated, treatment tasks: (1) relational reframe, (2) alliance building with the adolescent and then (3) with the parent, (4) repairing attachment, and finally (5) competency building. The general structure of these tasks (Diamond & Siqueland, 1998; Diamond, Diamond, & Liddle, 2000) and preliminary efficacy data (Diamond, Reis, Diamond, Siqueland, & Isaacs, 2002) have been presented elsewhere. Adolescent attachment theory (Kobak & Sceery, 1988; Allen & Land, 1999) provides the overarching theoretical framework, while structural (Minuchin, 1974) and multidimensional family therapy (Liddle, 1999) provide the clinical foundation for this approach. A number of other clinical traditions have also influenced the development of ABFT, including emotionally focused therapy (EFT; Greenberg & Johnson, 1988), contextual therapy (Boszormenyi-Nagy & Krasner, 1986), trauma and recovery theory (Herman, 1992), and research on the process of forgiveness (McCullough, Pargament, & Thoresen, 2000; Worthington, 1998). This chapter expands on findings from a task analysis of the attachment repairing task. Using one attachment episode as a case study, the current chapter provides the clinical and theoretical underpinnings of this task, which in many ways serves as the cornerstone of the entire ABFT model.

THEORY BASE

Attachment Theory

Attachment theory rests on the assumption that humans innately strive for connection with others (Bowlby, 1969, 1988). When a parent appropriately responds to this need in a child, the child generally develops a *secure* attachment style (i.e., the capacity to be autonomous yet intimate). When children's attachment needs are not effectively met, they may develop a variety of insecure attachment styles. Adolescents with a *dismissing* attachment style minimize the importance of attachment relationships by devaluing them or negating their influence. By contrast, adolescents with an *anxious* attachment style remain intensely focused on and overinvolved in their attachment relationships. Finally, adolescents with an *unresolved* attachment style are incoherent, disoriented, and disorganized, in describing their attachment relationships (Allen & Land, 1999). Insecure attachment styles are common among adolescents with a history of trauma and depression (Cole-Detke & Kobak, 1996; Kobak, Sudler, & Gamble, 1991; Rosenstein & Horowitz, 1996). Patients we have treated with ABFT seem to display elements of both dismissive and anxious–insecure attachment strategies. Most patients presented with indifference to and rejection of parental love and protection, yet remained fundamentally preoccupied with their parents, often conveying a deep-seated worry about their parents' welfare and capacities.

As in childhood, attachment security during adolescence rests on three perceptions: (1) that open communication with primary caregivers is possible, (2) that these figures are accessible, and (3) that they will provide protection and help if needed (Ainsworth, 1990; Kobak et al., 1991). While physical interactions between parents and children remain a determining factor in shaping early attachment security, given adolescents' increasing cognitive capacity, conversation increasingly becomes the vehicle through which attachment security is negotiated and experienced by teens (Kobak & Duemmler, 1994).

Repairing Attachment

An underlying assumption of ABFT is that family conversations may also serve a reparative function in families where the attachment bond has been compromised. We propose that the conditions for promoting secure attachment (e.g., positive parent–adolescent interactions) can be reestablished through family conversations that directly address adolescents' felt injustices and trauma experiences. This reparative function rests on the principle that attachment styles are open to revision based on new experience across the lifespan (Bowlby, 1969). While research supports the plasticity of attachment style (Waters, Kondo-Ikemura, Posada, & Richters, 1991), most studies have examined how negative life events can lead to a discontinuity of secure attachment. However, Main and Goldwyn (1988) argue that improvements in felt security and self-perception can occur within the context of later secure relationships such as a romantic or a therapist–client relationship. Individuals with insecure attachment styles who can develop some understanding and coherence about the role of these experiences in their interpersonal relationships can recover a sense of secure attachment and develop an "earned security." ABFT facilitates adolescents earning security by helping them work through problems or negative life experiences with their caregivers, who are often partially responsible for these traumas. Successful conversations can also promote new and positive caregiving behaviors, thus creating a mutually reinforcing experience of family growth.

In early childhood, having a secure base allows for developmentally appropriate independence and exploration of the environment (Bowlby, 1969). In adolescence, a secure attachment relationship promotes the developmental task of individuation. Throughout childhood and adolescence, the parent's ability to act as a *container* for the child's negative or difficult feelings plays a critical role in appropriate development (Winnicott, 1969). Securely attached adolescents can assert their autonomy (i.e., express their point of view) without the fear of criticism or abandonment. In contrast, insecurely attached adolescents often lack confidence in the stability of interpersonal relationships, and therefore are unable to make appropriate claims of reparation for past wrongs. Consequently, they harbor anger about attachment failures (e.g., "You did not protect me"; "You did not admire me") or become preoccupied with preserving fragile and dysfunctional relationships. They may go to great lengths to "protect" their parents from their angry or sad feelings, worrying that their concerns would drive their parents further away or overburden them. In such cases, many adolescents develop a negative self-schema that makes them vulnerable to depression (Cicchetti, Toth, & Lynch, 1995; Kobak et al., 1991).

In contrast, families that have or can acquire the capacity to tolerate and resolve conflict can liberate adolescents to develop a more differentiated sense of self, which forms the foundation for establishing the capacity for intimacy (Erikson, 1950). If the parent can remain loving during the process of differentiation, the adolescent retains a sense of feeling lovable, while achieving individuality (Kohut, 1971). When properly structured and prepared for, the expression of adolescent anger (and ultimately sadness) about parenting failures promotes adolescent autonomy, while strengthening rather than weakening the attachment bond. Appropriate autonomy and attachment build on one another. While secure attachment allows for appropriate individuation, the open, honest, and genuine expression of difficult feelings also allows for a closer parent–adolescent relationship.

Trauma and Forgiveness

As indicated throughout the text, there are many parallels between our conceptualization of the attachment repairing task and models of trauma recovery and forgiveness. Many of the depressed adolescents in our study experienced trauma through physical or sexual abuse or by witnessing violence. Others suffered emotional abuse that had a traumatic impact on their felt security in their family and their sense of safety in the community. Herman's (1992) model of trauma recovery delineates several steps toward working through these experiences. These steps include helping the patient (1) restore a sense of control, (2) establish safety, (3) tell the trauma story in detail, (4) mourn losses, and (5) reconnect with self and community. Forgiveness researchers have identified similar processes, including (1) experiencing strong emotions, (2) giving up the need for redress from the perpetrator, (3) seeing the offenders as distinct and separate from one's needs and identify, and (4) developing empathy for an offender (Enright, Santos, & Al-Mabuk, 1989; McCullough et al., 2000; Worthington, 1998). Several individual, family, and couple therapy models have turned to these frameworks to help understand core therapeutic processes (Johnson, Makinen, & Millikin, 2001; Gordon & Baucom, 1998; Hargrave & Sells, 1997). In many ways, the attachment-repairing task in ABFT can be thought of as a forgiveness process for resolving past trauma.

The Attachment-Repairing Task

The ABFT model provides a treatment methodology to help adolescents work though attachment failures and repair the parent–child attachment bond. ABFT therapists assume that depressed adolescents have a history of perceived (or real) attachment failures that have damaged adolescent–parent trust. These failures may be characterized by specific traumas such as neglect, physical abuse, or sexual abuse, or by more psychological processes such as criticism, rejection, or emotional abandonment. Regardless of the type of injustice, helping adolescents identify and address these experiences—and helping parents listen to and acknowledge them—can reduce family tension and rebuild trust. When these conversations are successfully facilitated, they enact the essential attachment caregiver behaviors that foster secure attachment (e.g., adolescents seeking help, parents providing support and protection). In this regard, during the attachment-repairing task, family members practice interpersonal skills that will hopefully generalize to future interactions. Additionally, focusing on adolescents' grievances early in treatment helps engage them (Liddle, 1995) and diffuses their feelings of revenge, anger, or rejection associated with these events. If avoided, these negative emotions can derail relationships and treatment (Diamond & Liddle, 1999).

ABFT relies heavily on the *enactment* methodology described by Minuchin and Fishman (1981). The ABFT therapist interrupts deleterious interactional sequences between family members by engineering or promoting new, successful conversations. In this regard, learning new relational skills is strengthened through experience and practice. During these sequences, the therapist functions as a coach, monitoring and shaping each family member's affect, cognition, and behavior in order to increase the likelihood of a successful conversation. Generally, the therapist directs family members to talk directly to each other rather than "through" the therapist. The therapist encourages reworking past and current conflicts directly with the family members that caused and perpetuated them (Minuchin & Fishman, 1981).

Based on a previous task analytic study, the attachment-repairing task appears to have three main phases, with several subtasks within each phase (Stern & Diamond, 2003). Phase A, "Adolescent Disclosure," consists of expressions of the adolescent's anger and vulnerable emotions, along with an exploration of attributions about past trauma. Parents remain primarily empathic and receptive. Phase B, "Parent Disclosure," involves a parent telling his or her side of the story and the adolescent deepening his or her understanding of these events. In Phase C, "Parent–Child Dialogue," the conversation becomes more mutual, mature, and reciprocal than in the previous phases.

Even in successful attachment sessions, all three phases are not always present, nor necessarily follow this order. Session structure and content are very family-dependent. However, an extended period of adolescent disclosure is essential for even a modest degree of attachment repair. Still, when appropriate, facilitating the parent disclosure and mutual dialogue phase seems to enhance the thoroughness and effectiveness of this task.

CASE EXAMPLE

Background and Case Formulation

The attachment-repairing event presented in this chapter involves a 16-year-old adolescent, Sandra, who on repeated occasions witnessed her mother being physically abused by her substance-abusing father.[1] The core conflict between the mother and the adolescent revolved around the

---

[1]Names and details have been changed to protect confidentiality.

mother's failure to protect herself from her abusing husband and to protect her children from witnessing the abuse and its associated problems. Additionally, the mother's parenting failures placed inordinate responsibility on Sandra to be the primary emotional caretaker for her three younger siblings. The burden of parentification reinforced Sandra's depression and resentment. The father, currently in jail for aggravated assault, was due to return home in 6 months, prompting the onset of the girl's depressive episode and the family's pursuit of treatment at our clinic.

Preparatory Tasks

The ABFT model must be tailored and flexibly applied to take into account the structure, strengths, resources, and history of the particular family being treated. ABFT can be applied to families who have experienced a wide range of traumas and interpersonal injuries as well as to a variety of family structures (e.g., one- or two-parent families). Application of the intervention, however, must be guided by good clinical judgment about who should participate in the sessions, the strength of the marital system, and the contribution that different family members can make to the reattachment process. Some families can complete this task during one session while other families may take several sessions, yet even modest gains can set the stage for further growth. Admittedly, in some families trust has been so damaged and betrayed that this intervention may not be appropriate. In such cases, alternative therapeutic strategies may be sought, such as accepting and grieving loss or a planned separation.

Three prior tasks lay the foundation for the attachment event. Task 1, the relational reframe task, usually done in the first session, focuses on helping the family define relationships and trust building between family members as the initial goal of therapy. To accomplish this, the session builds around the following question to the adolescent: "When you feel so depressed and think about hurting yourself, why don't you turn to your mother for help and comfort?" Development of this question leads to the recommendation that repairing trust and attachment may act as a buffer against current and future depression. In the case presented here, the mother readily agreed to trust building as an initial treatment goal, but Sandra expressed little interest in being closer to her mother.

In Task 2, the therapist meets individually with the adolescent and concentrates on alliance building. The therapist focuses on building closer bonds, developing meaningful goals, identifying core family conflicts that have damaged trust, and preparing the adolescent to discuss these issues with his or her parent. In this case, Sandra was quite reserved, giving mostly one-word answers, yet was able to identify some core family conflicts. She described years of parentification, along with resentment about her mother's dependence on an abusive husband. However, Sandra clearly refused to discuss any of this with her mother, fearing that doing so would burden her mother and change nothing. She did, however, agree to attend the next conjoint session where some of these issues might be discussed.

Task 3 focuses on alliance building with the parent(s). Meeting alone with the parent, the therapist focuses on current stressors or attachment failures in the parent's family of origin. The therapist empathizes with the parent's own experiences of loss, abandonment, and neglect in his or her current and/or past relationships. As parents become more empathic toward themselves, they are more receptive to appreciating the grievances of their adolescent. For example, the therapist might say, "Sounds like you know how painful it is for a child to have no one to turn to for help. Do you think your daughter might feel this way sometimes?" In the case presented here, the mother readily recognized how naïve she had been to think that martial violence and other problems had no impact on her daughter. She eagerly agreed to discuss this with her daughter in the next session. Anticipating the daughter's resistance, we prepared the mother to share her own thoughts about how past family events had affected the family.

Initiating the Attachment-Repairing Task

Given the preparation of the previous sessions, the therapist can begin this task with a clear plan for the session. The therapist usually begins with a brief summary of earlier sessions, clarifies the goals of the current session, reaffirms each family member's commitment to the task, and conveys optimism and support.

> "So far, I'm very impressed with both of you. There are a lot of admirable strengths in this family, and I am feeling very optimistic that we can help you (*to daughter*) start to feel better. I have met with both of you alone and I think we have identified many important things that the two of you have agreed to discuss. I understand, Sandra, that you feel hesitant about this, but I do think your mother has some important things that she would like to say. So my job is to support both of you and make sure the conversation goes well. OK? Any questions? Good. Mom, would you like to start?"

This opening statement represents the clarity, focus, and explicitness that therapists can use to initiate the attachment-repairing task when appropriate groundwork has been laid. In ABFT, enactments of conversations focused on attachment failures are not capricious and happenstance, but rather well crafted, timed, and prepared, thereby increasing the likelihood of success. Furthermore, therapists need to be creative and flexible in planning this task. For example, while ideally the adolescent initially presents his or her grievances, in this case the therapist modified this expectation by asking the mother to take the lead in acknowledging the daughter's felt injustices. This alternative strategy approximated the session goal, yet responds to the particular needs of the family (e.g., Sandra's stated unwillingness to talk).

Phase A: Adolescent Disclosure

Phase A of the attachment repairing task focuses primarily on the adolescent telling her or his story and the parents listening and acknowledging the adolescent's experience. This phase consists of three distinct yet interrelated processes: the disclosure of perceived attachment failures, the expression of a wide range of emotions (particularly direct anger and vulnerable emotions), and the exploration of attributions about these rupture events. Exploring each of these component processes helps both the adolescent and the parents construct a more coherent and honest understanding of the facts, feelings, and motives that contribute to family conflict and distrust. These three areas intermingle, but are often explored in the order proposed. More important than order, however, is the thoroughness with which the therapist explores each area. "Thoroughness" does not mean covering every aspect of a topic, but rather making coherent and new meaning from what is being explored. Have important topics been identified? Were powerful emotions expressed? Have avoided issues been uncovered? Do family members better understand the motives behind the adolescent's hostility or withdrawal? Asking these kinds of questions helps the therapist determine when to move on to the next topic or phase.

Adolescent Anger

Ideally, the adolescent begins the session by presenting the core conflicts identified in the prior adolescent alliance-building task. Usually these conflicts concern current or past experiences of neglect, abandonment, or abuse, but may also involve interpersonal dynamics between parent and child (e.g., adolescents feel disrespected, infantilized, or overcontrolled). Resentment about these specific betrayals or negative interactions, and the adolescent's inability to identify and effectively address these issues, inhibits an adolescent from turning to his or her parents for help.

Although anger may not be the first emotion expressed, it is often essential for a full working through of rupture events. Many depressed adolescents feel too protective of or loyal to their parents and worry about burdening them with these concerns. Others feel self-protective, expecting criticism and denial of their concerns (i.e., emotional abandonment). Still others don't feel entitled to have their needs met. Therefore, the expression of anger, when linked to core felt injustices, energizes and motivates adolescents to make more direct claims of reparation. Direct anger is a more productive and healthy coping strategy than withdrawal, self-punishment, or self-harm and is indicative of adolescents with a secure attachment style (Allen & Land, 1999). In the sequence below, Sandra reveals for the first time her anger about past negative family events.

MOM: So Dad would often take you out of school to watch the kids? And how did you feel about that?

SANDRA: I didn't like it. I didn't like takin' care of young kids all the time. I mean I wasn't that old of a kid myself.

MOM: And, um . . . you didn't feel that you could come to me and say anything about it?

SANDRA: I thought you knew.

MOM: While I was at work?

SANDRA: I mean I thought . . . I don't know . . . I just thought you knew.

MOM: Um, so . . . OK. You didn't like it, right? And you started feeling like that he was imposing on you too much because you were a child yourself?

SANDRA: (*Nods head yes.*)

MOM: So that's when you started resenting him?

SANDRA: (*Nods head yes.*)

MOM: And you resented me also?

SANDRA: Mmmm . . . no, I resented you for staying with him.

MOM: OK, OK. And um . . . Ok. So you resent me staying with your father because . . .

SANDRA: Because he hit you.

MOM: OK . . . (*pause*). Well, let me . . . let me tell you a little about how I was feeling at that time.

THERAPIST: Actually (*to mother*), I think you're doing a very nice job at listening to your daughter right now. I think we should hear a bit more from her before you say some of the things that you have been thinking about.

MOM: OK.

   Much to our surprise, Sandra decided to actively participate in this conversation. This was the first time Sandra had expressed these memories and feelings to her mother, the first time she had felt entitled and safe enough to tell the truth. Instead of responding defensively, the mother responds with empathy and curiosity, thereby making it safe for the daughter to continue talking. The therapist meanwhile coaches the family in order to keep the conversation on track. For example, at the end of the segment, the mother, who had been primed to tell her side of the story in anticipation of the daughter's resistance, needs redirecting back to the stance of interviewing, listening, and empathizing. This posture keeps the daughter at "center stage" while she tells her version of the family history. The therapist aims to sustain this conversation as long as necessary for the family to gain a better understanding of these events and to experience success at addressing difficult issues. At this point in the session, the therapist merely asks for more descriptive detail and tries to keep the negative affect level contained. This is not a formal testimony or "flooding" experience. However, as Herman (1992) notes, the mere act of telling a story in the safety of a protected relationship facilitates the working through of trauma memories. Having the perpetrator (e.g., the mother) as the witness further intensifies the significance of the conversation.

THERAPIST: Maybe Sandra could talk a bit more about what she actually saw, because you always thought that nobody saw or knew about these fights.

MOM: Yeah. What . . . what did you see?

SANDRA: Like what?

MOM: Like what . . . ? Everything!

SANDRA: Well I saw him hitting you. I mean, that's basically all he did.

MOM: And what else? Did you hear things?

SANDRA: I don't know. Him cussing and you screaming "Stop!"

THERAPIST: Where were the other kids during all this?

SANDRA: In the room with me. All together upstairs.

THERAPIST: Cause you were told to bring the kids upstairs?

SANDRA: Sometimes, yeah. Most of the time.

THERAPIST: Do you think they heard all this also?

SANDRA: (sarcastically) What do you think?

MOM: Did you ever talk about it with your sisters?

SANDRA: Why would I? That wasn't my job!

Sandra's indictment of her mother was long in coming. With the mother's genuine openness, Sandra finally came forth and expressed core conflictual concerns. At this point, the goal is modest: help the adolescent tell the truth without being too attacking or too hostile. Escalation of negative emotion or blaming behavior could destabilize the parent's ability to sustain supportive attention on the adolescent. However, exposing the deepest, most painful aspects of these seminal rupture events gives the therapist better access to the adolescent's schema of core negative emotions and attributions.

The correct parenting style during this phase is essential to the success of this task. If parents become impatient, critical, or defensive, the adolescent will regress back to blaming or withdrawal. Ideally, parents should show receptivity, interest, and concern, making the communication open and safe. The parents remain focused on the adolescent, freeing the adolescent from the need to protect, monitor, or take care of the parents. In this regard, the conversation serves as a corrective attachment experience.

However, parents' feelings of contrition and culpability can either motivate them to remain empathic or activate defensiveness. Preparation in the parent alliance-building session targets these possibilities. In that session, the therapist addresses parents' philosophy of emotions, helping them appreciate the importance of eliciting painful emotions, regulating intense affect, and putting feelings into words (Gottman, Katz, & Hooven, 1997). Once they accept these values, the therapist teaches parents to become better emotional coaches, developing the skills of empathy, admiration, support, and acknowledgment. Two motives help parents to embrace this new approach to problem solving. First, exhausted by adolescent indifference, withdrawal, or irritability, most parents hunger for direct and clear communication (albeit painful) from their depressed child. Second, uncovering parents' own history of attachment losses helps rekindle their desire and instinct to protect their child from similar traumas (Diamond et al., 2000).

Adolescent Vulnerable Emotions

If parents maintain a nondefensive, listening, and curious posture, the adolescent's anger often dissipates, giving way to softer, more vulnerable feelings (Johnson & Greenberg, 1988; Johnson, Maddeaux, & Blouin, 1998). While the expression of anger amplifies the request for autonomy and motivates self-defining actions, the expression of vulnerable emotions signals the desire for greater connection and inspires increased affiliative behavior from others (Greenberg & Safran, 1987). These vulnerable feelings are often denied or ignored and instead expressed through behavioral disruptions or self-punishment (Blechman, 1990). However, in the attachment-repairing task, the adolescent finally expresses powerful feelings of loss, abandonment, and rejection in an articulate and nonblaming manner. The adolescent's expression of sadness signals a new openness and receptivity (e.g., "Protect me!"), thereby evoking the parent's innate caregiving instincts of protection, comfort, and love (Bowlby, 1988). Consequently, parents become more affectivity attuned and usually, at least momentarily, more effective caregivers. In this regard, the attachment repairing task helps promote in the session the behaviors indicative of a secure attachment caregiver system.

In addition to these interpersonal benefits, helping the adolescent successfully navigate a conflictual conversation provides an opportunity to improve affect regulation skills. These skills involve being aware of one's emotional state and associated cognitions, monitoring and controlling one's expressions, discovering an emotional vocabulary to communicate them, and exercising self-soothing skills that can modulate these emotions (Lindahl & Markman, 1990). Therefore, accessing these underlying, more primary emotions deepens the adolescent's awareness of, comfort with, and capacity to verbalize conflictual emotional states.

If vulnerable emotions do not emerge, the therapist may try to elicit them. However, parents' empathic probes for these emotions are often more successful. The therapist restrains parents from overidentifying with the adolescent or from excessively focusing on or sharing their own pain. The therapist guides parents to concentrate on affirming and understanding as well as nurturing and protecting (Stern & Diamond, 2003). Helping the parents name simple vulnerable emotions facilitates this goal.

THERAPIST: You seem a bit upset now just talking about this.

SANDRA: I'm OK.

THERAPIST: Were you worried about Mom? Did you ever think she could get hurt or killed or anything like that?

SANDRA: Yeah! She did get hurt!

THERAPIST: Did you see those things? Her getting hurt?

SANDRA: Yeah (*irritated*).

THERAPIST: Mom, what do you think Sandra was feeling when she was upstairs in the bedroom protecting the kids and listening to your fights?

MOM: I don't know. Mad, I suppose.

SANDRA: I was mad. I was *really* mad!

THERAPIST: But I wonder what else Sandra was feeling?

MOM: You mean like worried or scared?

THERAPIST: Those are good guesses. Why don't you ask about that?

MOM: (*to daughter*) Well . . . besides being mad, how were you feeling when you were in your room?

SANDRA: Worried, scared. Angry with myself for not doing more to protect you.

MOM: Wow . . . (*pause*). That's a lot to deal with for a little girl.

SANDRA: (*Starts to cry.*)

Adolescent Attributions

The therapist and parent may elicit not only details of past grievances, but also probe the adolescent's attributions about attachment ruptures. Ideally adolescents will articulate their implicit assumptions about fault and responsibility regarding these attachment failures—theories that have a direct bearing on their emotions and behaviors. Research on attributions in marriage suggest that negative relationships are characterized by attributions of selfishness, blame, and malicious intent, as well as stable, global, and internal causes (Fincham, Bradbury, & Scott, 1990). The ABFT therapist tries to assess and alter similar attributional domains. In the current session, this process involves an exploration of the adolescent's attributions regarding her mother (was she incompetent or indifferent?), her father (was he malicious or on drugs?), and herself (was she to blame or a victim?).

THERAPIST: Why do you think your mother didn't leave him . . . get rid of your father?

SANDRA: I don't know, ask her!

THERAPIST: Well, for now, I am more interested in how you thought about this. What is your theory?

SANDRA: I don't know. She has always been a bit of a pushover.

THERAPIST: So you think she was just too weak to leave him?

SANDRA: Yeah! I suppose.

THERAPIST: Is she also then too weak to help you with your problems?

SANDRA: Something like that.

Phase B: Parent Disclosure and Apology

Prior to this phase, the therapist delicately blocks the parents' attempts to explain, defend, or apologize for their past behavior. Once the adolescent's memories, feelings, and attributions have been thoroughly explored, however, the therapist encourages parents to briefly present their own perspective of the identified trauma events or grievances. Parents' statements may include descriptions of mitigating circumstances or personal weaknesses. Statements of remorse and contrition are common. Therapists block parents from defending their actions or working through their own pain and loss. Instead, they are encouraged to share information that will help acknowledge the adolescent's experience (e.g., "Yes, it *did* happen"), give the adolescent new information about the events (e.g., "Yes, your father *was* using drugs"), and disclose some of the parents' own weaknesses and vulnerabilities (e.g., "I was scared too"). During this phase, parents do shift slightly away from the primarily supportive and nurturing posture held in Phase A, and instead do more disclosing and expressing of personal experiences and feelings (Stern & Diamond, 2003). This confessional, however, often helps parents face up to bad decision making and take responsibility for past actions.

During Phase B, the adolescent is not expected to adopt the validating posture her parents held in Phase A. However, in the most successful episodes, adolescents do extend some momentary active listening toward parents (and away from their own concerns). More importantly, the therapist encourages and supports the adolescent to use appropriate assertiveness and communication skills (e.g., affect regulation) and to ask parents difficult questions about past behaviors. These problem-solving skills are reflective of a secure attachment style (Allen & Land, 1999). However, the therapist must balance the goal of skill building for the adolescent and addressing important content. If an adolescent can not provide leadership in this phase, the therapist may actively address the most difficult issues her- or himself. In the following sequence, Sandra's mother begins with disclosing her own despair regarding these events, which, after questions from the therapist and the adolescent, results in a direct apology from the mother to Sandra.

MOM: Mainly life for me back then was bleak. I had no self-esteem. I was sad all the time and afraid most of the time. . . . Not knowing if your father was going to suddenly walk in the door and what mood he would be in.

(*A few moments later . . .*)

THERAPIST: (*to Sandra*) Why didn't she throw him out after he got back on drugs again?

SANDRA: (*to mother*) Yeah?

MOM: I couldn't even give you an answer for that. Because . . . I suppose I was in love with your father. Even though it was hard on me, I was trying to help him.

SANDRA: (*Silent*)

THERAPIST: Did you know how the kids were feeling about all this?

MOM: I thought I was concealing that from them. With them in the other room, I assumed they were asleep. I was trying to protect them.

THERAPIST: Tell Sandra. (*Directs mother to look at and talk directly to Sandra.*)

MOM: I was so much trying to protect you and your sisters. Even though I was the one being hurt, my priority was all of you. I didn't want anything to happen to you or your sisters. But I was sad all the time and afraid most of the time. And when you're really afraid of something . . . you feel like you don't have any out. I felt like nothing would help the situation. You kinda understand what I'm saying?

SANDRA: No.

MOM: I was afraid to leave him and I was afraid to stay with him. And so because I was afraid of that, my main priority was to make sure that nothing happened to you kids. Whatever the consequences or whatever happened to me, that didn't matter. The only thing that mattered was you and the other kids.

(A few moments later . . .)

MOM: And Sandra, I am really sorry for whatever part I played in making you unhappy, because that was not my intention at all. I wanted to make sure that you were happy. Do you understand that?

SANDRA: (Nods head yes.)

The parents' confessional statement can be powerful for several reasons. First, this acknowledgment offers the adolescent a new perspective of him- or herself and his or her parents. Parents are momentarily viewed as mortal, independent human beings with their own vulnerabilities and challenges. This is particularly important for older adolescents who have to begin demythologizing their parents and start accepting them for who they are. Simultaneously, by learning that they share similar experiences of victimization, many adolescents feel a new affiliation with their parents. This new realization further decreases the motivation for revenge and rejection and instead promotes empathy and the desire for closeness. In this regard, the attachment-repairing task brings family members emotionally closer, while also promoting a more articulated, coherent, and positive sense of self (Mikulincer, 1995). This helps reestablish a more normative balance of attachment and autonomy while building the skills and confidence to continue negotiating this developmental challenge (Allen & Land, 1999).

Second, abused and neglected adolescents are at high risk for repeating these and other destructive behaviors in the relationships they form as adults (Howard, 2000). Abused boys are more likely to become abusive men and abused girls are more likely to enter into victimizing relationships or to become self-injurious (Carmen, Reiker, & Mills, 1984). When one's sense of trust and fairness has been violated, one feels entitled to treat others poorly or not entitled enough to be treated fairly (Boszormenyi-Nagy & Krasner, 1986). In contrast, receiving acknowledgment and contrition from one's perpetrator can begin to repair that sense of injustice (Herman,

1992). Research on forgiveness suggests that when the "victimizer" takes responsibility for hurting the victim, it frees the victim from the tendency to blame him- or herself for, or to feel ashamed about, traumatic events (Worthington, 1998).

Because the process of adolescent disclosure coupled with parent nondefensive listening is so fundamental to the attachment-repairing task, the importance of the parent's disclosure may at first appear counterintuitive. Nevertheless, data from a previous study suggest that a discrete period of the parent "disclosing and expressing" constitutes a crucial turning point in the session and correlates strongly with attachment-repairing task success (Stern & Diamond, 2003). For example, during and after Phase B, parent communication was more differentiated (e.g., more respectful of the adolescent's autonomy). As in many trauma/recovery and forgiveness models, an apology from a perpetrator, though rare, expedites the victim's ability to resolve the past traumas (Herman, 1992).

Phase C: Mutual Dialogue

The adolescent and parents disclosure phases appears to lay the foundation for a more mutual dialogue and developmentally appropriate family interaction. As each family member feels heard and acknowledged, the conversation becomes more of a give-and-take exchange. The parents continue with the more independent posture that they established in Phase B, which help prevent the self-disclosure from becoming a burden to the adolescent. Yet, in contrast to previous phases, the parents' attention remains more equally divided between listening and disclosing. It is as if momentarily, adolescents and parents transform into three adults sharing (and possibly bonding around) the stories of their difficult lives. This dialogue is characterized by mutual respect, appreciation of each other's point of view, and greater empathy and acceptance of each other's strengths and weaknesses.

Like Phases A and B, Phase C also consists of several component processes. First, the therapist often takes this opportunity to help adolescents explore their reactions to their parents' disclosure. Parents' explanations and apologies often act as a catalyst for the adolescent to express even deeper and more vulnerable emotions (e.g., sadness, remorse) than they do in Phase A (e.g., fear, worry). Second, the conversation may focus on helping adolescents explore and accept mixed or ambivalent feelings (e.g., empathy and resentment) and struggle with when and how to accept their parents' apologies. The articulation and acceptance of ambivalent thoughts or feelings can increase self-efficacy (Shapiro, 1989) and is more reflective of the thought processes of adolescents with secure attachment (Allen & Land, 1999). Third, therapists may try to link new information regarding relational ruptures and grievances to current conflicts and symptoms. This can refocus the family on repairing relationship failure as a means to reducing and buffering against adolescent depression (Diamond & Siqueland, 1998).

In addition to exploring some of the Phase C themes mentioned above, Sandra showed clear signs of better understanding her mother's perspective. Sandra began to see her mother as a unique person with her own strengths and weaknesses, not simply as a mother who failed to protect her. In fact, Sandra gleaned comfort from the fact that her mother was trying to protect her, as if her good intentions helped make up for her ineffectiveness.

THERAPIST: Sandra, you cringed and turned away when Mom talked about wanting to provide you a two-parent family. What was that reaction about?

SANDRA: I don't know. You just don't find too many people with a mother and father and happy. Like I said, he was in and out of my life since I was young. So his being there did not make things any better. In fact, it made them worse.

THERAPIST: So you don't understand why your mother held onto that fantasy?

SANDRA: (*Shakes head no.*) But maybe that's what made her wake up every morning, that picture.

MOM: What do you mean?

SANDRA: You know. Somehow this kept you going . . . taking care of him, thinking you were protecting us. At least you were trying.

Sandra's statements exemplify one of the overarching goals from this task: increasing adolescents' capacity to understand another person's perspective. Greater empathy toward the perpetrator is a critical step in the process of forgiveness (e.g., McCullough, Worthington, & Rachael, 1997; Malcolm & Greenberg, 2000). This involves the victim's ability to recognize the perpetrator's limitations, while maintaining and insisting the perpetrator accept responsibility for his or her own actions (e.g., Hargrave & Sells, 1997). The ability to have perspective constitutes a kind of moral maturation (Kohlberg, 1994) in which (at least momentarily) the adolescent's egocentricity diminishes. As parents appear more mortal and adolescents show more maturity, the two become more like peers, sharing strengths and weaknesses and accepting responsibility for their own contributions to the current tension. Worthington (1998) refers to this stage as "humility." The victim comes to accept that she or he may have similar weaknesses or potential for harm as the victimizer. Among our depressed adolescents, many began to see how their own excessive rage or withdrawal had also contributed to damaging the relationship. For example, at one point Sandra says to her mother, "Maybe I have been too hard on you as well."

Wrap Up

Ending the session with an intellectualized explanation of what happened (e.g., summing up) should be avoided. Instead, the therapist should compliment the family members for sustaining such an intense, honest, and revealing conversation. The therapist punctuates the integrity shown by each family member as well as the collective mood of intimacy, vulnerability, and strength. Statements like "This has been a profound conversation. I was honored to be part of it" move the process toward closure while keeping the intense mood alive. The therapist might also check in with the family to try and limit any negative consequences from the conversation.

THERAPIST: (*to mother*) Do you have any concerns about having had this conversation with your daughter?

MOM: Well, I'm hoping it will bring us closer together, and that you (*to daughter*) can understand a little bit what I was going through as well.

THERAPIST: (*to mother*) But are you at all worried about how Sandra might feel after this conversation?

MOM: Sure. I worry that you might feel that I was a weak person cause I stayed with your father and I didn't get out. That I was stupid.

THERAPIST: (*to daughter*) Are any of those things true?

SANDRA: I used to think you stayed with him because you were weak. But now I see you were just scared and confused.

THERAPIST: Do you think you lost any respect for your mother tonight? Did this conversation make you think any less of her?

SANDRA: No. I'm glad she said what she said. But it did make me think less of him.

CONCLUSION

The attachment-repairing task represents a reparative conversation where relational failures are overtly addressed between parents and their adolescent. From the adolescent's perspective, past family experiences of threats to his or her physical integrity (e.g., abuse, neglect) or ongoing negative interactions (e.g., criticism, psychological control) have damaged the family's capacity to function as a secure base. Unaddressed, these traumas motivate adolescents' resentment and distrust. Consequently adolescents either attack or withdraw (Worthington, 1998). The attachment-repairing task by itself will not resolve years of mistrust. It must be followed up with new and consistent interactions that promote respect, protection, and commitment. Nevertheless, helping families successfully address these ruptures significantly increases the possibility of healing the relational fabric of family life.

To accomplish this in ABFT, therapists help adolescents identify and express these grievances while helping their parents bear witness and acknowledge them. When adolescents' feelings and needs are recognized by parents, adolescents more willingly accept them as allies and authority figures. Further, adolescents who can understand and come to accept their own and their parents' vulnerabilities and limitations may develop the earned security that can protect them from the depressogenic impact of early interpersonal trauma and loss (Kobak et al., 1991).

Parents simultaneously learn that listening and affective attunement increase communication more effectively than criticism and control. Although statements of apology and forgiveness are infrequently overt or complete, even the partial success of this process can profoundly reduce family tension and help strengthen family cohesion (Worthington, 1998). In addition to working through the content, the very enactment of the caregiver attachment system during the attachment-repairing task provides an experiential learning situation that helps solidify learning from previous sessions (Diamond & Diamond, 2001). With additional reinforcement in future sessions and at home, new positive parent–adolescent interactional behavior develops a new sense of mutual trust and dependability. In this regard, ABFT seeks to reestablish a healthy, normative developmental context that can promote secure attachment, thereby reducing and/or buffering against future depression.

ACKNOWLEDGMENTS

This work was supported by research awards to Guy Diamond from the National Institute of Mental Health (R21MH52920), the National Alliance for Research on Schizophrenia and Depression, and the American Suicide Foundation.

REFERENCES

Ainsworth, M. D. S. (1990). Some considerations regarding theory and assessment relevant to attachments beyond infancy. In D. Cicchetti, M. Greenberg, & M. Cummings (Eds.), *Attachment in the preschool years* (pp. 463–488). Chicago: University of Chicago Press.

Allen, J. P., & Land, D. (1999). Attachment in adolescence. In J. Cassidy & P. R. Shaver (Eds.), *Handbook of attachment: Theory, research, and clinical applications* (pp. 319–335). New York: Guilford Press.

Blechman, E. A. (1990). *Emotions and the family: For better or for worse*. Hillsdale, NJ: Erlbaum.

Boszormenyi-Nagy, I., & Krasner, B. R. (1986). *Between give and take: A clinical guide to contextual therapy*. New York: Brunner/Mazel.

Bowlby, J. (1969). *Attachment and loss: Vol. I. Attachment*. New York: Basic Books.

Bowlby, J. (1988). *A secure base*. New York: Basic Books.

Carmen, E. H., Reiker, P. P., & Mills, T. (1984). Victims of violence and psychiatric illness. *American Journal of Psychiatry, 141*, 378–383.

Cicchetti, D., Toth, S. L., & Lynch, M. (1995). Bowlby's dream come full circle: The application of attachment theory to risk and psychopathology. *Advances in Clinical Child Psychology, 17*, 1–75.

Cole-Detke, H. E., & Kobak, R. (1996). Attachment processes in eating disorders and depression. *Journal of Consulting and Clinical Psychology, 64*, 282–290.

Diamond, G. M., Diamond, G. S., & Liddle, H. A. (2000). The therapist–parent alliance in family-based therapy for adolescents. *Journal of Clinical Psychology, 56*(8), 1037–1050.

Diamond, G. S., & Diamond, G. M. (2001). Studying a matrix of change mechanisms: An agenda for family-based process research. In H. L. Liddle, D. A. Santisteban, R. Levant, & J. Bray (Eds.), *Family psychology: Science-based interventions* (pp. 41–66). Washington, DC: American Psychological Association Press.

Diamond, G. S., & Liddle, H. A. (1999). Transforming negative parent–adolescent interactions: From impasse to dialogue. *Family Process, 38*(1), 5–26.

Diamond, G. S., Reis, B. F., Diamond, G. M., Siqueland, L., & Isaacs, L. (2002). Attachment-based family therapy for depressed adolescents: A treatment development study. *Journal of the American Academy of Child and Adolescent Psychiatry, 41*, 1190–1196.

Diamond, G. S., & Siqueland, L. (1998). Emotions, attachment and the relational reframe: The first session. *Journal of Systemic Therapies, 17*(2), 36–50.

Enright, R. D., Santos, M., & Al-Mabuk, R. (1989). The adolescent as forgiver. *Journal of Adolescence, 12*, 95–110.

Erikson, E. H. (1950). *Childhood and society*. New York: Norton.

Fincham, F. D., Bradbury, T. N., & Scott, C. K. (1990). Cognition in marriage. In Frank D. Fincham & Thomas N. Bradbury (Eds.), *The psychology of marriage* (pp. 118–148). New York: Guilford Press.

Gordon, K. C., & Baucom, D. H. (1998). Understanding betrayals in marriage: A synthesized model of forgiveness. *Family Process, 37*(4), 425–449.

Gottman, J. M., Katz, L. F., & Hooven, C. (1997). *Meta-emotion: How families communicate emotionally*. Hillsdale, NJ: Erlbaum.

Greenberg, L. S., & Johnson, S. M. (1988). *Emotionally focused therapy for couples*. New York: Guilford Press.

Greenberg, L. S., & Safran, J. D. (1987). *Emotion in psychotherapy: Affect, cognition, and the process of change*. New York: Guilford Press.

Hargrave, T. D., & Sells, J. N. (1997). The development of a forgiveness scale. *Journal of Marital and Family Therapy, 23*(1), 41–62.

Herman, J. L. (1992). *Trauma and recovery*. New York: Basic Books.

Howard, J. (2000). Working with child abuse and neglect issues. *CSAT Treatment Improvement Series, 36*, 1–9.

Johnson, S. M., & Greenberg, L. S. (1988). *Emotionally focused therapy for couples*. New York: Guilford Press.

Johnson, S. M., Maddeaux, C., & Blouin, J. (1998). Emotionally focused family therapy for bulimia: Changing attachment patterns. *Psychotherapy: Theory, Research, and Practice, 35*, 238–247.

Johnson, S. M., Makinen, J., & Millikin, J. (2001). Attachment injuries in couples relationships: A new perspective on impasses in couples therapy. *Journal of Marital and Family Therapy, 27*, 145–156.

Kobak, R., & Duemmler, S. (1994). Attachment and conversation: Toward a discourse analysis of adolescent and adult security. *Advances in Personal Relationships, 5*, 121–149.

Kobak, R., & Sceery, A. (1988). Attachment in late adolescence: Working models, affect regulation, and representations of self and others. *Child Development, 59*, 136–146.

Kobak, R., Sudler, N., & Gamble, W. (1991). Attachment and depressive symptoms during adolescence: A developmental pathways analysis. *Development and Psychopathology, 3*, 461–474.

Kohlberg, L. (1994). Stage and sequence: The cognitive-developmental approach to socialization. In B. Puka (Ed.), *Moral development: A compendium* (Vol. 1). New York: Garland.

Kohut, H. (1971). *The analysis of the self*. New York: International University Press.

Liddle, H. (1995). Conceptual and clinical dimensions of a multi-dimensional, multisystems engagement strategy in family-based adolescent treatment. *Psychotherapy: Theory, Research, and Practice, 32*, 39–58.

Liddle, H. (1999). Theory development in a family-based treatment for adolescent drug abuse. *Journal of Clinical Child Psychology, 28(4)*, 521–532.

Lindahl, K. M., & Markman, H. J. (1990). Communication and negative affect regulation in the family. In E. A. Blechman (Ed.), *Emotions and the family: For better or for worse* (pp. 99–115). Hillsdale, NJ: Erlbaum.

Main, M., & Goldwyn, R. (1988). *Adult attachment classification system. Version 3.2*. Unpublished manuscript, University of California, Berkeley.

Malcolm, W. M., & Greenberg, L. S. (2000). Forgiveness as a process of change in individual psychotherapy. In M. E. McCullough, K. I. Pargament, & C. E. Thoresen (Eds.), *Forgiveness: Theory, research, and practice* (pp. 179–202). New York: Guilford Press.

McCullough, M. E., Pargament, K. I., & Thoresen, C. E. (Eds.). (2000). *Forgiveness: Theory, research, and practice*. New York: Guilford Press.

McCullough, M. E., Worthington, E. L., & Rachal, K. C. (1997). Interpersonal forgiving in close relationships. *Journal of Personality and Social Psychology, 73*, 321–336.

Mikulincer, M. (1995). Attachment style and the mental representation of the self. *Journal of Personality and Social Psychology, 69*, 1203–1215.

Minuchin, S. (1974). *Families and family therapy*. Cambridge, MA: Harvard University Press.

Minuchin, S., & Fishman, H. C. (1981). *Family therapy techniques*. Cambridge, MA: Harvard University Press.

Rosenstein, D. S., & Horowitz, H. A. (1996). Adolescent attachment and psychopathology. *Journal of Consulting and Clinical Psychology, 64(2)*, 244–253.

Shapiro, D. (1989). *Psychotherapy of neurotic character*. New York: Basic Books.

Stern, R., & Diamond, G. S. (2003). *A task analysis of repairing attachment ruptures in families with depressed adolescents*. Unpublished manuscript.

Waters, E., Kondo-Ikemura, K., Posada, G., & Richters, J. E. (1991). Learning to love: Mechanisms and milestones. In M. R. Gunnar & L. A. Sroufe (Eds.), *Self processes and development: The Minnesota symposia on child psychology*. (Vol. 23, pp. 217–255). Hillsdale, NJ: Erlbaum.

Winnicott, D. W. (1969). *The child, the family, and the outside world*. Harmondsworth, UK: Penguin Books.

Worthington, E. L. (1998). An empathy–humility–commitment model of forgiveness applied within family dyads. *Journal of Family Therapy, 20*, 59–76.

PART III

USING AN ATTACHMENT PERSPECTIVE IN INTERVENTIONS WITH PARTICULAR POPULATIONS

11

The First Couple
Using Watch, Wait, and Wonder to Change Troubled Infant–Mother Relationships

NANCY J. COHEN
ELISABETH MUIR
MIREK LOJKASEK

Optimally, adults in a relationship provide one another with affection, emotional support, and a base from which the individuals in the relationship can continue to develop a sense of themselves as individuals in their own right as well as partners in a relationship. But this does not always happen. Adult couples come to therapy with complaints about each other in their relationship—often ones that involve being unable to stand up for and be oneself. Not infrequently, they go something like this: "He [she] only loves me if I am who he [she] wants me to be. If I don't go along with it, he [she] is angry and cold toward me and I begin to feel as if I don't exist. I worry that if I assert myself and my own feelings he [she] will leave me. That scares me because I need him [her]. But if I am always going along with what he [she] wants me to be, I lose my sense of who I am. And that is terrible too." If infants who are brought by their parents to mental health clinics could talk, they might have something similar to say. It is the relational struggles of the infant–parent couple that are the focus of this chapter.[1]

---

[1]In the remainder of the chapter, we will be referring to the parent as "mother" because this is usually who is most often seen and to the infant as "he," just to keep the pronouns straight.

Infants obviously cannot use words to express their anxieties and distress about their relationships. Accordingly, referral in infancy occurs when this relational distress emerges in the nonverbal realm of problematic interactions. Symptoms typically manifest as functional problems in the infant involving feeding, sleeping, and behavioral regulation such as extreme tantrums or difficulty being soothed. While not apparently relational, these problems commonly reflect difficulties in the relationship between mother and infant. For example, sleeping problems may reflect the infant's separation anxiety resulting from an anxious attachment (Benoit, Zeanah, Boucher, & Minde, 1992; Cassidy, 1994). In other cases, the reasons for referral are more directly related to a mother's depression or her expressed difficulty in becoming attached to or bonded with her infant. That makes meeting her infant's needs more difficult.

Although it is the infant who is the greatest clinical concern, the actual focus of treatment is usually the mother (Lojkasek, Cohen, & Muir, 1994). It is a challenge to find ways to intervene that address the infant's dilemma directly while also working with the mother. In our work we have focused on how best to include the infant in infant–parent dyadic therapy directly through the infant's activity. In this chapter, we describe the theoretical underpinnings and therapeutic techniques of an infant-led psychotherapy: Watch, Wait, and Wonder (Wesner, Dowling, & Johnson, 1962). Watch, Wait, and Wonder is a dyadic psychotherapy that works directly and immediately with the relationship by empowering the infant in the therapy. In this form of therapy, the mother is asked to follow her infant's spontaneous and undirected activity in much the same way that a therapist observes and follows the lead of an adult patient. Although this infant-led approach centers on the infant–parent relationship, it is guided by the infant activity. The therapeutic process in Watch, Wait, and Wonder is best formulated using attachment theory. In this context we touch on intergenerational transmission of attachment relationships. We also describe our research on the outcome of Watch, Wait, and Wonder, which compares it to a more traditional psychotherapeutic intervention with the mother with the infant present. Although this chapter focuses on the infant–mother relationship, it is important to point out that we do use this infant-led approach with fathers, with more than one parent, and with children beyond infancy. Moreover, one of us (E. M.) has successfully adapted this approach for use with adult couples where the focus is on each partner following the other's lead in their conversations during therapy sessions.

SETTING THE STAGE FOR THE INFANT–MOTHER
RELATIONSHIP TO UNFOLD

For most couples, having a baby is a source of both happiness and anxiety. There is, of course, the excitement of bringing a new life into the world and the sense of a fresh start in the formation of relationships. At the same time, pregnancy and childbirth precipitate a psychological crisis in the family due to the activation in family members of internalized relational patterns from their own infancies (Menzies, 1975; Notman & Lester, 1988). While this occurs to a certain extent in all mothers, some mothers are more vulnerable. In particular, some mothers have difficulty with unresolved mourning related to their own deprivations in their early attachment relationships, such as abandonment or the threat of it, rejection, too early and frequent separations, or family loss and/or trauma. The resulting insecure attachment restricts the mother's own development, autonomy, and relational patterns. These mothers, who were unable to grieve as infants or children, can be overwhelmed by an activation of disavowed intense feelings and frustrations associated with those early experiences. Fraiberg and colleagues (Fraiberg, Adelson, & Shapiro, 1987) describe how these unresolved issues haunt the mother–infant pair as if there are "ghosts" residing in the nursery. These ghosts powerfully influence the mother's relationship with her own infant, thereby affecting, in turn, the infant's attachment security and relational repertoire.

Infants' inherently normal attachment needs and developmental striving are powerful activators of their mothers' disavowed infantile feelings related to their infants' striving for secure attachment. Thus, some mothers can be very threatened by the activity or the mere presence of their infants, even though their infants' behavior is developmentally appropriate. Inevitably, these mothers must defend themselves against any painful reemergence of their own grief. This grief is often accompanied by rage over what they did not get from their own mothers. When infants are brought to the clinic, we view their symptoms as a joint outcome of their mothers' struggles with the source of these painful feelings in conjunction with the infants' individual temperamental characteristics and specific components of the context in which the infant–mother dyad lives, including the marital relationship and the wider social milieu. From this perspective, we regard the developmental problems of infants to be *relationally derived*. By this we mean that whether the problem resides more or less in the mother or in the infant, it is how infant and mother negotiate their respective needs, including their "fit" with each other, that determines whether or not a problem will develop. The respective needs of mother and infant may vary in nature and involve developmental, psychological, physical, and emotional issues.

Many problems in infancy can then be understood as emerging when a stifling compromise occurs in the relational connection between the mother and the infant. Infant symptomatology represents a way of simultaneously coping with and protesting against what is for the infant a relational and developmental dilemma related to his own attachment and autonomy. Looking back to the kind of relational dilemma for adult couples that introduced this chapter, the infant compromises in an attempt to find a way to fit in with his mother, restricting his self-differentiation, exploration, and elaboration of potential self (Muir, Lojkasek, & Cohen, 1999). Our goal in therapy is to intervene in this cycle in order to help the dyad achieve both greater autonomy and relational harmony.

Infancy provides a good opportunity to intervene. The family system is already unsettled by the arrival of a baby, requiring a readjustment of all members. This is usually accompanied by the parents' hope that they can provide the new infant with a life better than their own—the apparent excitement of a new beginning and accompanying hope. Clinicians from various disciplines who work with the problems of infancy and early childhood generally agree that changes in the relationship between mother and infant have to occur. Consistent with much of the current work in the area of infant mental health, the theoretical framework of attachment guided our clinical work in delineating the critical relational components and goals of therapy. Our research and the essential hypotheses we tested relied on attachment theory, which guided our systematic examination of treatment outcome. Before proceeding, we will discuss attachment theory and how it may be related both to the evolution of infant–parent relational problems and to approaches to treatment.

ATTACHMENT THEORY AND ITS ASSOCIATION WITH INFANT–PARENT RELATIONAL PROBLEMS

The term *attachment* refers specifically to a biologically primed behavioral system that operates under threatening conditions and enables infants to seek safety and comfort from distress through proximity to their mothers. Bowlby (1980, 1988) suggested that attachment security develops through the experience that infants have with their mothers in relation to their mothers' emotional responsivity and physical proximity. Considerable evidence has accrued to indicate that for secure attachments to form, mothers must perceive their infants' emotional signals accurately, respond to them sensitively, display affection, accept their infants' behavior and feelings, and be physically and psychologically available when their infants are distressed. In turn, development appears to proceed more optimally for infants who are securely attached. These infants are able to regulate their emotions and have a sense of inner confidence and efficacy (Goldberg, 2000). Feeling safe, securely attached infants can express their curiosity and are eager to explore their environment. It is presumed that these activities, in turn, support social and cognitive development. Securely attached infants enjoy more relational pleasure and harmony with their mothers, which in turn fosters infants' openness to other relational experiences. As they get older, securely attached infants have the capacity to have secure and enduring relationships, which ultimately provide the foundation for their own children's secure attachment. Thus, generally, development appears to proceed more optimally for infants who are securely attached.

In contrast, infants who are not securely attached have mothers who are unpredictable, who either provide minimal or inconsistent care, and who may even be frightening to their infants. In a problematic relationship, an insecurely attached mother interprets her infant's normative bids to gain access to her and to explore and master the environment negatively, thus promoting insecurity in the infant. Paradoxically, insecure attachment patterns can actually be viewed as adaptive in the sense that the infant is at least learning a strategy for fitting in with his mother's representations of him and for getting his needs at least minimally met. In some cases, this requires the infant to seem very independent, thus making minimal demands on a rejecting or unresponsive mother. In other cases, the infant expresses his distress and frustration behaviorally to gain the attention of an inconsistently responsive mother. Despite the adaptive aspects of the infant's behavior, these strategies are not optimal. Insecurely attached infants are less able to regulate their emotions and behavior and may appear to be withdrawn or easily distressed. Still other infants exhibit an attachment pattern that is not adaptive in that the infant is disorganized and lacks a consistent strategy for getting needs met, a pattern that develops in infants who are maltreated or whose mothers are struggling with unresolved loss (van IJzendoorn, 1995). This pattern is commonly observed in clinical samples (van IJzendoorn, Schuengel, & Bakermans-Kranenberg, 1999). Without consistent access to care, insecurely attached infants tend to be preoccupied with getting their attachment needs met and are less likely to exhibit the curiosity and exploration of securely attached infants.

Although empirical evidence is sparse, it has been postulated that through repeated interactions with attachment figures, *representations*, or "internal working models" of self in relation to others, are set down and thereafter unconsciously guide and filter attention and processing of experiences in regards to attachment and thus impact the course of future relationships (Bowlby, 1980). Infants who become securely attached develop internal working models of their mothers as sensitively responsive and available and themselves as worthy of care and love. In contrast, infants who become insecurely attached see caregivers as rejecting, unreliable, or even frightening and view themselves as unworthy of care (Thompson, 1999).

Based on the above discussion, an intervention consistent with attachment theory would need to meet a number of criteria:

- Provide emotional and physical access to the mother.
- Focus directly on maternal sensitive responsiveness to the infant's behavior and emotional signals.
- Place the mother in a nonintrusive stance, which allows for the evo-

lution of the infant's initiative, curiosity, self-expression, and mastery of the environment.

- Provide a space in which the infant can work through relational struggles through play and interaction with the mother.
- Provide a therapist who can function as a secure base for the dyad working through their relational difficulties.

THERAPEUTIC INTERVENTIONS AND ATTACHMENT THEORY

Not all infant–parent therapies explicitly use attachment theory. However, most therapeutic endeavors focus on enabling the mother to accurately read her infant's emotions, to accept her infant's behavior and feelings as distinct from her own, and to respond sensitively. In order to put Watch, Wait, and Wonder into perspective, it is important to first briefly review two other forms of psychotherapy predominant in the literature on infant mental health and their assumptions regarding how such changes in the infant–mother relationship can be effected. This is not intended to be a comprehensive review of all infant–mother interventions; a more thorough review can be found in Lojkasek et al. (1994).

Psychodynamic psychotherapy assumes that therapy modifies the mother's mental representation of her relationship with her infant by exploring her assumptions derived from her relationships with her own parents (Cicchetti, Toth, & Rogosch, 1999; Cramer et al., 1990; Fraiberg et al., 1987; Lieberman, Weston, & Pawl 1991; Robert-Tissot et al., 1996). In this approach it is regarded as essential that the mother gain insight. The primary work is between the mother and the therapist. The infant is present during therapy but participates largely as a motive for change and a catalyst for the psychotherapeutic work. The basic process is similar to adult psychotherapy except that the therapy focuses on the current difficulties the mother is experiencing with her infant. The focus is not on the infant himself using the session therapeutically. Through the mother's relationship with the therapist, and fueled by the new experience of motherhood and her current difficulties with the infant, insights are assumed to be facilitated by the reenactment or repetition of the mother's early and other past relationships in her current relationship with her infant. These relationships also emerge in enactments with the therapist through the transference. Shifts in maternal sensitivity and responsiveness come about as a result of the mother's increasing capacity to differentiate her infant from herself, which enables her to perceive her infant more objectively and to respond accurately to her infant's needs.

Interventions that focus on the behavioral aspects of the mother–infant relationship are represented by therapies such as interactional guidance (McDonough, 1992). In this approach, videotaped interactions of mother and infant are used by the therapist to help the mother to recognize her own positive responses and interactions with her infant and thus to elaborate appropriate responsiveness. Mutual enjoyment is emphasized and new, more pleasurable interactions between mother and infant are encouraged, which is presumed to help the mother build confidence in her parenting role. Again, the infant is involved only indirectly. That is, his communications about himself and his mother, revealed in interactions with her, are used to guide the mother's perceptions. It is the therapist's role to guide the mother to selected infant cues and characteristics to which she is encouraged to attend and respond. To achieve this, a degree of parental guidance and direction is used. Again, although the aim is to achieve maternal sensitivity and the capacity to read, accept, and accurately respond to the infant's behavior, this type of intervention does not make it an explicit goal that the infant use the time therapeutically himself or be an active force in his own right in the treatment process.

It is understandable that descriptions of therapeutic interventions recount the *content* of the infant's play as a stimulus for discussion or to provide cues for guidance and do not address how infants themselves use the activity and play to work through their own experience or their developmental and relational struggles. This is because it has been hard to conceptualize and devise techniques for directly involving the infant in therapeutic work. Selma Fraiberg and colleagues summed up the situation as follows:

> A baby has none of the conventional attributes of a psychiatric patient. He can't form a therapeutic alliance. He has no capacity for insight. Such patients are usually labelled not suitable for treatment in the language of psychotherapy. (Fraiberg, Shapiro, & Cherniss, 1983, p. 56)

Finding a way to directly involve the infant in therapy is important because an infant cannot wait until his mother addresses the difficulties between them through individual work. He too is anxious, depressed, or distressed and needs assistance, although he is unable to directly ask for help. It is true that the mother is in the more powerful position in the dyad and has more freedom to change her behavior compared to the relatively helpless infant. She also brings with her past relational experiences, while the infant is just embarking on his relational path. However, it does not necessarily follow that because the mother's contributions to the difficulties may be greater, or because she is in a better position to adapt to the infant's temperament than the infant is to adapt to her personality, that the infant, himself, should not be an active contributor in therapy.

WATCH, WAIT, AND WONDER

The focus of our work has been on developing ways of including the infant more fully in relational psychotherapy. Specifically, we have been exploring an infant-led psychotherapeutic procedure called Watch, Wait, and Wonder. Watch, Wait, and Wonder allows the infant to become an active partner in the therapeutic process and works at both the behavioral and the representational levels. The history and theoretical and technical aspects of Watch, Wait, and Wonder are presented in greater detail by Muir (1992), Muir and Thorlaksdottir (1994), and Muir, Lojkasek, and Cohen (1999, 2000). Watch, Wait, and Wonder aims to intervene in the mother–infant relationship in a way that fosters the development of a secure relational connection between mother and infant and that facilitates the infant's exploration and differentiation of his potential self, self in relation to other, and self-efficacy. This is achieved by creating a space where the attentive mother allows the infant to engage in unimpeded sensorimotor activity and play in order for the infant to explore his relationship with her and his surrounding environment in his own way.

When used with infants, it is best to start Watch, Wait, and Wonder no earlier than the age of 4–6 months when infants can regulate emotional and behavioral states to some extent and are mobile to explore. Adaptations may be made for younger infants, but they will not be discussed here.

We delineate the Watch, Wait, and Wonder space physically with a heavy-duty blue plastic mat. The toys are always arranged in the same order. These are toys that the infant can manipulate and include both construction toys and representational toys. Typically, some of the toys are chosen to promote emotional and relational themes central to the infant's presenting symptoms. For instance, an infant with eating problems is often drawn to the feeding utensils such as bowls and spoons, and an infant with sleeping problems to the dolls and doll bed.

This is how Watch, Wait, and Wonder works. The mother is given instructions at the outset of treatment that she engage in a form of play with her infant that includes as essential elements that she:

- Get down on the floor.
- Follow her infant's lead.
- Not initiate any activities herself.
- Be sure to respond when the infant initiates but not to take over his activities in any way.
- Allow the infant freedom to explore—whatever the infant wants to do is OK as long as it is safe.
- Remember to watch, wait, and wonder.

The mother engages in this form of activity for half the session (20–30 minutes). She is thus put in the position of being physically accessible to her infant and observing, accepting, and responding to his spontaneous and undirected behavior. This fosters an observational and reflective stance in the mother and potentially encourages her to become more sensitively, even, optimally, responsive. This process assumes that there is an innate human striving for a secure relational connection when a space is created that enables a connection to be made. It also is assumed that because this relational connection derives from an affective experience, it cannot simply be taught. In fact, mothers are encouraged to believe that they and their infants are able to and will need to find their own way of connecting with each other. This watching, waiting, and wondering by the mother parallels the role of the therapist.

The therapist's role in Watch, Wait, and Wonder is less interactive than in other forms of psychotherapy. In a way it is more psychoanalytic. Just as the mother is asked to watch, wait, and wonder with her infant, the therapist sits slightly off to the side of the area defined by the blue mat and watches, waits, and wonders, reflecting on the interactions of mother and infant. He or she shows interest and curiosity in the relationship and inner life of the dyad, and supports and validates the mother's experience. This parallels the task of the mother, since the mother is also placed in the position of being curious about and accepting of her infant's evolving inner life.

As mentioned earlier, infant symptomatology is in a sense a communication about the relational dilemma. A free-play assessment commonly reveals the interactive transmission of a relational pattern. The following case example illustrates how a 9-month-old boy's symptoms may be linked to qualities of an intrusive maternal interactive style.

At the time of referral, Mrs. G. described her infant son, Sam, as "passive." She was concerned that he was unresponsive and "never played." His behavior sharply contrasted with that of an older brother born 2 years earlier who was described as "exuberant" in his interactions with objects and people. The mother–infant play sequence that follows took place during the 15 minutes of free play that was part of the assessment preceding treatment.

Sam sat placidly on the blue mat with legs spread wide to maintain balance, with his hands remaining by his side. Mrs. G. initiated the play by holding a toy telephone receiver to Sam's ear and saying, "Do you know what this is?" When he turned away, she went to his other side, that is, to where she assumed he was looking, and pushed a small car toward him. Sam turned away again. Mrs. G. then proceeded to present various toys to Sam in rapid succession: a plastic animal, a doll, a block, and so on. With each presentation, she would say "What about that?" or "How do you like that?" in a soft but tense voice intended to entice Sam to play but also betraying her anxiety. His demeanor continued to be passive and unresponsive during each of his mother's attempts to engage him and throughout he never vocalized once. Finally, when presented with a bowl of toys, Sam reached out tentatively and chose a rolling pin. Mrs. G. immediately took the rolling pin from Sam's hand and began to roll it on the floor saying, "Do you want to have a look at that?" Sam returned to his impassive state without reaching out again. He looked blankly first at his mother and then at the rolling pin without making a move or a sound.

In this sequence one can see that Mrs. G.'s anxiety about her son's inability to play led her to take the lead in the play. She was inattentive to Sam's signals of either interest or avoidance of her intrusive style and did not allow him the time or the space to explore the one toy he had chosen. The sequence reflects the interactional manifestation of Mrs. G.'s anxieties and concerns. Indeed, Sam appears quite passive for a 9-month-old baby and shows little initiation or affect. It seems that the two were stuck in a particular way of interacting that was not satisfying to either member of the dyad. Circumstances changed noticeably in the first Watch, Wait, and Wonder session. Although shifts in mother and infant behavior do not always occur so rapidly, we have been struck by how in some dyads both problems in the relationship and their solution come to the forefront in the first few treatment sessions.

After Mrs. G. was given the Watch, Wait, and Wonder instructions, she sat at the edge of the blue mat, leaning forward with interest to look at Sam. Although not instructed specifically where to sit, Mrs. G. chose a position distant enough so that it would be impossible for her to initiate play without moving herself closer to Sam. Initially, Sam sat in his placid unmoving position, alternating his gaze between his mother and the toys. He appeared to us to be somewhat puzzled by the change in his mother's behavior. Finally, after what seemed like a very long 30 seconds, he dropped to his hands and knees and tentatively began to explore the toys just inches from where he had been sitting. He then picked up a toy animal and waved it about while vocalizing at length. Then he put the animal down on the mat again. After a pause, while he sat quietly looking repeatedly toward and then away from his mother, Sam again began to crawl. This time he explored farther afield and, one after another, picked up various toys as if to test out the array of possibilities before settling on a specific activity. All the time he vocalized and cooed happily.

This sequence following the Watch, Wait, and Wonder instructions suggested to us that Sam was not inherently passive. Rather, he had not been given the time and space to explore on his own. Initially he was cautious and checked back with his mother to see if what he was doing was acceptable to her. When her interested but nonintrusive posture signaled her permission, his own developmental agenda rapidly became apparent. We noted that his mother positioned herself to make it difficult for her to intrude in his play. It often happens that at some level mothers who tend to be overly active and intrusive seem to sense the necessary position they must adopt in order to avoid becoming intrusive when asked to follow their infant and not initiate activity.

The earlier practice of Watch, Wait, and Wonder focused primarily on the infant-led play. In the 1980s, Muir, Stupples, and Guy (1989) developed a modification of this earlier approach by dividing the sessions into two parts. The first part of the session was the infant-led activity. The second part involved an essentially psychotherapeutic discussion of the mother's observations and experiences of her infant's activity. It is this adaptation of Watch, Wait, and Wonder that we have continued to develop and research in Toronto (Muir et al., 1999). The modification to include a discussion was stimulated by the realization that mothers often became extremely anxious when asked to follow their infant's lead. The discussion was intended to address this anxiety. During the discussion, the therapist asks the mother to describe what she observed, to talk about what she imagines her infant's experience was during the play and what she thinks his play was about, and to discuss her own thoughts and feelings. The therapist does not instruct, give advice, or interpret the infant's activity or play but rather provides a safe, supportive environment, that is, a sensitive and responsive environment, so that the mother can express her own observations, thoughts, feelings, and interpretations of her infant's activity and their relationship. The mother and the therapist discuss the mother's observations of her infant's activity and attempt to understand the themes and relational issues that the infant is trying to master, focusing on the inevitable problems that emerge as the mother begins to struggle with following her infant's lead. Uncomfortable or painful experiences are raised, whether directly or indirectly, by the mother when she makes her observations or describes how she feels. Here the therapist helps the mother to focus on what made it difficult for her to stay with her infant's activity. Through exploring and working through her uncomfortable or puzzling feelings, the mother gradually disentangles her own and her infant's feelings and experiences, enabling her to recognize what her infant represents in her internal world. This frees her to differentiate her infant's needs from her own and to see him more clearly, that is, less distorted by her own representations. Through play she comes to see her infant in his own right. This encourages his exploration, autonomy, and differentiated sense of self. As a result, the mother and the infant are presumed to respectively modify or to revise their working models to be more in line with their new mutual experiences together in therapy. This permits the mother to examine her internal working models of herself in relation to her infant and vice versa.

THERAPIST: So, what did you observe?

MRS. G.: (*tentatively*) Well, Sam did seem to play a little bit today. He's so quiet.

THERAPIST: Can you say a bit more about that?

MRS. G.: Well, I was a little nervous at first and thought this isn't going to be any different. He didn't seem sure what to do and at the beginning just sat there for the longest time.

THERAPIST: What was that like for you?

MRS. G.: Like I said, I was nervous. It was hard for me not to jump in and try to get him to play. But I remembered what you told me, the watch, wait, and wonder thing, so I held myself back. Then he started playing and I was sort of surprised.

THERAPIST: Surprised?

MRS. G.: Last time we played here Sam just sat there and didn't play, just like at home. I really tried to get him to play. So I didn't think it would be any different today.

THERAPIST: What do you imagine it was like for Sam?

MRS. G.: (*laughing softly*) He looked at me a few times, like what are you doing?

THERAPIST: What do you make of that?

MRS. G.: Well,'cause a lot of the time I try so hard to get him to play. I realized that maybe I don't give him a chance. He's so different from Tony [her other son] and when I look at Sam it's hard not to compare them.

It is important to emphasize that the primary work is experiential and takes place in the infant-led component. The goal of the discussion is to enable the mother to become better at following her infant's lead and immersing herself in her infant's life so that she can respond to his spontaneous gestures. Her observations are enhanced by her understanding of her relationship with her infant. Since this is not easy, it may take some time before the mother is finally able to observe her infant's behavior without becoming anxious. In this second example, it took many weeks for the mother of a 14-month-old boy to understand the intent of her child's play.

> Brian goes over to the beanbag chair and lies in it. He looks at his mother, then whines a little. His mother assumes that he needs a diaper change and picks him up to change him but finds that he doesn't need a diaper change. The following week he goes to the beanbag chair again and falls into it. He turns and gives his mother a look.

In the discussion, the mother says the following:

> "He really likes that beanbag chair . . . and he was looking at me like . . . almost like . . . 'Are you jealous?' "

The therapist had observed this interaction but had a different interpretation, which was that Brian wanted his mother to join him on the beanbag
chair. However, the therapist (with some difficulty) did not contradict the
mother's experience by offering an alternate interpretation. This play went
on for two more weeks. In the third session after this, the mother was talking more warmly about Brian and what they do at home.

MOTHER: He just loves to crawl up on the bed and just cuddle up with you
and fall into the duvet. (*After a brief pause she turns to the beanbag
chair, touches it.*) It's very similar . . . you know! (*She looks at the therapist.*)

THERAPIST: Oh, so maybe that's it? . . .

MOTHER: Yeah, that might be that . . . I never thought of that before!

THERAPIST: So maybe rather than just a kind of smug "Look! See!" that
might have been an invitation for you to join him [in the beanbag
chair].

MOTHER: Yeah! Yeah!

Not long after this session, Brian's mother, who had complained from
the start about Brian not wanting to cuddle, observes how cuddly he has
become.

The discussion segment of Watch, Wait, and Wonder is also an opportunity for some mothers to make links between the past and present and to
explore with the therapist intergenerational influences on parenting behavior, although this is not essential. The strongest difficulties for the therapist
occur around this issue, as was the case with Brian and his mother. Therapists are actively trained to help patients and, for many, simply being with
the dyad while they sort things out is experienced as doing very little. When
we feel uncertain about the dyad's capacity to work things through on their
own, we are bound to get busy and clever with suggestions and interpretations. Transference issues in relation to the therapist that are central in
other psychodynamic psychotherapies (e.g., Fraiberg et al., 1987) do
emerge in Watch, Wait, and Wonder. In Watch, Wait, and Wonder, although the transference is addressed, it is examined primarily with respect
to how it impacts on the interaction of the mother with her infant and how
it influences her capacity to follow her infant's activity.

RESEARCH ON WATCH, WAIT, AND WONDER

Until recently the outcome of Watch, Wait, and Wonder had not been
tested empirically. In fact, there have been relatively few studies of any psy-

chotherapeutic interventions with clinical infant populations generally or that have contrasted and compared different models of therapy that might help to elucidate applied and theoretical issues in infant–parent psychotherapy (Cohen et al., 1999; Cramer et al., 1990; DeGangi & Greenspan, 1997; Robert-Tissot et al., 1996). There has been one empirical study of Watch, Wait, and Wonder (Cohen et al., 1999) which has shown that this approach has more salutary outcomes than a psychodynamic psychotherapy (Cohen et al., 1999) similar in form to that used by Fraiberg et al. (1983) and more recently by Lieberman et al. (1991) and Cramer et al. (1990).

The recently published findings of the Cohen et al. (1999) study showed change in a range of behaviors in both infants and their mothers, many of which were predicted from attachment theory (Cohen et al., 1999; Cohen, Lojkasek, Muir, Muir, & Parker, 2002). The 58 10- to 30-month-old infants who participated in this study were primarily referred for problems manifested as functional symptoms in the infant or in behavioral or emotional regulation. In some other cases, referral was triggered by factors that impeded the mother's capacity for infant care, such as feelings of failure in the attachment process or maternal depression. In a few cases there was risk or allegations of abuse. Problems were long-standing, beginning in the infant's earliest months of life. Assessments were done before treatment began (pretreatment), at the end of treatment (posttreatment), and 6 months after treatment ended (follow-up).

At the end of the relatively brief treatment (averaging 14 sessions over approximately 5 months), we found that both psychotherapeutic interventions had positive effects on infants and their mothers. Specifically, at the end of treatment both forms of psychotherapy resulted in reducing infants' presenting problems, increasing mothers' confidence that they could manage these problems, and decreasing stress associated with parenting. As well, at the end of treatment mothers were observed to be less intrusive and to engage in less conflict with their infants in infant–mother play interactions. In many respects the results of this study were similar to those observed with other clinical and at-risk infant samples, particularly with regard to reduction of presenting problems, more sensitively responsive and harmonious infant–mother interactions, and lower stress and increased positive attitudes toward parenting (Cramer et al., 1990; DeGangi & Greenspan, 1997; Lieberman et al., 1991). This suggests some common salutary effects of treatment regardless of technique.

At the same time, we found differential treatment effects. In particular, infants in the Watch, Wait, and Wonder group were more likely to shift toward a more organized or secure attachment relationship than infants in the group whose mothers had psychodynamic psychotherapy. The infants in the Watch, Wait, and Wonder group also showed greater improvements in cognitive development and increased capacity to regulate their own emotions and behavior in order to engage in cognitive tasks. Although we do not know whether improvement in cognitive functioning resulted from increases in attachment security or organization, attachment theory does suggest that improved cognitive developmental functioning should be an outcome of increased attachment security. This variable has not been included in most studies of psychotherapeutic interventions, but obviously should be in future investigations. Moreover, at the end of treatment, mothers of children in the Watch, Wait, and Wonder group were significantly less depressed and reported more satisfaction and efficacy in parenting than mothers in the group receiving psychodynamic psychotherapy. The differential treatment effects that we observed cannot be attributed to differences in the quality of the therapeutic relationship because mothers' ratings of their therapeutic relationship with their therapist were not related to the type of therapy received.

When followed up 6 months later, effects of both psychotherapeutic interventions on presenting complaints and maternal and child functioning were maintained (Cohen et al., 2002). Moreover, in some respects, further gains were observed after treatment ended in that, at follow-up, there was continued improvement in infant symptoms and observational measures of maternal intrusiveness and dyadic reciprocity. Although this general conclusion applied to both treatment groups, the pathway for change for the two treatments had a different timeline. As reported above, greater gains were made from the beginning to the end of treatment in the Watch, Wait, and Wonder group than in the psychodynamic psychotherapy group on measures of infant attachment security, emotion regulation, and cognition and on maternal depression and parenting confidence. In the dyads receiving psychodynamic psychotherapy, these gains were also observed but not until the follow-up assessment was done 6 months after treatment ended. At the same time, an advantage persisted in the Watch, Wait, and Wonder group from the end of treatment to 6-month follow-up in that mothers in this group reported a further increase in comfort in dealing with the infant problems that brought them to treatment and a further decrease in their ratings of parenting stress.

What might account for the different timeline for changes to appear in the two treatments? In trying to understand this, we return to attachment theory. We think that Watch, Wait, and Wonder maximizes the requirements for forming a secure attachment relationship. The instructions to the mother to allow her infant to take the lead increase maternal sensitive responsiveness and make the mother uniquely physically accessible to her infant, creating the potential for a secure connection. Due to the need to find a way to establish a more secure relationship with the mother, when left to his own devices the infant will inevitably approach her. We have observed that at this point the infant will quickly bring forward the core issues in his relationship with his mother into the play situation, for example, the infant's desire for closeness when physical accessibility was previously restricted. Watch, Wait, and Wonder involves enhancing the mother's capacity to respond to the infant's initiations with a reciprocal gesture, by placing her in a nonintrusive stance that allows for the evolution of the infant's potentialities or "true self" (Winnicott, 1976). We speculate that when the mother observes her child without being able to intrude, her assumptions (representations) of herself, her infant, and her relationship with the infant are challenged. More importantly, the interaction will *feel* different and more pleasurable. Since as part of the process the mother begins to feel more competent in reading her infant's cues, she gains confidence to work things out with her infant on their own, resulting in enhanced confidence as a caregiver. Thus, it is the involving of the infant directly and the mother's nonintrusiveness that might account for the difference between Watch, Wait, and Wonder and the more traditional psychodynamic psychotherapy. Although the infant is involved in psychodynamic psychotherapy, the primary focus is on the mother's representations and her transference relationship with the therapist. This focus may delay changes because the mother needs to work through her earlier relationships before her new insights can influence the relationship with her own infant (see Goldfried & Wolfe, 1998, and Seligman, 1995, for work on the uncovering process in adults).

The therapist in Watch, Wait, and Wonder engages in a parallel process of watching, waiting, and wondering, that is, he or she does not intervene by modeling or directing for the mother or interpreting the infant's activity. Due to this, and to the expectation that the mother observe her infant's activity, she is enabled to become more knowledgeable about her own infant and not feel the same need to rely on the knowledge of the therapeutic "expert." At another level, working with her own observations allows the mother to reflect on her infant's inner experience or, in other words, to develop a reflective capacity (Fonagy, Steele, Steele, Moran, & Higgitt, 1991). It also allows her to work through those anxieties that are aroused while trying to follow her infant's lead, which are often manifested in her difficulties in being sensitive and responsive to her infant's emotional cues.

It is also important to take a closer look at the differential timing of the treatments on maternal depression in light of research that attests to the impact of continuing maternal depression on attachment (Egeland & Sroufe, 1981) and infant cognitive and language development (Murray, Hipwell, Hooper, Stein, & Cooper, 1996; NICHD Early Child Care Research Network, 1999). Many mothers who are depressed try to compensate for their lack of feeling connected with their infants by becoming falsely bright and overly active in engaging with them. In Watch, Wait, and Wonder the mother is relieved of having to take sole responsibility for the interaction. She comes to understand that she does not have to work so hard at the interactive level since the initiating infant is an active and stimulating contributor himself. In turn, the infant has the possibility of developing a sense of efficacy and mastery by impacting on the relationship with the mother. In these several ways, Watch, Wait, and Wonder would seem to reinforce in the mother a sense of competence and enjoyment in mothering and this may contribute to the lower levels of maternal depression in the Watch, Wait, and Wonder group. In line with this, it has been shown that mothers assessed as depressed were less depressed after an intervention that improved their feelings about their relationship with their infant (Murray & Cooper, 1994). It is possible that the relatively rapid decrease in maternal depression in the mothers in the Watch, Wait, and Wonder group will further buffer their children from mental health problems and improve their opportunities for developing a more secure attachment by reducing the risks associated with insecurity.

Stern (1995) suggests that there are a number of "ports of entry" into addressing relationship problems, for example, the overt infant–parent interactional behavior or parent representations. We recognize that both treatments that we studied aim to improve maternal sensitive responsiveness, but each approached this in a different way, and that both were successful. Thus, "all roads lead to Rome" (Stern, 1995), but taking some roads takes less time than others.

REFERENCES

Benoit, D., Zeanah, C. H., Boucher, C., & Minde, K. K. (1992). Sleep disorders in early childhood: Association with insecure maternal attachment. *Journal of the American Academy of Child and Adolescent Psychiatry, 31,* 86–93.

Bowlby, J. (1980). *Attachment and Loss: Vol. III. Loss: Sadness and depression.* New York: Basic Books.

Bowlby, J. (1988). *A secure base: Parent–child attachment and healthy human development.* New York: Basic Books.

Cassidy, J. (1994). Emotion regulation: Influences of attachment relationships. In N. A. Fox (Ed.), The development of emotion regulation. *Monographs of the Society for Research in Child Development, 59*(2–3, Serial No. 240), 228–249.

Cicchetti, D., Toth, S. L., & Rogosch, F. A. (1999). The efficacy of toddler–parent psychotherapy to increase attachment security in offspring of depressed mothers. *Attachment and Human Development, 1,* 34–66.

Cohen, N. J., Lojkasek, M., Muir, E., Muir, R., & Parker, C. J. (2002). Six month follow-up of two mother–infant psychotherapies: Convergence of therapeutic outcomes. *Infant Mental Health Journal, 23,* 361–380.

Cohen, N. J., Muir, E., Lojkasek, M., Muir, R., Parker, C. J., Barwick, M., & Brown, M. (1999). Watch, Wait, and Wonder: Testing the effectiveness of a new approach to mother–infant psychotherapy. *Infant Mental Health Journal, 20,* 429–451.

Cramer, B., Robert-Tissot, C., Stern, D. D., Serpa-Rusconi, S., De Muralt, G. B., Palacio-Espasa, F., Bachman, J., Knauer, D., Berney, C., & D'Arcis, U. (1990).

Outcome evaluation in brief mother–infant psychotherapy: A preliminary report. *Infant Mental Health Journal, 11,* 278–300.

DeGangi, G. A., & Greenspan, S. T. (1997). The effectiveness of short-term interventions in the treatment of inattention and irritability in toddlers. *Journal of Developmental and Learning Disorders, 1,* 277–298.

Egeland, B., & Sroufe, L. A. (1981). Attachment and early maltreatment in infancy. *Child Development, 52,* 44–52.

Fonagy, P., Steele, M., Steele, H., Moran, G. S., & Higgitt, A. C. (1991). The capacity for understanding mental status: The reflective self in parent and child and its significance for security of attachment. *Infant Mental Health Journal, 12,* 201–218.

Fraiberg, S., Adelson, E., & Shapiro, V. (1987). Ghosts in the nursery: A psychoanalytic approach to the problems of impaired infant–mother relationships. In S. Fraiberg (Ed.), *Selected writings of Selma Fraiberg* (pp. 100–136). Columbus: Ohio State University Press.

Fraiberg, S., Shapiro, V., & Cherniss, D. (1983). Treatment modalities. In J. D. Call, E. Galenson, & R. L. Tyson (Eds.), *Frontiers of infant psychiatry* (pp. 56–73). New York: Basic Books.

Goldberg, S. (2000). *Attachment and development.* London: Arnold.

Goldfried, M. R., & Wolfe, B. E. (1998). Toward a more clinically valid approach to therapy research. *Journal of Consulting and Clinical Psychology, 66,* 143–150.

Lieberman, A. F., Weston, D. R., & Pawl, J. H. (1991). Preventive intervention and outcome with anxiously attached dyads. *Child Development, 62,* 199–209.

Lojkasek, M., Cohen, N. J., & Muir, E. (1994). Where is the infant in infant intervention?: A review of the literature on changing troubled mother–infant relationships. *Psychotherapy: Theory, Research, and Practice, 31,* 208–220.

McDonough, S. (1992). *Interactional Guidance Manual.* Unpublished manuscript, Brown University, Providence, RI.

Menzies, I. (1975). Thoughts on the maternal role in contemporary society. *Journal of Child Psychotherapy, 4,* 5–14.

Muir, E. (1992). Watching, waiting, and wondering: Applying psychoanalytic principals to mother–infant intervention. *Infant Mental Health Journal, 13,* 319–328.

Muir, E., Lojkasek, M., & Cohen, N. (1999). *Watch, Wait, and Wonder: A manual describing a dyadic infant-led approach to problems in infancy and early childhood.* Toronto, ON: Hincks-Dellcrest Institute.

Muir, E., Lojkasek, M., & Cohen, N. (2000). Observing mothers observing their infants: An infant observation approach to early intervention. *PRISME, 31,* 154–170.

Muir, E., Stupples, A., & Guy, A. D. (1989). *Mother–toddler psychotherapy and change in patterns of attachment: Some pilot observations.* Unpublished manuscript, Child and Family Section, Department of Psychological Medicine, Otago University, Dunedin, NZ.

Muir, E., & Thorlaksdottir, E. (1994). Psychotherapeutic intervention with mothers and children in daycare. *American Journal of Orthopsychiatry, 64*(1), 60–67.

Murray, L., & Cooper, P. J. (1994). Clinical applications of attachment theory and research: Change in infant attachment with brief psychotherapy. In J. Richer (Ed.), *The clinical application of ethology and attachment theory* (pp. 15–24). Occasional papers no. 9. London: Association for Child Psychology and Psychiatry.

Murray, L., Hipwell, A., Hooper, R., Stein, A., & Cooper, P. (1996). The cognitive development of 5–year-old children of postnatally depressed mothers. *Journal of Child Psychology and Psychiatry, 37,* 927–935.

NICHD Early Child Care Research Network. (1999). Chronicity of maternal depressive symptoms, maternal sensitivity, and child functioning at 36 months. *Developmental Psychology, 35,* 1297–1310.

Notman, M., & Lester, E. P. (1988). Pregnancy: Theoretical considerations. *Psychoanalytic Inquiry, 8,* 139–159.

Robert-Tissot, C., Cramer, B., Stern, D. N., Serpa-Rusconi, S., Bachmann, J.-P, Palacio-Espasa, F., Knauer, D., De Muralt, M., Berney, C., & Mendiguren, G. (1996). Outcome evaluation in brief mother–infant psychotherapies: Report on 75 cases. *Infant Mental Health Journal, 17,* 97–114.

Seligman, M. E. P. (1995). The effectiveness of psychotherapy: The Consumer Reports Study. *American Psychologist, 50,* 965–974.

Stern, D. N. (1995). *The motherhood constellation: A unified view of parent–infant psychotherapy.* New York: Basic Books.

Thompson, R. A. (1999). Early attachment and later development. In J. Cassidy & P. R. Shaver (Eds.), *Handbook of attachment* (pp. 265–286). New York: Guilford Press.

van IJzendoorn, M. H. (1995). Adult attachment representations, parental responsiveness, and infant attachment: A meta-analysis on the predictive validity of the Adult Attachment Interview. *Psychological Bulletin, 177,* 387–403.

van IJzendoorn, M. H., Schuengel, C., & Bakermans-Kranenburg, M. J. (1999). Disorganized attachment in early childhood: Meta-analyses of precursors, concomitants, and sequelae. *Development and Psychopathology, 11,* 225–249.

Wesner, D., Dowling, J., & Johnson, F. (1962). What is maternal–infant intervention?: The role of infant psychotherapy. *Psychiatry, 45,* 307–315.

Winnicott, D. W. (1976). The capacity to be alone. In D. R. Winnicott (Ed.), *The maturational processes and the facilitative environment* (pp. 29–36). London: Hogarth Press.

12

The Journey of Adolescence
*Transitions in Self within the Context
of Attachment Relationships*

MARLENE M. MORETTI
ROY HOLLAND

> No variables, it can be held, have more far-reaching effects
> on personality development than have a child's experiences
> within his family: for, starting during the first months in his
> relation with his mother figure, and extending through the
> years of childhood and adolescence in his relations with
> both parents, he builds up working models of how
> attachment figures are likely to behave towards him in any
> of a variety of situations; and on those models are based all
> his expectations, and therefore all his plans, for the rest of
> his life.
>
> —BOWLBY (1973, p. 418)

Bowlby's theory of attachment has had a profound effect on how we understand the development of infants and young children, and, more recently, it has elucidated our understanding of adult romantic relationships (Shaver & Hazan, 1993). In contrast to these areas of investigation, the developmental period of adolescence has been relatively ignored by attachment researchers. Yet adolescence offers important opportunities to study the significance of attachment security over the course of important personal and social transitions. In the psychological literature, adolescence is commonly viewed as a period of identity crystallization, where childhood tendencies and proclivities become consolidated and deepened into an enduring internal sense of selfhood. Adolescence is the "developmental bridge" between childhood and adulthood, when children move from dependency to autonomy and from bonds shared primarily with family to bonds shared with close friends and intimate partners. Changes in the complexity of representational thought during adolescence allow for a richer understanding of social relationships. The sphere of important social relations broadens to include peers, school and work colleagues, and romantic partners. Bonds within the family must be balanced and reorganized to accommodate new significant relationships and social roles.

The complex changes of the adolescent period offer new opportunities and challenges for youth and their families. This period of transition can provide new avenues for parents and children to transform their relationships with each other and, in turn, their personal sense of selfhood. For many reasons, however, parents and children frequently struggle with this transition. Too often opportunities for the development of autonomy, balanced with connectedness to family, are lost and adolescents fail to establish a sense of self that is differentiated yet connected with family. Dysfunctional dependence or detachment is the result. In this chapter we discuss the transformation of self during adolescence and the role of social context and social-cognitive shifts that underlie this process. We use the term *self* to refer to the *self system*, an internal regulatory system that is based on relational experiences which over time become consolidated into internal representations of self and other (Moretti & Higgins, 1999a). The self system exists in a dynamic relationship within one's ecology, shaping and being shaped by interpersonal experiences. We emphasize that adolescent–parent attachment is the central interpersonal context in which self-development unfolds and is a significant determinant of adolescent adjustment. Attachment theory provides a theoretical structure for organizing systemic interventions for troubled adolescents and their families. Case examples are provided and attachment-based programs for high-risk adolescents and their families are described.

THE JOURNEY OF ADOLESCENCE: INTEGRATING MULTIPLE PERSPECTIVES ON THE SELF

The emergence of the self system is not restricted to any particular developmental period, but stretches across the lifespan. Adolescence, however, represents an important period of transition. Two factors underlie the transformation of the self system during adolescence: (1) rapid changes in social roles and interpersonal contexts; and (2) shifts in the capacity for representational thought and self-reflection. The social contexts in which adolescents function gradually broaden from late childhood to early adulthood

(Buhrmester & Furman, 1987; Selman, 1980). In most cultures, adolescence is recognized as a period of transition in personal bonds that involves broadening the scope of significant relationships and personal ties. In North American culture the period of adolescence is marked by dramatic decreases in the amount of time that youth spend with parents relative to peers. Time spent with family drops from 35% to 14% of waking hours between late childhood and midadolescence (Larson, Richards, Moneta, & Holmbeck, 1996). By grade 12—around the age of 17—the majority of adolescents spend more time with their peers than with their parents. They rely increasingly on peers for intimacy and support, although this does not displace the role of parents as important confidants (Furman & Buhrmester, 1992; Laursen & Williams, 1997; Levitt, Guacci-Franco & Levitt, 1993; Trinke & Bartholomew, 1997).

New social roles beyond the family also include first-time employment and romantic relationships. Most adolescents enter the work force at age 15 or 16 and many are employed for 15 to 20 hours per week (Bachman & Schulenberg, 1993; Greenberger & Steinberg, 1986). In North American society, adolescents typically exert some degree of control over how they spend their own income. Their employment status attenuates their financial dependence on family and alters their social identity by virtue of endowing them with the status of consumers. Dating relationships begin in early adolescence—around age 13 for girls, age 14 for boys (McCabe, 1984)—although it is not until late adolescence that these relationships are characterized by genuine intimacy and deep emotional involvement (Douvan & Adelson, 1966).

Importantly, social role changes occur in conjunction with developmental shifts in metacognitive and representational capacity from early to late adolescence (Case, 1985; Chalmers & Lawrence, 1993; Selman, 1980) and promote a more differentiated and complex view of self and others (Harter, 1990; Marsh, 1989; Moretti & Higgins, 1999a, 1999b). As children move into adolescence (13–16 years of age), they develop the capacity to simultaneously consider several perspectives on multiple attributes (Case, 1985; Selman & Byrne, 1974). One consequence of this cognitive shift is that adolescents form increasingly abstract and differentiated perceptions of themselves and others. They begin to simultaneously compare their evaluation of their own attributes with the evaluations that they believe several others hold of them (e.g., parents, peers, romantic partner), and the standards that they infer are important to them. This level of cognitive sophistication allows adolescents to consider the relation of actual-self attributes with several standards or self-guides (e.g., their own standards for the self; the inferred standards of each parent, peer standards, cultural norms), and to consider the relation of various self-guides to each other. Furthermore, adolescents can speculate about the self-representational structure of others: the type of attributes that others possess, would like to possess, and so on. The capacity of adolescents to represent complex self–

other scenarios provides them with the opportunity to imagine and act out alternative personas and to imagine being in different types of relationships.

As they move through adolescence, youth are increasingly concerned with the views that others hold of them, particularly their peers and romantic partners. They are strongly motivated to gain the acceptance of peers and may attempt to do so by presenting themselves "falsely." That is, they may present themselves as possessing attributes or beliefs that are not their own but are designed to impress others or to conceal attributes they feel are not accepted by others (Harter, Marold, Whitesell, & Cobbs, 1996).

Elkind (1967) proposed that the cognitive shifts that occur in adolescence result in a form of adolescent "egocentrism" in which the adolescent is overwhelmed by the sense that he or she is the focus of everyone's attention, coupled with the belief that his or her experiences are essentially unique. The capacity of adolescents to simultaneously consider multiple perspectives on the self, in concert with rapid transition in their social roles and relationships, provokes a period of intense self-preoccupation and pressure to consolidate a sense of self. Adolescents have new opportunities for experiencing the self in relation to others, and thus can better adjust to a range of social contexts. However, they are also more likely to experience discrepancy among the diverse ways that they experience self. Thus, adolescents may suffer because they are now able to perceive that who they are (i.e., the actual self) is incongruent with who they themselves wish to be (own standards), who they believe their parents wish them to be (parental standards), and who they believe their peers wish them to be (peer standards). The challenge of adolescence lies in integrating multiple views of the self that emerge from these varied and often conflicting social contexts (e.g., family, peer, romantic, work contexts).

Although the capacity to think about the self from multiple perspectives grows from early to midadolescence, the ability to integrate divergent views remains limited. It is not until late adolescence that seemingly contradictory aspects of the self can be incorporated (Harter & Monsour, 1992; Harter, Bresnick, Bouchey, & Whitesell, 1997). It is likely that a capacity to integrate divergent perspectives on others (e.g., parents, peers) follows a similar developmental trajectory. From early to midadolescence it may be difficult for youth to integrate opposing impressions or views of others. Only later in development can seemingly divergent characteristics of others be integrated and understood as part of the complexity of personality.

DIFFERENTIATION OF PERSONAL VERSUS PARENTAL STANDARDS FOR THE SELF DURING ADOLESCENCE

In parallel with changes in social relationships and representational capacity, adolescents transform their internal regulatory system in terms of (1) the degree to which they share standards or goals for the self with significant others (e.g., parents and peers), and (2) the psychological consequence of congruence or discrepancy between how adolescents view themselves and these standards or goals. Our research in this field is based on an extension of self-discrepancy theory (Moretti & Higgins, 1999a, 1999b; Moretti & Wiebe, 1999). This model of self-regulation assumes that internal representations of self are organized along two dimensions: domains of self-representation (i.e., the actual self, the ideal self, and the ought self) and standpoints on self-representation (i.e., one's own standpoint vs. the inferred standpoints of significant others). Together these self-state representations form a dynamic self-regulatory system that guides motivation and emotion. Self-state representations that include our hopes and wishes for self, or our sense of duty and obligation, provide important standards, or self-guides, that regulate emotion and behavior.

Our research has investigated developmental shifts in the differentiation of adolescents' standards for themselves from the standards that they believe their parents hold for them. In other words, we are interested in whether adolescents and parents change in how much they agree on the standards that adolescents should strive for and the goals that are important for them to achieve. In a study of high school students in grades nine to 12, we found that only 25% of the standards that adolescents believe parents hold for them are adopted as standards for themselves (Moretti & Wiebe, 1999). The remaining 75% of parental standards for the self were exactly that: parental standards that adolescents recognized but did not necessarily share for the self. These standards are not completely adopted as one's own but remain the "felt presence" of others in the self (Blatt & Behrends, 1987; Schafer, 1968). Thus, at this point in development, adolescents and their parents have only a limited "shared reality" (Moretti & Higgins, 1999a) about the adolescent's identity. It is not surprising, then, that many adolescents and their parents feel as if they live in "different worlds"; "different worlds" that involve the adolescent evolving into a person who may be different from what his or her parents wishes or hopes. These sentiments were aptly captured in one adolescent girl's description of her relationship with her mother: "We are like two people meeting from opposite ends of the world who don't know each other."

The question, then, is whether or not adolescents will indeed adopt parental standards, or a subset of these standards, as they move toward consolidation of their own identities. Needless to say, this process can engender considerable anxiety in both adolescents and their parents as adolescents work through which self-regulatory standards and guides will be accepted and which will not. Consistent with the view that adolescent identity begins to consolidate in early adulthood, our research shows substantially greater overlap between standards for the self and parental standards in early adulthood as compared to adolescence. In a study of undergraduate university students around 25 years of age, we found that 40% of the standards that young adults believed their parents held for them were adopted as their own standards (Moretti & Higgins, 1999b). Thus, although not all parental standards for the self come to be adopted by young adults, results show a greater "shared reality" between parents and young adults about identity.

Our next question focused on the psychological consequence of congruence or discrepancy between how adolescents view themselves and their standards or self-guides for the self. Consistent with the bulk of research on self-discrepancy theory (Moretti & Higgins, 1999a), we found that both adolescents and young adults suffered from psychological distress when they perceived their actual self as discrepant from their own standards for self (Moretti & Wiebe, 1999; Moretti & Higgins, 1999b). That is, when youth felt that they failed to live up to who they themselves wished to be or felt they should be, they universally reported distress. Interesting differences between girls and boys, and between younger and older adolescents, were apparent. Girls in midadolescence suffered from distress *regardless of the source of perceived discrepancy*: discrepancy with their own standards, discrepancy from parental standards (regardless of whether they were adopted as their own or not), and discrepancy from peer and romantic partner standards all predicted psychological problems. These results underscore the significant challenges for early to midadolescence girls in consolidating a sense of identity and may explain why rates of depression and other psychological disorders, such as eating disorders, rise dramatically for girls with the onset of adolescence. For late adolescent girls and young adult women, discrepancy with their own standards continued to be a source of distress, as was discrepancy with standards that were shared with parents. Beyond this, however, only discrepancy with maternal standards that were not adopted by daughters was predictive of psychological problems.

In contrast to the results with girls, adolescent boys and young adult men suffered from distress *only* when they perceived discrepancy with their own independent standards for the self. These findings suggest that the process of identity consolidation may be different for girls and boys, with girls' development being more strongly influenced by their interpersonal context and relationships than boys (Cross & Madson, 1997; Jordan, Kaplan, Miller, Stiver, & Surrey, 1991; Moretti, Rein, & Wiebe, 1998). Yet it is too early to conclude that this is the case, as the role of significant others in the development of self in boys and young men may require examining this process through a different lens. From a developmental perspective, it makes sense that significant others play as important a role in the development of boys' as compared to girls' self-representation, although *how* significant others influence self-development may be gender-specific.

WHAT IS UNIQUE ABOUT AN ATTACHMENT
PERSPECTIVE ON ADOLESCENCE?

The model of adolescent self-development that we have sketched thus far mirrors elements of Erikson's (1963, 1968) classic ego development theory. For example, both views share the assumption that identity development involves the differentiation or exploration of values and standards that are important to the self, followed by a period of consolidation. For Erikson (1963), the search for identity serves the function of the consolidation of *fidelity*, an ego strength that can then be brought forward into young adulthood to support intimacy and commitment in sexual relationships and to further procreation. From this perspective, youth need to distinguish themselves from their historical and cultural context and set forth their uniqueness and integrity as a prerequisite for identity consolidation and entrance into adulthood.

An attachment perspective casts the process of adolescent self-development in a unique light. From an attachment perspective, the rapid change in social contexts and relationships coupled with the cognitive shifts in representational capacity create not only a cognitive–emotional dilemma for youth to resolve—that of integrating the diverse and conflicting experiences of the self in different social contexts—but also an attachment dilemma. The attachment dilemma is classic: to maintain a sense of connectedness and a secure base in attachment relationships with parents while simultaneously exploring new ways of experiencing the self and others. As adolescents work toward consolidation of their internal sense of self, so must they work in their close relationships to alter, modify, and renegotiate their place within these relationships and the attachment functions that they serve. This is a transactional process with internal representations influencing experiences within relationships, which in turn shape internal self–other representations of both the adolescent and their significant others. The process of adolescent transition in self-identity is thus nested within the sphere of close interpersonal relationships. The quality of these relationships prior to adolescence will therefore have a profound impact on how this period of development unfolds.

Importantly, from an attachment perspective, the successful transition of adolescence does not assume that youth detach themselves from their parents (Lamborn & Steinberg, 1993; Ryan, Deci, & Grolnick, 1995). *In fact, the transition to autonomy and adulthood is facilitated by secure attachment and emotional connectedness with parents* (Ryan & Lynch, 1989). This is important because it emphasizes that connection (secure attachment) and separation (autonomy) are two sides of the same attachment coin. In the same way that attachment security fosters exploration and the development of new competencies for toddlers, so too does it facilitate development of autonomy in adolescents.

What is most critical to youth during this period is the enduring availability and responsivity of parents in providing a secure base and a safe haven while simultaneously entering into a process of identity negotiation and relationship transition that inherently involves conflict. Thus, from an attachment perspective, the transition of adolescence simultaneously involves sustaining connectedness while moving toward individuation. Adolescents who feel secure in the availability and empathy of their parents, despite the conflict that is inherent in this development phase, can confidently move forward in exploring their own identity and the meaning of their emerging identity in terms of their relationship with their parents. These adolescents do not avoid exploration and individuation, nor do they force independence and form a fragile sense of selfhood in opposition to their parents. Indeed, some researchers have argued that the successful balancing between autonomy and relatedness—particularly in the context of adolescent–parent disagreements—is a stage-specific manifestation of attachment security (Allen, Moore, & Kuperminc, 1997).

Like earlier periods of development, then, the hallmark of security in adolescence is the successful and age-appropriate balancing of autonomy and dependence. Yet the uniqueness of the adolescent period must not be underestimated. What is unique about adolescence is that younger children will rarely, if ever, physically leave their family of their own accord and go off on their own. Many adolescents, in contrast, possess—or believe they possess—sufficient life skills to leave their family and forge ahead in their lives. For many families, adolescence becomes a period of attachment crisis because separation and loss are now a concrete reality that for the first time can be initiated through the efforts of the child. The significance of leaving home was identified by Kobak and his colleagues (Kobak, Ferenz-Gillies, Everhart, & Seabrook, 1994) as provocative of attachment issues, both in adolescents and in their mothers. Although Kobak et al.'s study suggested that leaving home plays a more significant role in adolescent–parent interactions during late rather than midadolescence, this issue arises earlier in families with a history of conflict and disruption. It is also likely to be more provocative for parents who themselves left home at an early age.

There are other implications of an attachment perspective on adolescence. From this viewpoint, adolescence is not viewed as a period of potential personality arrest and distortion, but as a station along a continuous route of development from childhood to adulthood. Experiences within the parent–child relationship up to the point of adolescence form internal representations that guide how this developmental period will be negotiated. Although earlier experiences and the working models that have formed in their aftermath influence the direction in which adolescence is likely to unfold, these experiences are not entirely deterministic. What is critical is the "fit" between parents and children as they move through this period of development and the capacity of each to sustain connectedness and dialogue so that the meaning of past experiences and future directions can be coconstructed.

Adolescence, then, can be a period of continued development along the same path or it can be an opportunity to change course and follow a new direction. Attachment theory offers a rich framework from which to understand the dynamic, transactional relationships between self-development and interpersonal context during adolescence. Given the fact that the transformation of the self in adolescence occurs in the "crucible" of adolescent–parent attachment relationships (Harter, 1999), it is obvious that they are best considered together, within a dynamic framework of mutual influence.

PARENT–ADOLESCENT RELATIONSHIP
QUALITY AND SELF-DEVELOPMENT

What role does the quality of adolescent–parent relationships play in determining the psychological impact of these transitions in the self system? In a recent study (Moretti & McKay, 2000), we examined whether adolescent daughters who perceived their mothers as autonomy-supportive were protected from the negative psychological consequences of perceived discrepancy with their mothers' standards for them. Consistent with our past research, we found that girls who perceived themselves as discrepant from who they believed their mothers wished them to be had lower self-esteem than did girls who perceived themselves as congruent with their mothers' standards for them. Importantly, however, the relationship was moderated by maternal autonomy support. Girls who perceived themselves as discrepant from their mothers' standards for them and who also experienced their mothers as low in autonomy support had the lowest level of self-esteem. In contrast, girls who perceived themselves as discrepant from their mothers' standards for them but experienced their mothers as high in autonomy support had the highest level of self-esteem, higher even than girls who perceived themselves as congruent with their mothers' standards for the self. In other words, differentiation of standards for the self—that is, differences between adolescent girls' and their mothers' desires regarding the shaping of identity—enhanced self-esteem for girls who felt they could embark on this exploration of identity within a relationship where their mothers were supportive of this process. Another way of thinking of these results is that the mother–daughter relationship could tolerate and support differentiation—that is, the relationship provided a secure base for self-exploration.

To summarize, these studies suggest that the process of *differentiation* in self-representation that is the hallmark of adolescence peaks in mid-adolescence, followed by greater *integration* between adolescent and parent perspectives on the self in late adolescence/early adulthood. The results also point to the importance of specific factors within the adolescent–parent relationship—in this case, autonomy support—as moderating or changing the psychological meaning of adolescent–parent discrepancy regarding goals for the self and emerging identity. Thus, even in the context of provocative parent–adolescent disagreement about identity, autonomy support is the crux of ensuring continued emotional connection and support. As one young woman put it, "My mom and I argue about lots of stuff . . . but she respects my opinion and most of my choices, so I know she cares about me no matter what."

Autonomy support is, however, only one component of the attachment relationship between adolescent and parent. Our recent work extends our previous investigations by specifically examining the importance of adolescent–parent attachment in understanding severe emotional and behavioral problems in adolescents. Youth who participated in this research were selected from consecutive referrals to a center designated to provide assessment and intervention to the most severely behaviorally disturbed adolescents in the province of British Columbia, Canada. All youth referred to this facility were involved in significant antisocial and delinquent activity, including aggression and violence toward others (e.g., family, peers, teachers), refusal to follow parental and school rules (e.g., staying out all night, hanging around with delinquent peers, skipping school), and delinquent behavior (e.g., vandalism, theft, drug use). In addition, the majority of youth (particularly girls) suffered from a range of psychiatric disorders (i.e., attention-deficit/hyperactivity disorder, generalized anxiety disorder, posttraumatic stress disorder) as diagnosed through structured interview (Moretti, Reebye, Wiebe, & Lessard, 2002; Reebye, Moretti, Wiebe, & Lessard, 2000). Some adolescents were intermittently suicidal and some had been exploited through prostitution. Chronic exposure to multiple forms of maltreatment of varying degrees was common.

In terms of family relationships, almost half of these adolescents were no longer living with their families on a regular basis. This is not to imply, however, that they were psychologically disconnected from their families. In fact, these adolescents reacted strongly to discussing family issues and to having contact with their parents. Often their interactions were marked by intense conflict, interspersed with aggressive and sometimes violent exchanges. Their feelings ranged from extreme anger and rage to deep despair. Not surprisingly, parents of these adolescents often reported a similar history of conflict and trauma with their own parents; they frequently expressed a deep sense of loss and frustration that they were unable to prevent their own children from having the same experiences that marred their lives. Despite these extremely difficult circumstances, invariably there was an intense desire to continue to maintain connection and to "make things right."

Our research examined attachment patterns and links to psychopathology in these youth using Bartholomew and Horowitz's (1991) family attachment interview. This system identifies four prototypes of attachment—secure, anxious–preoccupied, avoidant–fearful, and dismissing–avoidant—and assumes that individuals rely to varying degrees on strategies that represent each of the prototypes. Dominant patterns are coded by identifying the most frequently used or characteristic attachment strategies. Of the 170 adolescents we assessed, 38% were predominantly avoidant–fearful, 25% were anxious–preoccupied, and 22% were dismissing–avoidant. Only 7% were secure; the remaining 8% of the adolescents could not be coded with a dominant attachment pattern. Attachment patterns differed by gender: although an equal percentage of girls and boys were classified as avoidant-fearful, significantly more girls than boys were classified as anxious-preoccupied and more boys than girls were classified as dismissing–avoidant.

Examination of the relationship between attachment ratings and measures of emotional and behavioral functioning showed that attachment security was associated with significantly less emotional distress and significantly lower levels of engagement in aggressive and delinquent behavior (e.g., theft, threats to hurt others). These results are consistent with how securely attached adolescents describe their ability to cope with difficulties by using parents for support or by relying on their own resources. For example, one adolescent stated: "I can talk to my mom when I'm upset, when she's in the right mood, or I can do other things to feel better like drawing. I like spending time with her when I can." Avoidant–fearful tendencies, on the other hand, were associated with symptoms reflecting painful avoidance coupled with desire for connection—that is, feeling unloved, lonely, depressed, worthless, and suicidal. In their interviews, youth who were high on avoidant–fearfulness often spoke of their family relationships with great despair, as illustrated in the following excerpt: "I'm homesick. I look forward to seeing my parents on visits, but I don't think they miss me because they hate me. They're not proud of me. I don't think they would even miss me if I were dead. I'm not the little girl they wanted."

Anxious–preoccupied tendencies were linked with symptoms of anxiety and to aggressiveness toward others. Frequently adolescents high on anxious–preoccupied tendencies provided idealized portrayals of their family, expressed the desire to be close to others, and described coercive and controlling social behavior. One girl whose father had been charged with abuse described her father as "funny, lovable, and really nice—I wouldn't change anything about him, he's great." She described intense friendships that were often tumultuous, as in the following excerpt: "I really trusted this new girl that I met but I found out she spread rumors about me. . . . I went crazy and beat her up so now it's OK because we're friends." In contrast, dismissing–avoidant tendencies were negatively correlated with youth endorsing items that indicated any form of internalized distress such as depression, anxiety, guilt, unhappiness, or suicidality. These findings are consistent with the presentation of dismissing–avoidant youth in interview.

One boy who was high on dismissingness stated: "I don't really talk to my parents, I don't need them. They're [parents] are just idiots. I just do whatever I want." The dismissing–avoidant adolescents' intellectualized presentation is inconsistent with the extremely difficult circumstances of their lives, which shows in their inability to integrate periods of emotional upset as illustrated by this boy's acknowledgment: "Sometimes I cry by myself . . . I don't know why . . . I don't really feel upset before it happens."

Overall our results are consistent with previous research showing that attachment security is linked with adaptive functioning in adolescence while insecure attachment predicts a broad range of poor psychological outcomes, the nature of which depends on the type of attachment insecurity (Doyle & Moretti, 2001; Doyle, Moretti, Brendgen, & Bukowski, 2001; Kerns & Stevens, 1996; Kobak & Sceery, 1988).

Our examination of the quality of internal self–other representations in these adolescents revealed marked differences in content and structure as compared to adolescents from our normative samples (Moretti & Wiebe, 1999). Not only was the content of self and other (mother and father) representations in troubled adolescents significantly more negative, but these representations were also impoverished. That is, adolescents in our clinical sample had difficulty describing how they saw themselves, how they believed others viewed them, what their own goals were for themselves, and what their parents' or peers' goals were for them. Furthermore, the negativity of self–other representations was a robust predictor, particularly for girls, of multiple forms of aggressive behavior, including relational and overt aggression and assault (Moretti, Holland, & McKay, 2001).

In summary, our research showed that adolescents with severe behavioral problems typically showed insecure attachment patterns in relation to their parents. These adolescents held a fundamental and deep mistrust in the interest and/or capacity of adult caregivers to be available and responsive to their attachment needs. Relative to nonclinical samples, their internal view of self was impoverished and negative. The insecurity of their attachment patterns and the lack of integrated and positive self-representation would make autonomy development extremely challenging.

What can attachment theory offer to guide intervention with these youth and their families? We believe the value of attachment theory lies in making the attachment needs that underlie "problem behavior" visible. These attachment needs are often extremely difficult to decipher in the context of aggressive, threatening, and risk-taking behavior. These behaviors typically become the focus of therapeutic attention because, as mental health professionals and parents, we wish to prevent danger and harm to our children. Rarely do we look at these behaviors as symbolic of unmet attachment needs and as strategies to maintain connectedness, yet protect against anticipated rejection. It is only by understanding and responding to these underlying attachment issues, however, that we can tailor interventions to promote curative attachment experiences and avoid further alienation and detachment.

ATTACHMENT-BASED SYSTEMIC PERSPECTIVES ON INTERVENTION

For many years, clinicians believed that delinquent youth were unresponsive to psychological intervention; in fact, many held the view that "nothing works" and that these youth were doomed to a future of incarceration and marginal functioning (Shamsie, 1981). The development of multimodal systemic interventions has offered hope in altering this developmental trajectory (Moretti, Holland, & Moore, 2002; Henggeler, 1991; Fisher & Chamberlain, 2000; US Department of Health and Human Services, 2001). The efficacy of systemic interventions lies in the appreciation of multiple levels of the ecology that influence child development and adjustment. Intervention strategies can be individually tailored to address a range of factors that have been shown to contribute to problem behavior.

Attachment theory enhances a systemic perspective on intervention because it helps clinicians *understand the unique meaning of disruptive behavior within the context of the child–parent relationship* (Byng-Hall, 1991; Byng-Hall & Stevenson-Hinde, 1991). With this understanding in hand, interventions can be tailored so they fit with the unique set of factors that contribute to problem behavior and with the attachment dynamics that operate in conjunction with these factors. For example, all troubled adolescents that we worked with were oppositional, hostile, and aggressive, yet their displays of aggressive behavior stemmed from different attachment-related sources and strategically functioned in different ways to engage caregivers. The value of attachment theory is illustrated in the following case examples of adolescents who shared similar types of disruptive behavior yet differed in their attachment patterns and the family dynamics associated with these behaviors.

Peter was a sullen but anxious 13-year-old boy. He was oppositional at home, skipped school, and was involved with older peers who used drugs. He sometimes stayed out all night and refused to accept the authority of his parents. Peter had been charged with breaking into a neighbor's home and stealing a number of items. From a diagnostic perspective, he clearly met criteria for conduct disorder.

Peter spoke openly about his disrespect for his stepmother—in his words, she was not his mother so she had no authority to parent him. On the other hand, Peter expressed superficial but unwavering respect for his father. After some probing, Peter revealed that his father "saved" him. When asked what that meant, he disclosed that his father came back for him and got custody when it was discovered that his biological mother was involved in extensive criminal activity. Peter was ambivalent toward his biological mother—although angry toward her for exposing him to abusive experiences and then relinquishing him, Peter harbored the hope that someday she would return for him. Despite his displaced anger toward his stepmother, Peter desperately wanted to remain in the family. He was extremely anxious that he had crossed the line and this time would be kicked out.

Peter had developed a very negative view of himself. He described himself as a "loser"; the few concrete goals he held for himself were highly discrepant from how he viewed himself, leaving little hope that these goals were achievable. The only place Peter felt good about himself was with his peer group; these youth were similar to Peter and he felt accepted by them.

Peter's attachment interview revealed a predominantly avoidant–fearful pattern. Intimacy and closeness were extremely anxiety-provoking for him. He longed for connection with his parents and so wished to be taken care of, yet he feared rejection. His anger and fear of rejection stemmed from his experiences of rejection and neglect by his biological mother. Yet he could not direct these feelings toward her because his connection with her was so tenuous that it could not withstand his rage. Instead his feelings were redirected toward his stepmother, whom he feared but wished to be close to. It was extremely anxiety-provoking for this boy to allow closeness with his stepmother; whenever he experienced more intimacy than he could manage, he would "self-destruct" by acting out in ways that were sure to distance his stepmother and father. On a positive note, he could sometimes accept his father's authority, yet this placed a wedge between his father and stepmother. Peter's father seemed strangely comfortable with this situation, suggesting that he shared his son's distrust of women and fear of commitment because he had also been traumatized in his relationship with Peter's mother.

Attachment theory helped us to understand both Peter's behavior and the family dynamics in which it occurred. Interventions focused on helping Peter's parents understand the attachment issues underlying their son's behavior and supporting their use of structure and consistency in meeting his needs. Peter needed to hear, both verbally and in other ways, that he would not be abandoned even if his behavior was problematic and limits were enforced. This helped to soothe his anxiety and reduce the intensity of his disruptive behavior. Peter's parents benefited from couple therapy that focused on attachment issues that undermined intimacy and trust in their own relationship. This work allowed each parent to forge a more secure relationship with Peter, knowing that neither parent would be displaced through this process. Despite the need for Peter to work through issues of loss and anger in relation to his biological mother, he was not ready to enter into this work. Instead, Peter was able to connect with a childcare worker who offered him empathy and support in his day-to-day struggles. This was useful in providing Peter with guidance around social skill issues, but more importantly it reinforced the notion that adults cared about him and could be trusted for support.

Although Peter's aggressive and delinquent behavior is similar to that of the adolescent in our next case example, Mary, her attachment pattern is distinctive, as are the family dynamics related to her behavior problems.

Mary was the first child born to her parents, both of whom were unable to care for her due to their entrenched drug dependence. Her father disappeared from her life early on and his whereabouts were unknown. Mary's mother attempted to care for her daughter, but at age 4 Mary was placed in a foster home due to concerns of neglect and possible sexual abuse. Mary's mother continued to be involved in her daughter's life and genuinely cared for her daughter, yet she was unable to follow through on her commitments. Her fear of losing her daughter to other caregivers often led her to undermine Mary's development of a connection with new foster parents. Consequently Mary had spiraled through over 25 placements within 10 years.

When Mary first came into contact with our service her behavior was an enigma. She expressed her desire for closeness with her foster mother through peculiar behaviors, including patting, stroking, and hitting her. She often tried to please her stepmother and to be the "perfect" child, only to fall suddenly into a rage and destroy things around her. Mary was extraordinarily sensitive to any behavior that even remotely suggested abandonment or rejection; she became very distraught when separated from her foster mother and would do whatever it took to keep her nearby.

Mary's relationships with her peers were similarly volatile. She was highly dependent on them and developed intense connections quickly. But inevitably she became enraged with them for seemingly minor events and sometimes this led her to assault her peers.

Mary struggled to integrate her experiences of herself and others in her life. Despite her very difficult relationship with her mother and her mother's obvious failure to provide adequate and consistent care, Mary idealized her. She continued to hope that "this time" her mother would come through for her and consequently her pain when her mother failed to follow through was overwhelming. Mary's sense of herself was also fragmented; how she felt about herself was directly a function of how she believed others felt toward her. Therefore, her self-esteem was like a roller coaster, temporarily reaching heights only to plunge quickly into despair.

Mary was characterized by a predominantly anxious–preoccupied attachment pattern. From an attachment standpoint, Mary's extreme dependency and aggressive behavior achieved the same goal: to ensure and maintain intense connectedness with others. Despite this goal, her behavior typically led others to feel overwhelmed by her needs and afraid for their own well-being; consequently they pushed her away. Separation for Mary was unbearable because her sense of self was almost entirely dependent on whomever she was with. Attempts to limit her "attention seeking" and "manipulative" behavior only resulted in escalation until ultimately she secured someone's attention, even if it was only the brief attention that her self-harm behavior brought her in emergency rooms. It was important to work with Mary in a "matter-of-fact" manner and to avoid falling into the struggle and path to rejection that Mary was so familiar with. Offering Mary opportunities to connect with others *before* she became agitated and coercive proved helpful in allowing Mary to experience connection without having to force it upon others. Helping Mary structure her emotional experiences and offering empathy and support for her attempts to establish autonomy were also important. Mary was able to accept empathic reflections from her caregivers about how frightening it was to feel alone, and over time she became more comfortable spending small amounts of time by herself, trusting that her caregivers would not disappear if she relaxed her constant monitoring and attempts to control their behavior.

Our last case example illustrates an attachment pattern that is assumed to be present in most delinquent youth, but that was found to be present in less than 25% of adolescents we assessed. The defining quality of this attachment pattern is the profound deactivation of the attachment system.

Paul seemed unperturbed by his separation from his family. From his point of view he could not understand why his parents and teachers were so "bent out of shape" by his behavior. Paul openly admitted to involvement in drug trafficking. He didn't think it was such a big deal and viewed it as a reasonable way to make a few bucks. Paul had been charged with assault. He explained that it was not his fault—the kid he beat up was just in the wrong place at the wrong time and should have known better.

Paul described life in his family as fairly chaotic. From an early age he had to fend for himself because his parents were either not around or they were too "wasted" to be of much good. Yet Paul did not think his childhood was that bad; he displayed no direct feelings of anger toward his parents except for cool and distant irritation. He talked about very disturbing events as if they were happening to someone else. Paul stated that he was able to take care of himself. He thought he was smart and good-looking, and he wanted to have lots of money and a great car. He claimed to have lots of friends. He thought he was "good" with people and could get them to do pretty much anything he wanted.

Paul showed a classic dismissing–avoidant profile. From an attachment perspective, Paul had worked hard to ensure that he would no longer have to rely on his parents for his physical or emotional well-being. In doing so, he also learned to close the door to others and to his own emotional life. It was important for us to respect Paul's fragile sense of competence while at the same time offering him tolerable doses of empathy and demonstrating our usefulness to him. Initially, Paul could only accept that staff were useful in getting things he wanted, yet over time he began to develop interest in others as mentors from whom he could learn new skills. Paul was always careful to limit his feelings of dependency, but he was gradually able to feel that others could be interesting and valuable additions to his rather barren psychological life.

Interestingly, our experience parallels the observations of Holmes (1997) who noted that therapists working with avoidant clients (avoidant–fearful and dismissing–avoidant) are likely to experience a sense of disengagement and rejection. In contrast, those working with anxious–preoccupied clients typically feel stifled, overwhelmed, and coerced into taking on more and more of their clients' problems. These cases illustrate that even though these youth shared a diagnosis of conduct disorder and equally engaged in aggressive and delinquent behavior, they differed in ways that are relevant to developing a therapeutic plan. By focusing only on the behavior problems that defined these adolescents, we would have missed the issues of most relevance to treatment. Their unique attachment issues required appropriately tailored interventions. For example, both the avoidant–fearful and the anxious–preoccupied adolescent require an empathic and supportive approach. However, too much empathy, too quickly, overwhelms the avoidant–fearful adolescent. In contrast, not enough proactive engagement leads to abandonment anxiety in the anxious–preoccupied adolescent and can increase acting-out behavior designed to aggressively provoke engagement by others. The dismissing–avoidant youth, on the other hand, requires that others prove their "value" in concrete terms as a prerequisite for any relationship building whatsoever and that their fragile sense of self-competence be supported and respected.

By understanding the unique attachment issues underlying the behavior problems of these youth, systemic interventions can be tailored to enhance their effectiveness. In British Columbia, two programs have been developed for high-risk youth based on attachment theory: the Response Program (Holland, Moretti, Verlaan, & Peterson, 1993; Moretti et al., 1997; Moretti et al., 2002; Moretti, Holland, & Peterson, 1994) and the Orinoco Program (Moore, Moretti, & Holland, 1998). The Response Program provides a comprehensive evaluation of the attachment dynamics underlying the development and maintenance of child adjustment problems in the family. To achieve this goal, a multidisciplinary team works with each youth and his or her family—both on site and in the community—to gather information at each level of the ecology (cultural, community, family, and individual). The multidisciplinary team, community, family, and youth come together to share information and develop a "care plan" that provides an understanding of the attachment pattern of the youth and the attachment dynamics underlying interactions with parents and other important people within his or her ecology. Strategies are provided that are most likely to support adaptive functioning within the home community. Outreach staff working with community teams support the implementation of the care plan within the youth's home community. Respite care for up to 2 weeks is provided to ensure that systems of care remain intact over time.

Consistent with research supporting the efficacy of systemic intervention, evaluation of the Response Program has shown reductions in problem behavior (e.g., aggressive and delinquent behavior, anxiety, depression) from both caregiver and youth perspectives for up to 18-months follow-up (Moretti et al., 1994). Although this was not a controlled evaluation, reductions in problem behavior were noted for even the most highly aggressive youth in this study. Spontaneous remission is atypical in this population. The pattern of change found in the evaluations was revealing. Caregivers were first to shift in their perception of youth problem behavior; youth reported fewer problems months later. One interpretation of these findings is that by shifting caregivers' understanding of the attachment dynamics underlying problem behavior, the quality of the caregiver–youth relationship changes and thus reduces the functional need for problem behavior.

The Orinoco Program is an extension of the Response Program (Moore et al., 1998). This program admits both youth and their caregivers into an intensive 3-month multimodal program based on attachment theory. Program components include family therapy, parenting groups, a work shadowing program, and milieu therapy, all of which focus on attachment issues. Each childcare staff member works closely with only two youth during the entire duration of the program, working within the relationship and using ongoing experience to help youth develop skills in resolving interpersonal conflict in adaptive ways and to increase attachment security. Rather than "manage" difficult behavior through increased control and containment, staff attempt to use their connection with youth to influence the youth's behavior. This approach does not mean that all forms of behavior are acceptable and that there are no limits or consequences. However, empathy goes hand-in-hand with limit setting and social consequences. The benefits of an attachment approach are twofold: the quality of relationships is improved and internal self-organization is enhanced. Youth in the program learn to trust others as potential sources of support and nurturance, and through growing security they are able to integrate their internal psychological experiences and move forward in autonomy development. This work may or may not occur in conjunction with changes in family patterns of relating to each other, depending on the capacity of each family member to engage in the change process. Change in family functioning is certainly desirable and always occurs to some degree. However, even when it is minimal, youth can work in other relationships and gain a greater sense of trust in adults as potential sources of security and support, and a greater degree of internal integration and identity development.

How well does this program work? Based on youth, family, and community support for the program, it has been extremely successful. Youth often remain connected with the program through their alumni association for years. They do not "run away" as they did when the units were "lockdown" facilities. The door has been removed from the seclusion room; staff have found other ways of keeping kids safe by working within the relationship. It is important to recognize, however, that this is extremely difficult and challenging work; staff require ongoing support and supervision regarding attachment issues and therapeutic strategies. Yet most report that they feel they are doing the best work they have ever done—they are more real in their relationships and adolescents respond positively to their authenticity.

FUTURE DIRECTIONS

Adolescence can be a period of psychological and relational expansion in which a child and his or her family celebrate the exploration and inclusion of a wider and richer world of attachment relationships. This growth is mirrored internally in the adolescent's development of richer, more complex, and integrated representations of self and other. Divergence or conflict between adolescents and their parents can be opportunities for growth rather than evidence of dysfunction. Together, and in relation to each other, adolescents and their parents can be positively transformed through this process.

In this chapter we focused our attention on the dynamic relationship between transitions in the self system and attachment. The evidence we presented suggests that the quality of adolescent–parent relationships shapes the psychological meaning of differentiation between parents and adolescents. Identity differentiation and autonomy development enhances self-esteem in securely attached adolescents, but it is threat for adolescents who are insecurely attached. Our research also shows that adolescents with insecure attachment to their parents generally have more negative and less elaborated internal self–other representations. We need to examine the complexity of self-representation much more deeply and in relation to specific qualities of adolescent–parent attachment, following some important research strategies that have been developed in adult samples (Mikulincer, 1995).

The troubled and aggressive youth we discussed in this chapter are characteristically insecure in their attachment to parents. Are insults to the attachment system truly a cause of aggressive behavior? Bowlby (1973) believed so; indeed, he noted that "the most violently angry and dysfunctional responses of all, it seems probable, are elicited in children and adolescents who not only experience repeated separations but are constantly subjected to the threat of being abandoned" (p. 288). Furthermore, he underscored the importance of threats to attachment as a determinant of aggression by drawing on Burnham's (1965) observations of violent adolescents: one adolescent who murdered his mother exclaimed afterward, "I couldn't stand to have her leave me." Another, a youth who placed a bomb in his mother's luggage as she boarded an airliner, explained: "I decided that she would never leave me again" (p. 290, as cited in Bowlby, 1973).

The research we presented in this chapter lends support to the view that insecure attachment is characteristic of aggressive adolescents. Yet our understanding of *how* insecure attachment is linked to aggression, and what types of attachment insecurity may be tied to different *types* and different *patterns* of aggressive behavior is limited. Future research is required to understand the specificity in link between attachment insecurity and aggression. We also need to evaluate whether Bowlby's (1973) distinction between functional versus dysfunctional anger is valid. He argued that dysfunctional anger—such as uncontrollable rage and destructive attacks on caregivers—weakens relational bonds. This may be true of some forms of extreme aggression but in our experience we find that aggressive behavior in youth often functions to *strengthen* bonds, but in a manner that compromises the psychological and physical well-being of all involved. Similar observations have been made by Dutton (1999) in men who assault their wives.

There are many issues that space did not permit us to address in this chapter. We focused only on attachment relationships with parents, yet during adolescence other important peer and romantic pair bonds emerge. As these relationships develop, the attachment functions served by parental relationships change (Trinke & Bartholomew, 1997). Although we know that parents continue to remain important attachment figures well into adulthood, we do not fully understand how children who are exposed to traumatic attachment experiences balance the emergence of peer and romantic relationships. Our guess is that these children are likely to prematurely shift toward peers and romantic partners in the hope that these new relationships will meet attachment needs that could not be met in their relationships with their parents. Thus, peers may strongly influence their behavior and contribute more to the development of antisocial and delinquent behavior for children with insecure attachment patterns.

Finally, although attachment theory has led us to be more aware of systemic and transactional influences on child development, much of our thinking remains deeply entrenched in understanding individuals apart from their interpersonal contexts. Recently Cook (2000) developed a methodology for looking at attachment from a "social relations theory" perspective. In his research he asks the question: How internal are internal working models? To what degree is attachment security related to individual differences versus family systems that are themselves embedded within complex ecologies? Only by understanding that attachment is *both* an emergent process within relationships and a relatively enduring individual difference characteristic can we move forward in understanding how each influences and shapes the other.

REFERENCES

Allen, J. P., Moore, C. M., & Kuperminc, G. P. (1997). Developmental approaches to understanding adolescent deviance. In S. S. Luthar & J. A. Burack (Eds.), *Developmental psychopathology: Perspectives on adjustment, risk, and disorder* (pp. 548–567). New York: Cambridge University Press.

Bachman, J., & Schulenberg, J. (1993). How part-time work intensity relates to drug use, problem behavior, time use, and satisfaction among high school seniors: Are these consequences or merely correlates? *Developmental Psychology, 29*, 220–235.

Bartholomew, K., & Horowitz, L. M. (1991). Attachment styles among young adults: A test of a four-category model. *Journal of Personality and Social Psychology, 61*, 226–244.

Blatt, S. J., & Behrends, R. S. (1987). Internalization, separation–individuation, and the nature of therapeutic action. *International Journal of Psycho-Analysis, 68*, 279–297.

Bowlby, J. (1973). *Attachment and loss: Vol. II. Separation.* New York: Basic Books.

Buhrmester, D., & Furman, W. (1987). The development of companionship and intimacy. *Child Development, 58*, 1101–1113.

Byng-Hall, J. (1991). The application of attachment theory to understanding and treatment in family therapy. In C. M. Parkes, J. Stevenson-Hinde, & P. Harris (Eds.), *Attachment across the life cycle* (pp. 199–215). New York: Routledge.

Byng-Hall, J., & Stevenson-Hinde, J. (1991). Attachment relationships within a family system. *Infant Mental Health Journal, 12*, 187–200.

Case, R. (1985). *Intellectual development: Birth to adulthood.* New York: Academic Press.

Chalmers, D., & Lawrence, J. A. (1993). Investigating the effects of planning aids on adults' and adolescents' organization of a complex task. *International Journal of Behavioral Development, 16*, 191–214.

Cook, W. L. (2000). Understanding attachment security in family context. *Journal of Personality and Social Psychology, 78*, 285–294.

Cross, S. E., & Madson, L. (1997). Models of the self: Self-construals and gender. *Psychological Bulletin, 122*, 5–37.

Dutton, D. G. (1999). The traumatic origins of intimate rage. *Aggression and Violent Behavior, 4*(4), 431–448.

Douvan, E., & Adelson, J. (1966). *The adolescent experience.* New York: Wiley.

Doyle, A. B., & Moretti, M. M. (2001). *Attachment to parents and adjustment in ado-*

lescence: Literature review and policy implications (File No. 032ss. H5219–9–CYH7/001/SS). Ottawa, ON: Health Canada.

Doyle, A. B., Moretti, M. M., Brendgen, M., & Bukowski, B. (2001). *Attachment to parents and adjustment in adolescence: Findings from the HBSC and NLSCY Cycle 2 studies* (File No. 032ss. H5219–00CYH3). Ottawa: Health Canada Childhood and Youth Division.

Elkind, D. (1967). Egocentrism in adolescence. *Child Development, 38,* 1025–1034.

Erikson, E. (1963). *Childhood and society* (2nd ed.). New York: Norton.

Erikson, E. (1968). *Identify: Youth and crisis.* New York: Norton.

Fisher, P. A., & Chamberlain, P. (2000). Multidimensional treatment foster care: A program for intensive parenting, family support, and skill building. *Journal of Emotional and Behavioral Disorders, 8,* 155–164.

Furman, W., & Buhrmester, D. (1992). Age and sex differences in perceptions of networks of personal relationships. *Child Development, 63,* 103–115.

Greenberger, E., & Steinberg, L. (1986). *When teenagers work: The psychological and social costs of adolescent employment.* New York: Basic Books.

Harter, S. (1990). Self and identity development. In S. S. Feldman & G. R. Elliott (Eds.), *At the threshold: The developing adolescent* (pp. 352–387). Cambridge, MA: Harvard University Press.

Harter, S. (1999). *The construction of the self: A developmental perspective.* New York: Guilford Press.

Harter, S., Bresnick, S., Bouchey, H. A., & Whitesell, N. R. (1997). The development of multiple role-related selves during adolescence. *Development and Psychopathology, 9,* 835–853.

Harter, S., Marold, D. B., Whitesell, N. R., & Cobbs, G. (1996). A model of the effects of perceived parent and peer support on adolescent false self behavior. *Child Development, 67,* 360–374.

Harter, S., & Monsour, A. (1992). Development analysis of conflict caused by opposing attributes in the adolescent self-portrait. *Developmental Psychology, 28,* 251–260.

Henggeler, S. W. (1991). Multidimensional causal models of delinquent behavior and their implications for treatment. In R. Cohen & A. W. Siegel (Eds.), *Context and development* (pp. 211–231). Hillsdale, NJ: Erlbaum.

Holland, R., Moretti, M. M., Verlaan, V., & Peterson, S. (1993). Attachment and conduct disorder: The response program. *Canadian Journal of Psychiatry, 38,* 420–431.

Holmes, J. (1997). Attachment, autonomy, intimacy: Some clinical implications of attachment theory. *British Journal of Medical Psychology, 70,* 231–248.

Jordan, J. V., Kaplan, A. G., Miller, J. B., Stiver, I. P., & Surrey, J. L. (1991). *Women's growth in connection: Writings from the Stone Center.* New York: Guilford Press.

Kerns, K. A., & Stevens, A. C. (1996). Parent–child attachment in late adolescence: Links to social relations and personality. *Journal of Youth and Adolescence, 25*(3), 323–342.

Kobak, R., Ferenz-Gillies, R., Everhart, E., & Seabrook, L. (1994). Maternal attachment strategies and emotion regulation with adolescent offspring. *Journal of Research on Adolescence, 4,* 553–566.

Kobak, R. R., & Sceery, A. (1988). Attachment in late adolescence: Working models, affect regulation, and representations of self and others. *Child Development,* *59*(1), 135–146.

Lamborn, S. D., & Steinberg, L. (1993). Emotional autonomy redux: Revisiting Ryan and Lynch. *Child Development, 64,* 483–499.

Larson, R. W., Richards, M. H., Moneta, G., & Holmbeck, G. C. (1996). Changes in adolescents' daily interactions with their families from ages 10 to 18: Disengagement and transformation. *Developmental Psychology, 32,* 744–754.

Laursen, B., & Williams, V. A. (1997). Perceptions of interdependence and closeness in family and peer relationships among adolescents with and without romantic partners. In S. Shulman & W. A. Collins (Eds.), *Romantic relationships in adolescence: Developmental perspectives. New directions for child development No. 78* (pp. 3–20). San Francisco: Jossey-Bass.

Levitt, M. J., Guacci-Franco, N., & Levitt, J. L. (1993). Convoys of social support in childhood and early adolescence: Structure and function. *Developmental Psychology, 29,* 811–818.

Marsh, H. W. (1989). Age and sex effects in multiple dimensions of self-concept: Preadolescence to early adulthood. *Journal of Educational Psychology, 81,* 417–430.

McCabe, M. P. (1984). Toward a theory of adolescent dating. *Adolescence, 19,* 159–170.

Mikulincer, M. (1995). Adult attachment and the mental representation of the self. *Journal of Personality and Social Psychology, 72,* 1217–1230.

Moore, K., Moretti, M. M., & Holland, R. (1998). A new perspective on youth care programs: Using attachment theory to guide interventions for troubled youth. *Residential Treatment for Children and Youth, 15,* 1–24.

Moretti, M. M., Emmrys, C., Grizenko, N., Holland, R., Moore, K., Shamsie, J., & Hamilton, H. (1997). The treatment of conduct disorder: Perspectives from across Canada. *Canadian Journal of Psychiatry, 42,* 637–648.

Moretti, M. M., & Higgins, E. T. (1999a). Own versus other standpoints in self-regulation: Developmental antecedents and functional consequences. *Review of General Psychology, 3,* 188–223.

Moretti, M. M., & Higgins, E. T. (1999b). Internal representations of others in self-regulation: A new look at a classic issue. *Social Cognition, 17,* 186–208.

Moretti, M. M., Holland, R., & McKay, S. (2001). Self–other representations and relational and overt aggression in adolescent girls and boys. *Behavioral Sciences and the Law, 19,* 109–126.

Moretti, M. M., Holland, R., & Moore, K. (2002). Youth at risk: Systemic intervention from an attachment perspective. In M. V. Hayes & L. T. Foster (Eds.), *Too small to see, too big to ignore* (pp. 233–252). Victoria, BC, Canada: Western Geographic Series, University of Victoria.

Moretti, M. M., Holland, R., & Peterson, S. (1994). Long term outcome of an attachment-based program for conduct disorder. *Canadian Journal of Psychiatry, 39,* 360–370.

Moretti, M. M., & McKay, S. (2000, August). *Self-discrepancy in adolescents: Parental autonomy support and self-esteem in girls.* Paper presented at the annual meeting of the American Psychological Association, Washington, DC.

Moretti, M. M., Reebye, P., Wiebe, V. J., & Lessard, J. C. (2002). *Comorbidity in ado-*

lescents with conduct disorder. Unpublished manuscript, Department of Psychology, Simon Fraser University, Burnaby, BC, Canada.

Moretti, M. M., Rein, A. S., & Wiebe, V. J. (1998). Relational self-regulation: Gender differences in risk for dysphoria. *Canadian Journal of Behavioural Science, 30,* 243–252.

Moretti, M. M., & Wiebe, V. J. (1999). Self-discrepancy in adolescence: Own and parental standpoints on the self. *Merrill-Palmer Quarterly, 45,* 624–649.

Reebye, P., Moretti, M. M., Wiebe, V. J., & Lessard, J. C. (2000). Symptoms of posttraumatic stress disorder in adolescents with conduct disorder: Sex differences and onset patterns. *Canadian Journal of Psychiatry, 45,* 746–751.

Ryan, R. M., Deci, E. L., & Grolnick, W. S. (1995). Autonomy, relatedness, and the self: Their relation to development and psychopathology. In D. Cicchetti & D. J. Cohen (Eds.), *Developmental psychopathology: Vol. 1. Theory and methods. Wiley series on personality processes* (pp. 618–655). New York: Wiley.

Ryan, R. M., & Lynch, J. H. (1989). Emotional autonomy versus detachment: Revisiting the vicissitudes of adolescence and young adulthood. *Child Development, 60,* 340–356.

Schafer, R. (1968). *Aspects of internalization.* New York: International Universities Press.

Selman, R. L. (1980). *The growth of interpersonal understanding: Developmental and clinical analyses.* New York: Academic Press.

Selman, R. L., & Byrne, D. F. (1974). A structural developmental analysis of levels of role-taking in middle childhood. *Child Development, 45,* 803–806.

Shamsie, S. J. (1981). Antisocial adolescents: Our treatments do not work—Where do we go from here? *Canadian Journal of Psychiatry, 26,* 357–364.

Shaver, P. R., & Hazan, C. (1993). Adult romantic relationships: Theory and evidence. In D. Perlman & W. Jones (Eds.), *Advances in personal relationships* (Vol. 4, pp. 29–70). London: Jessica Kingsley.

Trinke, S. J., & Bartholomew, K. (1997). Hierarchies of attachment relationships in young adulthood. *Journal of Social and Personal Relationships, 14,* 603–625.

U.S. Department of Health and Human Services. (2001). *Youth violence: A report of the Surgeon General.* Rockville, MD: U.S. Department of Health and Human Services, Centers for Disease Control and Prevention, National Center for Injury Prevention and Control; Substance Abuse and Mental Health Services Administration, Center for Mental Health Services; and National Institutes of Health, National Institute of Mental Health.

13

Implications of Adult Attachment for Preventing Adverse Marital Outcomes

REBECCA J. COBB
THOMAS N. BRADBURY

Although attachment is a relatively stable attribute with possibilities for change across time (e.g., Hamilton, 2000; Waters, Merrick, Treboux, Crowell, & Albersheim, 2000; Weinfield, Sroufe, & Egeland, 2000), surprisingly little is known about the mechanisms of change in attachment and whether it is possible to effect change through intervention. Examining whether and how individual attachment can be changed is important because security of attachment is known to be associated with happier and better functioning relationships (e.g., Collins & Read, 1990; Carnelley, Pietromonaco, & Jaffe, 1996; Kobak & Hazan, 1991). Thus, if we can foster security in people's relationships, we may be able to reduce negative marital outcomes, such as dissatisfaction and divorce, and the harmful effects on the physical and mental health of the adults and their children from these marriages.

One form of couple therapy, emotionally focused therapy (EFT), demonstrates that it is useful to focus on attachment processes in therapy to improve maritally distressed relationships (Greenberg & Johnson, 1988; Johnson, 1996; Johnson, Hunsley, Greenberg, & Schindler, 1999; Johnson & Talitman, 1996). In this chapter, we offer an analysis that is conceptually similar to EFT, but with a focus on prevention rather than on therapeutic intervention. We do so under the assumptions that the majority of couples

seek therapy once they (and perhaps their children) are experiencing significant distress, that marital treatment is a difficult undertaking (e.g., Jacobson & Addis, 1993), and that many couples do not seek therapy prior to divorcing. We therefore join numerous other researchers who are focusing
their energies on earlier stages of relationships, particularly with engaged
and newlywed couples, and designing interventions with the purpose of improving relationship functioning before the development of serious problems (Bradbury, 1998). Because attachment security is associated with positive outcomes in relationships, we propose that it may be useful to apply
the attachment framework to understanding the mechanisms of change in
current marital prevention programs, and to develop new programs as couples move into committed relationships.

The purpose of this chapter is to explore the links between attachment
and prevention of marital distress with couples in the early stages of their
relationship. Research on instability in attachment models over time is
reviewed, with a specific focus on possible mechanisms of change. A framework for understanding the reciprocal influences of attachment and interactional processes targeted in premarital intervention programs is proposed. We also explore how attachment theory may clarify mechanisms of
influence of existing premarital interventions.

ATTACHMENT AND RELATIONSHIP FUNCTIONING

Attachment patterns have been linked to relationship functioning and outcomes, and as such, attachment models and behaviors may be important
areas to target in an intervention. Attachment models are presumed to be
relatively enduring cognitive schemas, or beliefs about the self and others,
and to influence and also to be influenced by interpersonal interactions. Although attachment models may be considered an individual characteristic,
it is supposed that people may have differing levels of security within specific relationships. Also, the models may change due to experience within a
particular relationship. Attachment security may be understood as the degree to which individuals hold positive models of themselves and of others,
or to which they see themselves as worthy of others' love and affection, feel
comfortable with intimacy, are able to depend on others, and see others as
accepting and willing to offer help and support when needed. The intersection of these two dimensions, models of self and other, yield four prototypes of attachment: secure, fearful, preoccupied, and dismissing (Bartholomew & Horowitz, 1991). The *secure* prototype describes individuals who
have a positive model of self and others. They are comfortable being close
to others and relying on them for help and support, and generally feel as
though they are worthy of others' love and expect to be treated well in
close relationships. *Fearful* individuals have negative models of self and

others. They desire closeness with others, but are afraid to seek it for fear of rejection. They consider themselves as unworthy of love and affection, and expect others to be distant and or rejecting. *Preoccupied* individuals have a positive model of others, but a negative model of self. They crave attention and closeness, and may be seen as clingy and intrusive in close relationships. However, they generally feel that they value others more than they themselves are valued. *Dismissing* individuals have a positive model of self and a negative model of others. They neither want nor feel that they need intimacy in relationships, and they generally avoid relying on others for emotional support or comfort.

Attachment security has been associated with greater relationship satisfaction (e.g., Collins & Read, 1990; Senchak & Leonard, 1992), better communication, and problem-solving skills (Cohn, Silver, Cowan, Cowan, & Pearson, 1992; Kobak & Hazan, 1991), more adaptive social support processes (Carnelley et al., 1996; Feeney, 1996; Simpson, Rholes, & Nelligan, 1992), and greater self-reported commitment and relationship investment (Simpson, 1990). Insecure attachment is also associated with the dissolution of dating relationships (Kirkpatrick & Davis, 1994) and marriages (Davila & Bradbury, 2001). Kirkpatrick and Davis (1994) found that anxious women and avoidant men tend to have negative views of their relationships, but that their relationships tend to be relatively stable. In a study of married couples, Davila and Bradbury (2001) also found that anxious attachment was associated with stable but unhappy relationships. Of note, in the Davila and Bradbury study, couples who would go on to remain in unhappy marriages could be differentiated from the happy or divorced couples early in their marriages by their degree of insecurity: those spouses who had the highest degrees of insecurity at the beginning of their marriage were the most likely to remain in unhappy marriages through 4 years.

In sum, security of adult attachment is associated with many positive features of relationship functioning, and secure spouses in stable marriages are happier than insecure spouses in stable marriages (Davila & Bradbury, 2001). Findings from Davila and Bradbury also indicate that we can identify couples who are at risk early in their marital trajectory on the basis of attachment pattern (see also Davila, Chapter 7, this volume). The next obvious question is whether or not we can actually effect change in attachment models that will have consequences for the long-term outcomes in relationships.

THEORY AND RESEARCH ON ATTACHMENT CHANGE

Bowlby (1982, 1988) hypothesized that attachment models would exhibit continuity across the individual's lifetime, but at the same time proposed developmental pathways whereby attachment models might undergo revision in light of new experiences. To date, four longitudinal studies have assessed attachment in infancy using the Ainsworth Strange Situation paradigm and again in late adolescence–early adulthood using an attachment interview (Hamilton, 2000; Lewis, Feiring, & Rosenthal, 2000; Waters et al., 2000; Weinfield et al., 2000). These studies, along with a host of shorter longitudinal studies focusing on attachment stability in both childhood (e.g., Egeland & Sroufe, 1981; Thompson, Lamb, & Estes, 1982; Vaughn, Egeland, Sroufe, & Waters, 1979; Waters, 1978) and adulthood (e.g., Baldwin & Fehr, 1995; Davila, Karney, & Bradbury, 1999; Fuller & Fincham, 1995; Kirkpatrick & Hazan, 1994; Scharfe & Bartholomew, 1994), indicate that there is substantial continuity in attachment across time when there is continuity in the environment. However, there are a significant number of individuals who either report changes in attachment or who are assessed (through behavioral observation or interview) as having a different attachment pattern, or style, from one point to another. In longitudinal studies of changes in adult attachment, approximately 30% of individuals report change. In the longitudinal studies examining change from childhood to adulthood, reports of change range from 23 to 50%. However, changes in attachment over time were consistently related to changes in the family environment, such as maternal depression and parental divorce, that would be expected to impact attachment security.

These studies support Bowlby's premise that attachment patterns can change over time; however, the question of mechanisms of change remains. One theory is that attachment change may occur in the context of changing life circumstances (e.g., beginning a supportive relationship, experiencing a life transition, entering therapy). New interpersonal experiences may challenge existing models of attachment and require the updating of models in order to allow the individual to function adaptively within the new context (Bowlby, 1973). A model whereby attachment change occurs when there are changes in life circumstances has been referred to as the *contextual model* (cf. Davila et al., 1999), and has been explored with children (e.g., Sroufe, 1988) and adults (e.g., Bartholomew, Cobb, & Poole, 1997; Davila et al., 1999; Scharfe & Bartholomew, 1994).

Although the contextual model has received mixed support, there is some evidence to suggest that attachment fluctuates depending on changing life circumstances (e.g., Kirkpatrick & Hazan, 1994; Davila et al., 1999). These data provide us with some idea as to the mechanisms of change of attachment, that is, changing the nature or quality of the attachment caregiving bond allows for some change in the individual's beliefs about him- or herself and others. This suggests that a way to create change within a therapeutic context is to alter attachment-relevant behaviors within the relationship in order to affect the quality of the attachment bond rather than focusing exclusively on beliefs and cognitions as the way to effect change.

CHANGING BEHAVIOR IN MARITAL INTERVENTIONS
AND THE ROLE OF ATTACHMENT

Getting married is a transitional time for individuals, and as such was hypothesized by Bowlby (1982) to be a time when working models of attachment may be more open to revision. Thus, it will be important to determine whether or not security of attachment may be fostered through direct interventions focusing on changing attachment behaviors within relationships during this transitional period. Furthermore, targeting couples that we know are at higher risk for adverse marital outcomes would maximize the effect of our intervention efforts. The available evidence does suggest that couples who go on to separate or divorce can be distinguished on the basis of attachment pattern from couples who remain married and satisfied fairly early in their marriage. Also, Pasch and Bradbury (1998) were able to distinguish between couples who remained satisfied from those who were either unhappy or divorced over 4 years based on social support behaviors within the first 6 months of marriage. Although it is possible that it is a lack of caring reflected in the social support tasks that is responsible for negative outcomes, these couples were newly wed, and at the beginning of their marriages reported being very happy in their relationships. Thus, the results may be interpreted as meaning that spouses who respond negatively to their partner's expressed attachment needs, or who lack competence in expressing their own needs, will be at higher risk for negative outcomes. From research on attachment and social support, we know that the inability to seek or to offer support when feeling anxious or threatened covaries with insecurity of attachment (Simpson et al., 1992; Carpenter & Kirkpatrick, 1996). Therefore, targeting support-seeking and support-giving behaviors within the marital context is suggested by both basic research on attachment and on marriage.

Researchers have suggested that social support seeking in adulthood may correspond with the proximity-seeking function of the attachment system in childhood (Bartholomew et al., 1997; Cotterell, 1992). Among insecure individuals this function has developed, or failed to develop, in such a way that they are unable to adequately seek support. These behaviors can be seen as an adaptation to difficult circumstances that is no longer functional in later relationships (Bowlby, 1973). Thus, a pattern of not seeking support when experiencing distress could result due to fears of rejection or abandonment (fearful). Conversely, it is supposed that dismissing (avoidant) individuals tend not to seek support because of their belief that they would not benefit from it (Bartholomew et al., 1997). Individuals who are ambivalent, or preoccupied, about relationships may show a much different pattern. They may be chronic seekers of support, but they do not derive the same satisfaction from received support as do secure individuals (Bartholomew et al., 1997). Thus, insecure attachment manifests itself as either not seeking social support or being dissatisfied with the amount and quality of the support received. Continually denying one's need for support, failing to seek support, or never feeling as though one has received enough support could lead to interactional patterns that would only strengthen the existing insecure attachment models. Not seeking support, or not letting attachment figures know how they can be supportive, never allows the insecure individual to reap the benefit of comfort or help from others. Nor does it allow them to see others as being helpful and experience themselves as deserving of that comfort. Being overly demanding of others for support in times of distress may result in attachment figures becoming "burned out," and ultimately rejecting the insecure individuals' needs as too overwhelming. In both of these situations, insecure individuals have inadvertently created the very outcome that confirms, and presumably reinforces, their existing insecure views of themselves and others.

Attachment theory would suggest that a partner who could respond sensitively and appropriately to the insecure individual's attachment signals might promote a greater sense of felt security. Thus, learning to provide social support effectively may supply the feedback needed to disconfirm the insecure partner's negative self–other models. Furthermore, if we can teach insecure individuals to seek the support they desire in more adaptive ways—to help them transform their "distorted" attachment signals into behaviors that would elicit the desired responses—we may help couples create situations where attachment needs would be better met and thus provide the sense of felt security the insecure person is trying to achieve. Over time, if learning to seek and to provide social support successfully could be integrated into each spouse's behavioral repertoire, insecure partners should have a multitude of experiences within the marriage that are inconsistent with their existing models. If, as Bowlby suggested, these models remain open to revision in order to remain useful, we should eventually observe change in attachment models and in attachment behaviors. Ideally, a positive feedback loop would be activated whereby the positive and adaptive caregiving and support-seeking responses would be strengthened and would become more congruent with the newly revised attachment models. Thus, we would propose that there is a reciprocal relationship between attachment models and the individual's behaviors, and we suggest that the starting point for change be within the dyad, rather than within the individual. It seems reasonable to assume that helping couples change and shape their behavior in more appropriate ways (e.g., asking each other for help and support rather than being overly demanding or avoiding help seeking; responding to each other with empathy and validation rather than with minimization or blame) would be easier than attempting to change individual beliefs and expectations directly. In other words, helping couples to have different experiences in the context of the relationship is expected subsequently to influence the way spouses think about each other and their marriage. It is particularly important to note that the efforts to change behaviors occur with both spouses simultaneously—targeting both support seeking and caregiving. Thus, having the partner receive immediate and genuine feedback about his or her behavior may make the new experience more powerful and credible, resulting in real change of attachment models. Couples who are encouraged to try something different in their interactions, for example, asking for emotional support rather than avoiding distressing issues, or responding with empathy rather than minimization or problem solving, may find that these alternatives provide them with experiences that are inconsistent with their expectations. At the same time, the couple may talk about the emotional impact that the new behaviors have, and this feedback may strengthen adaptive support seeking and caregiving, which may lead to enduring changes in attachment beliefs.

Although attachment theory prompts a focus on supportive behaviors, a focus on conflict behaviors is also indicated. Spouses tend to experience heightened emotion during conflict (Burman, Margolin, & John, 1993; Margolin, John, & O'Brien, 1989), and conflict may also be experienced as a threat to the security within the relationship, which would then activate the attachment system (e.g., prompt attachment behaviors designed to restore felt security). Thus, the spouses would attempt to manage their fears about the state of the relationship and other distressing emotions inherent in the conflict situation. In attempting to regulate these emotions, spouses may be likely to seek reassurance and comfort from the very person who is seemingly causing such distress. The spouse's attempts to seek reassurance and to gain comfort from the partner may be enacted in various ways according to their attachment pattern, and insecurity may prevent the clear signaling needed to fulfill these attachment needs.

Kobak, Ruckdeschel, and Hazan (1994) have suggested that symptoms of marital distress, such as anger, blaming, and reciprocation of negative affect, may be viewed as distorted expressions of normal attachment emotions that arise when individuals see their partner as unavailable or withdrawing. These distortions prevent accurate understanding about partners' concerns and thus hinder effective communication. This perspective is supported by Kobak and Hazan's (1991) findings that insecurity and relatively inaccurate perceptions of one's partner are associated with more negative behaviors and less effective communication (e.g., being attacking or blaming) in problem-solving interactions, and also with lower marital satisfaction. This would suggest that helping couples to communicate clearly (e.g., to accurately describe their feelings and desires without being blaming or defensive) while focusing on empathic understanding of their partner's distress would foster the safe environment needed to discuss emotionally charged topics.

PREMARITAL INTERVENTION AND THE ROLE OF ATTACHMENT

Up to this point, we have emphasized how, in theory, an attachment perspective and related research might inform preventive intervention. Yet it might also prove useful to evaluate existing preventive interventions through the lens of attachment theory. Interventions that specifically target problem-solving skills, communication, and social support skills may serve to create an atmosphere of safety in the relationship that will provide a sense of trust in the partner and thus foster an increasing sense of felt security. Prevention programs have been hailed as important in improving couple communication to prevent discord and divorce and the attendant costs of marital distress (e.g., Bradbury & Fincham, 1990; Stanley, Markman, St. Peters, & Leber, 1995). Researchers have begun to shift their focus to include prevention programs because of the high rate of divorce, the finding that most divorces happen within 5 years of marriage, and speculation that most couples do not seek therapy until their relationships have deteriorated to a point where recovery is difficult (e.g., Markman, Floyd, Stanley, & Lewis, 1986). The relative lack of success of behavioral marital therapies (see Jacobson & Addis, 1993) and the high relapse rate of recovered couples who have been treated within a cognitive-behavioral framework (e.g., Jacobson & Truax, 1991) has led some researchers to investigate the efficacy of programs that are designed to maintain and enhance marital satisfaction *before* couples become distressed (e.g., Markman et al., 1986; see Bradbury & Fincham, 1990).

The vast majority of interventions available to couples entering marriage have not been subjected to serious empirical scrutiny. One clear exception is the Prevention and Relationship Enhancement Program (PREP) developed by Howard Markman, Scott Stanley, and colleagues (Markman, Renick, Floyd, Stanley, & Clements, 1993; Markman, Floyd, Stanley, & Storaasli, 1988; Renick, Blumberg, & Markman, 1992) to teach couples basic skills designed to improve communication, to manage marital conflict, and to target negative communication patterns presumed to be destructive in relationships. Research on PREP has demonstrated that couples are able to learn these skills, that they have improved communication immediately following the workshop, and that they maintain these gains over 3 years (Markman et al., 1988). Although marital satisfaction and stability may be enhanced over at least 3 years (Hahlweg, Markman, Thurmaier, Engle, & Eckert, 1998), these gains decay over longer time periods. In a study by Markman et al. (1993), 4- and 5-year follow-up data indicated that few of the benefits of PREP are maintained past the 3-year assessments. The only significant finding was that husbands who participated in the intervention had significantly higher marital satisfaction and continued to have more positive and less negative communication than did husbands in the control group. Overall, there were no differences in dissolution rates, and there were no significant differences in communication or marital satisfaction between wives in the intervention group as compared to wives in the control group.

PREP was originally based on a manual for behavioral couple therapy developed by Gottman, Notarius, Gonso, and Markman (1976) and it focuses primarily on improving communication behavior during conflict and problem solving. Because the workshop is based on a behavioral perspective, changes in these behaviors are emphasized as the means for improving relationship functioning. Although the program does include components on fun, friendship, sensuality, and forgiveness, research and theory suggest that it could be further expanded to include other important domains of marital functioning that may provide more durable effects. There has been a similar shift in the marital therapy field to incorporating a focus on affect in therapy in addition to the more traditional focus on behavioral processes (see Davila, Chapter 7 this volume, for a discussion). Focusing on aspects of marital functioning from an attachment perspective may improve the long-term outcomes of prevention programs. Theoretically, improved understanding, social support, forgiveness, and empathy would foster security within the marital relationship, which in turn may promote increasingly secure models of attachment. While PREP focuses on one important aspect of marital functioning, it could benefit from incorporating an attachment perspective that suggests how spouses solicit and provide social support and communicate about feelings are important domains to target within an intervention.

In an attempt to address some of these concerns, an intervention was developed at the University of California–Los Angeles (UCLA) with a focus on aspects of marriage in addition to conflict and problem solving. Compassionate and Accepting Relationships through Empathy (CARE; Rogge, Cobb, Johnson, Lawrence, & Bradbury, 2002) aims to enhance prosocial behaviors that may improve marital outcomes, rather than focusing on specific behavioral communication skills and conflict management. Although CARE was not developed explicitly from the perspective of attachment theory, it does address several relationship processes that the theory would suggest be targeted. These include promoting empathy and focusing on affective expression in the context of three important processes in marriage: social support, conflict, and forgiveness. Many ideas and techniques presented in CARE are adapted from integrative behavioral couples therapy (IBCT; Christensen, Jacobson, & Babcock, 1995; Jacobson & Christensen, 1996), which combines some aspects of traditional behavioral couple therapy with a focus on emotions, empathy, and acceptance of differences within the relationship.

The first CARE module helps couples to explore supportive behaviors within the relationship. Couples are encouraged to become better support seekers and support providers. Partners are asked to discuss a problem they are having outside the marriage or something they would like to change about themselves. This gives the couple an opportunity to practice discussing their vulnerabilities about issues not related to the relationship, which may be less threatening. When describing the problem to their partners, spouses are encouraged to be clear about the nature of the problem and the effect it has on them emotionally. Their partner is guided in *amplifying*, or responding with empathy and compassion. Amplification differs from simple paraphrasing in that it requires a deeper level of analysis on the part of the support giver; participants are asked to "play detective" and to try and argue their partner's side while focusing on showing their understanding of the emotions involved. Spouses are taught to see the problem from the partner's perspective, to avoid criticizing and "playing devil's advocate," and to show that they have understood the partner by responding in a way that demonstrates understanding and validation. Thus, the couple is encouraged to explore their negative affect and express their needs to each other in a safe environment where they can be sure their partners will at least attempt to respond in a validating and empathic manner.

One couple, Andrew and Kathryn, discussed her feelings of disappointment with her bridesmaids in her upcoming wedding. Kathryn started out talking about her frustration and anger that her bridesmaids were not providing her with the support she needed for the wedding arrangements. At first, Andrew responded by playing "devil's advocate" and suggested that maybe her friends were busy with their own lives, that they probably did not mean to be unsupportive, and that Kathryn should "just get over it." With help from their coach, the couple changed the way they communicated about this issue. Kathryn was encouraged to explain the reasons for her frustration and to tell Andrew how he could be helpful, and Andrew was prompted to respond with empathy and not to try and make Kathryn feel better by helping her to see her friends' side. Kathryn then went on to talk about how she felt let down and hurt that her friends weren't helping her as much as she wanted. And she explained to Andrew that she didn't want him to *do* anything but rather she just wanted him to listen and to understand her point of view. Andrew was able to amplify her feelings, and he also noted that she probably felt even more disappointed because Kathryn had been really helpful when one of her friends had married last year. The purpose of the exercise was not to solve any problems or to offer advice, but rather to simply understand and to provide emotional support. Upon completing the exercise, Kathryn remarked that Andrew's usual response was to offer solutions, and that hearing him amplify her feelings was more helpful and satisfying.

The social support exercises allow spouses to express their needs for help and support openly and clearly with the encouragement of a workshop coach, and in turn the partners' empathic response will serve as a powerful reinforcement for effective support seeking. The role of the coach is quite different from that of a therapist; in CARE, the coach is not offering reflections, interpretations, or support regarding the issues. The coach's role is to encourage each spouse to offer support and understanding so as to facilitate expression of emotions and to promote understanding of the issue being discussed. Encouraging this behavior could be seen as helping the spouses function as each others' safe haven. Similarly, the coach encourages the use of skills that facilitate the expression and experience of emotion within a discussion; however, there is not a direct evocation of emotion on the part of the coach, as there is in EFT (Johnson, 1996).

The second CARE module, conflict management, teaches couples to discuss relationship conflicts in a nonjudgmental way, focusing on soft feelings (e.g., hurt and sadness) rather than hard, or hostile and attacking emotions (e.g., anger, disappointment) that often accompany relationship conflict. Couples also continue to practice amplification in the context of a conflict discussion; spouses are encouraged to see the issue from their partner's perspective and to convey their empathy through amplification. Again, this is intended to create a safe environment in which spouses are better able to provide a sense of security for each other that allows them to explore the conflict without blaming or attacking the partner. As an additional way to explore the nature of conflicts in their relationship, spouses are encouraged to build acceptance and tolerance of each other's behaviors by exploring the origins of their typical behaviors in conflict and *reformulating* their views of each other's behaviors. Through reformulation, spouses are encouraged to see their partners' habits and behavior patterns as not simply annoying idiosyncrasies, but rather to understand the context within which the behaviors developed and how they may have been useful in previous relationships. Through discussions of these origins, the aim is to increase empathy and tolerance on the part of the partner. Although not the original intention, this exercise encourages couples to understand the roots of their own and each other's attachment patterns by discussing the original genesis and function of the behaviors. This may help spouses to better understand their own motivations and distorted attachment signals, which may in turn lead to changes in the context of the current relationship.

During the conflict exercise, Angie and John talked about their way of handling conflict. John had become increasingly frustrated when Angie verbally attacked him whenever she felt scared or threatened in some way. This left John feeling as though it was dangerous to talk about relationship problems with Angie, and made Angie feel like she needed to be more aggressive in bringing up problems in order to maintain a sense of control over the relationship. The two had become trapped in a cycle where the more Angie pushed John to discuss problems, the more he backed off for fear of igniting an argument, which left her feeling helpless and wondering if he cared about the things that mattered to her. During the reformulation exercise, Angie was able to tell John about her experiences growing up in a large family that she described as "cut-throat" and very competitive. She said that in her family, she had to be "up-front" with what was bothering her because otherwise her parents and siblings wouldn't notice. To Angie, talking, or yelling, about problems was a pretty normal way to get attention and make sure people cared about what was happening to her. John responded that his family was quite different. He had learned that it was easier not to talk about problems; his parents never brought things up and if there was anything wrong, everyone just ignored each other until enough time passed that they could forget about the problem. John noted that he felt particularly threatened whenever Angie was blaming or calling him names because the only time he had ever seen anything like that happen between his parents was when they had talked about separating. As this couple talked about the origins of their fears and behaviors, it became clear to both of them that although their actions may have been "normal" and adaptive in their own families, that they were creating a situation that was not providing either of them with what they really wanted from the other. Angie had interpreted John's lack of response as lack of caring, and John had interpreted Angie's aggressiveness as a sign that there were serious problems that if talked about might lead to a breakup.

As well as learning to understand each other's behaviors differently, couples also learn *detaching*, a skill that allows them to distance themselves from destructive emotions that may arise during conflict and that help them discuss the process of their communication. In this exercise, couples analyze the process of their communication, rather than talk about a specific marital issue. Thus, they are asked to describe to each other *how* they typically act and react to each other during conflict, rather than falling into the pattern and experiencing the intense, often negative, emotions associated with the problematic issue. In order to facilitate this experience, sometimes couples find it useful to describe the action in the third person, or as though describing a movie that they have watched, or talking about it as though it happened to another couple. This exercise is designed to reduce the emotional intensity associated with conflict issues. It allows the couple to examine how their particular negative pattern has evolved and is maintained in their relationship. Learning to reduce emotional reactions that interfere with discussing relationship issues is important because it allows couples to take a step back from the distressing emotions and understand how each other's frustrated attachment needs are contributing to possibly maladaptive behaviors. This may make spouses more consciously aware of their own needs and of ways to fulfill those needs and to understand how they may be ineffective in the current context. This awareness may be the first step in beginning to revise their views of the partner and the partner's availability, and may encourage the use of alternate strategies that may promote security and adaptation within the marriage.

Diane and Matt tried to detach from the intense emotion that was associated with discussions about the level of self-disclosure in their relationship. Diane thought that when Matt wasn't talking to her, or gave short answers to her questions, that he was mad at her for some unknown reason. Because Diane sees herself as very attuned to Matt, she saw herself as having big "feeling antennae" sticking out of her head trying to sense what was going on with Matt. When he wouldn't tell her how he felt, she would try to figure it out. She realized that she would usually assume something negative. Diane concluded by saying that when she asked Matt if he was mad, even when he said "no" it would just make her sure that he was. When Diane was sure Matt was angry and just not telling her, this made her mad and hurt that he wasn't sharing. This prompted her to make barbed comments to try and get a rise out of him (thus proving her assumptions to be correct!). Matt stated that Diane's barbed comments did make him mad and frustrated (even though he may not have been before) because they seemed to come out of the blue.

During this exercise Matt and Diane were able to detach successfully and to talk about their pattern without falling into having the argument. In this case, Diane was able to inject some humor into their discussion by introducing her metaphor of "feeling antennae," but couples often find it difficult to come up with metaphors for their own patterns, and at times had to be discouraged from coming up with metaphors for their partners. Diane and Matt found this exercise to be very useful because it allowed them, perhaps for the first time, to really understand how their behaviors were related to their fears about the relationship. They were able to see how their actions were not helping them to achieve the comfort and reassurance they desired from each other, but rather were causing them to feel hurt, frustrated, and confused about how to improve their situation.

In the third CARE module, forgiveness, the main aim is to present couples with a model for understanding forgiveness as a process in marriage that involves rebuilding trust and repairing empathy in the relationship when it has been damaged by the hurtful actions of one partner. In CARE, forgiveness is viewed as a process that involves decreasing motivation for retaliation, increasing positive feelings toward the offender, and conciliation (McCullough, Worthington, & Rachal, 1997). Additionally, spouses are encouraged to explore the attributions they make about their partner's behaviors, particularly when those attributions lead to hurt feelings or negative thoughts about the partner. Couples are asked to talk about a time within the marriage when their feelings have been hurt using amplification and revealing their soft feelings. This exercise focuses on examining past injuries within the relationship where one partner failed the other, where there was a breach of trust, that is, an action that was perceived as harmful. Johnson, Makinen, and Milliken (2001) conceptualize these situations as an *attachment injury*: a time when the partner fails to provide comfort and support when it is most needed. In CARE, couples are encouraged to discuss those injuries in a nonblaming manner that allows them to provide emotional understanding and support to each other rather than shifting into a defensive or attacking pattern.

Although couples were encouraged explicitly to explore their attributions for behaviors in this exercise, it is apparent from the example of Diane and Matt that understanding and checking assumptions was a theme throughout the CARE exercises. However, in this exercise there was a greater focus on how attributions, particularly negative ones, can play a very destructive role in relationships. Spouses were asked to think of a time when they had an argument or disagreement and to talk specifically about the assumptions they made about their partner's motivations and feelings both during the argument and during events that led to the argument.

Jayson and Michelle talked about her concern that he still kept in touch with an ex-girlfriend. Jayson had recently made a phone call to this woman after he and Michelle had a disagreement related to their wedding plans. Michelle assumed that Jayson was calling his ex-girlfriend to irritate her because she hadn't agreed with him over their plans. Michelle also thought that Jayson was talking to his ex-girlfriend about her, which made Michelle feel insecure and upset. When she made some angry comments about his "other girlfriend," Jayson assumed she was jealous and being petty so he ignored her comments, which made Michelle think he didn't really care about her feelings.

During the attributions exercise, Jayson and Michelle were able to talk about how Michelle's insecurity led her to make negative assumptions about Jayson's motivations. Jayson was also able to realize that Michelle wasn't being mean to punish him, but because she was feeling hurt and concerned that he was talking about her to another woman. Jayson was able to reassure Michelle that the timing of the phone call was coincidental, and the two agreed to spend some time discussing how Jayson could limit his contact with the ex-girlfriend and also to refrain from talking about personal details of their relationship with others.

It is intended that these core CARE skills, particularly the emphasis on social support and empathy, will foster the belief that the partner is understanding and can be depended upon, and that one's point of view is validated and accepted by the partner. Together, these skills seem most closely allied with the types of behaviors that would theoretically foster a sense of felt security within the relationship. If spouses can be taught to provide a safe haven for their partners, then, theoretically, this should provide experiences that would result in the dual processes of assimilation and accommodation of general working models of attachment. Thus, experiencing the partner as dependable, available, and accepting should enhance spouses' feelings of security, which in turn should result in increasingly positive models of others. Similarly, spouses who receive validation, support, and compassion from their partners should view themselves as worthy of the support and affection provided by the attachment figure, thus resulting in increasingly positive views of the self. These experiences will be assimilated into secure working models of attachment, or will cause updating, or accommodation, of insecure models and will be reflected in self-reports of increased attachment security. Additionally, these changes in attachment models should theoretically be related to positive changes in marital satisfaction over time.

Although PREP focuses mainly on the structure of communication in conflict and improving problem-solving skills, these behaviors can also help to create an environment where couples feel safe communicating their views and feelings. Thus, it is possible that changes in attachment pattern may be effected by participation in PREP as compared to not participating in any marital preparation program. However, because it targets support behaviors and affect more specifically, we predict that there is likely to be a greater benefit in terms of increasing security from participation in the CARE workshops.

THE UCLA MARRIAGE ENRICHMENT STUDY

The UCLA Marriage Enrichment study is a 3-year longitudinal study of 131 newlywed and engaged couples who were randomly assigned to one of three premarital interventions: CARE, PREP, or an attention-only control group (couples watched movies and responded to a questionnaire that guided them in a discussion of their own relationship based on themes portrayed in the film). Couples were recruited via newspaper and radio advertisements and through brochures mailed to bridal show attendees. Interested couples were screened over the phone in order to determine their eligibility. Couples were deemed eligible if (1) it was the first marriage for both spouses, (2) both spouses were between 18 and 45 years old, (3) they were married less than 6 months or engaged with a date set within the next year, (4) both spouses were willing to participate, and (5) couples were not maritally distressed.[1] Eligible couples were mailed a packet of questionnaires to complete at home. Once they returned the packet they were assigned to one of the treatment groups. The PREP and CARE workshops took place over the course of one weekend day (5 hours) and three evenings (3 hours each; all couples also participated in the Stop Anger and Violence Escalation program on the fourth evening [Neidig, 1989]). Couples completed packets again the first day of the workshop, then 6 months, 1 year, 2 years, and 3 years following the workshop. We are currently collecting fol-

---

[1]The study interventions were designed for nondistressed couples with the aim of *preventing* the development of problems; as distressed couples are thought to require a different treatment approach, they were referred for couple therapy where appropriate.

low-up data on these couples; thus, questions regarding changes in attachment and marital satisfaction as a result of participation in the workshops cannot yet be addressed.

However, in addition to the main questions of how attachment can be considered in the development of new interventions and in understanding the mechanisms of existing interventions, there are other ways that attachment may be important in the area of early marital intervention programs. For example, there is some data that indicate couples seeking premarital counseling are not necessarily the couples that might be in most need of treatment. Sullivan and Bradbury (1997) found that couples that were at risk for discord and divorce (e.g., because of lower marital satisfaction, age, income, and education at time of marriage; parental divorce; physical aggression; and higher neuroticism and stress at the time of marriage) are not necessarily the couples who are participating in premarital interventions; this effect was much stronger in a high-risk sample than in a low-risk sample. This indicates that there is some selection bias operating that keeps higher risk couples from seeking treatment prior to the onset of serious marital difficulties. It is possible that one such biasing variable is attachment pattern. If security of attachment is associated with the ability to clearly signal attachment needs, to seek support, and to be able to depend on others, then it could be that couples where one or both partners are relatively insecure may be less likely to seek interventions such as PREP or CARE. This would be a considerable problem if the very couples our research dictates we target with early intervention were the ones who choose not to participate.

To begin addressing this concern, we examined the relative distributions of attachment patterns of participants in the UCLA Marriage Enrichment Study. The relative frequencies of attachment patterns—secure, fearful, preoccupied, and dismissing—were very similar to those obtained in other samples (e.g., Whiffen, Kallos-Lilly, & MacDonald, 2001; Scharfe & Bartholomew, 1994). We also examined this question in another sample of 172 newlywed couples who answered questions about whether or not they had participated in counseling prior to their marriage (for a full description of this sample, see Davila et al., 1999). We found no significant association between attachment pattern and the tendency to seek premarital counseling. This indicates that the couples who are participating in premarital interventions are representative of general samples in terms of their attachment pattern.

A related question is whether attachment pattern is associated with attrition from premarital interventions. Again, it is possible that insecurity would represent a risk factor for dropping out. By definition, some insecure patterns reflect a reluctance to discuss emotions and conflicts within close relationships either due to a fear of rejection (fearful) or because such expressions are deemed as "weak" or unnecessary (dismissing). During the course of programs such as PREP and CARE, couples are required to spend considerable time discussing important relationship issues. This may be threatening to fearful spouses unaccustomed to the style of communication encouraged in the workshop and may result in one or both partners being unenthusiastic about continuing. Alternately, as seems to be the case with EFT, encouraging such a focus on expressing usually undiscussed material in a safe environment may be exactly what the fearful individual seeks and may encourage his or her participation. In considering dismissing attachment, it is possible that the general stance that confiding in others and discussing emotions is unnecessary or not useful may result in dismissing individuals seeing the program as being irrelevant to their relationship functioning, resulting in dropping out.

Again, we examined this question in the participants of the UCLA Marriage Enrichment Project. Of the 131 participants, 27 dropped out of the workshops (15.4% from CARE, 22% from PREP, 26% from attention-only control). Chi-square analysis indicated that there was no association between type of workshop and dropping out of the study. However, there was a trend for insecurity to be associated with attrition. Where possible, we grouped couples according to whether partners were secure (secure–secure) or having at least one insecure member (secure–insecure or insecure–insecure).[2] We then examined the association between couple insecurity and attrition. Chi-square analysis indicates that there was a trend ($p = .07$; one-tailed) for a greater number of couples where at least one member was insecure to drop out (24%) as compared to couples where both members were secure (10%). This provides some evidence that there may be an association between insecurity and the failure to complete a prevention program.

Another important question is whether insecure versus secure spouses might experience differential benefits from participation in premarital workshops. From the research on EFT, it is apparent that success in therapy that focuses on attachment processes is predicted to some extent by attachment pattern. Johnson and Talitman (1996) found that men who were initially less likely to seek their partner for comfort and support benefited most from the therapy in terms of changes in marital satisfaction. Thus, the experience of accessing usually unexpressed emotion within the marriage may have been particularly relevant and useful for individuals who generally feared that this would result in rejection of their attachment needs. If insecure spouses would gain the most from premarital interventions in comparison to secure spouses, it seems that we should consider this when recruiting couples to these types of programs. This is not to say that relatively secure couples should be excluded from interventions; there is no evi-

---

[2]Some participants rated two or more attachment dimensions (secure, fearful, preoccupied, dismissing) as describing themselves equally well. Thus, these individuals could not be placed into secure versus insecure groups. Couples where one member could not be classified as either secure or insecure were not included in the present analyses.

dence to show that having marital problems is specific to the insecure individual or couple, and strengthening marriages is the primary focus of interventions—a focus that may benefit any marriage.

FUTURE CONSIDERATIONS AND CONCLUSIONS

It is clear that insecure attachment is related to relationship distress (e.g., Senchak & Leonard, 1992), and may be one risk factor for deterioration of relationships over time (e.g., Davila & Bradbury, 2001). It is also apparent that interventions early in the marriage can, with varying degrees of success, prevent the erosion of happiness in marriage. There is evidence from EFT (Johnson et al., 1999) suggesting that a focus on the attachment bond between the spouses can be an effective way to create the changes (e.g., increasing availability and responsiveness of spouses) that will enhance satisfaction and alter negative interaction patterns. In this chapter, we have argued that using an attachment focus in the development of premarital programs may enhance the effectiveness of and provide a framework within which to understand the change processes of the currently available treatments. We propose that one such pathway of change may involve altering the affective exchanges between spouses, which may result in modification of attachment models, which may in turn strengthen "secure" behaviors within the marriage.

An interesting question related to the issues of change in attachment and behavior is whether it is attachment models or behaviors that change first. We propose that couples will learn skills that allow them to experience their relationship with their partners in new ways. They may learn to discuss and experience the softer emotions associated with marital conflict rather than blaming each other in hostile or frustrating exchanges. These new experiences and behaviors, if repeated and sustained over time, provide an accumulation of evidence that may eventually result in the reworking of insecure models of attachment. Likewise, these more secure perceptions and beliefs about the partner will affect the spouse's behaviors, which will serve to consolidate and solidify these new and more adaptive behavior patterns. It is possible that changing attachment behaviors within the context of the relationship will affect satisfaction, but not result in long-term change in attachment models. However, it is more difficult to imagine that these gains would be maintained in the long term if they were not accompanied by more fundamental alterations in the models of self and other that are presumed to guide interpersonal behavior over the lifespan. Answering these questions requires more long-term outcome research in order to understand if treatment gains are maintained when there is change not only in behavior, but in the underlying schemas that may direct spouses' behaviors within marriage.

Understanding the reciprocal relationship between interpersonal processes and attachment security requires us to look more closely at how the types of skills and experiences being targeted in our interventions are related to attachment behaviors and attachment patterns or models over time. If we can show that these two change processes are related, it will provide support for the proposal that interventions based on attachment theory can be useful and effective. Further, because attachment-based interventions may create changes not only in behaviors within the marriage, but also changes in beliefs about the self and others, they may demonstrate more promising long-term outcomes than what is currently being shown in the research on premarital interventions.

While the two premarital interventions discussed here address aspects of the attachment system and the attachment bond within the marriage, neither had attachment theory underlying its development. This does not necessarily mean that they cannot be understood in terms of the effects on attachment processes, but it does raise the possibility that more effective, or perhaps more streamlined, interventions could be delivered using a more specific focus on attachment behaviors and models.

Considering the high divorce rate and the negative circumstances that often accompany the end of a relationship, it is clearly important for researchers and clinicians to consider how we can intervene early in relationships. Continuing to evaluate the efficacy of our interventions in order to determine the most useful strategies to promote change will also be important. However, it will also be essential for us to begin to understand the nature and the mechanisms of change that occurs in the context of these early interventions. The abundance of research on dating and married couples suggests that attachment security is important for the well-being of individuals and their relationships. It is time to explore how this knowledge can be applied in the context of relationships early, prior to the development of serious relationship problems.

ACKNOWLEDGMENTS

Development of the CARE program and preparation of this chapter were supported by the John Templeton Foundation and by a Social Sciences and Humanities Research Council of Canada Doctoral Fellowship Award (No. 752-98-0293).

REFERENCES

Baldwin, M. W., & Fehr, B. (1995). On the instability of attachment style ratings. *Personal Relationships, 2,* 247–261.

Bartholomew, K., Cobb, R. J., & Poole, J. A. (1997). Adult attachment patterns and social support processes. In G. R. Pierce, B. Lakey, I. G. Sarason, & B. R. Sarason (Eds.), *Sourcebook of social support and personality* (pp. 359–378). New York: Plenum Press.

Bartholomew, K., & Horowitz, L. (1991). Attachment styles among young adults: A test of a four-category model. *Journal of Personality and Social Psychology, 61*(2), 226–244.

Bowlby, J. (1973). *Attachment and loss: Vol. II. Separation: Anxiety and anger.* New York: Basic Books.

Bowlby, J. (1982). *Attachment and loss: Vol. I. Attachment* (2nd ed.). New York: Basic Books. (First edition published in 1969)

Bowlby, J. (1988). *A secure base: Parent–child attachment and healthy human development.* New York: Basic Books.

Bradbury, T. N. (1998). *The developmental course of marital dysfunction.* New York: Cambridge University Press.

Bradbury, T. N., & Fincham, F. D. (1990). Preventing marital dysfunction: Review and analysis. In F. D. Fincham & T. N. Bradbury (Eds.), *The psychology of marriage: Basic issues and applications* (pp. 375–401). New York: Guilford Press.

Burman, B., Margolin, G., & John, R. S. (1993). America's angriest home videos: Behavioral contingencies observed in home reenactments of marital conflict. *Journal of Consulting and Clinical Psychology, 61*(1), 28–39.

Carnelley, K., Pietromonaco, P., & Jaffe, K. (1996). Attachment, caregiving, and relationship functioning in couples: Effects of self and partner. *Personal Relationships, 3,* 257–278.

Carpenter, E. M., & Kirkpatrick, L. A. (1996). Attachment style and presence of a romantic partner as moderators of psychophysiological responses to a stressful laboratory situation. *Personal Relationships, 3,* 351–367.

Christensen, A., Jacobson, N.S., & Babcock, J. C. (1995). Integrative behavioral couple therapy. In N. S. Jacobson & A. S. Gurman (Eds.), *Clinical handbook of couple therapy* (pp. 31–64). New York: Guilford Press.

Cohn, D. A., Silver, D. H., Cowan, C. P., Cowan, P. A., & Pearson, J. (1992). Working models of childhood attachment and couple relationships. *Journal of Family Issues, 13*(4), 432–449.

Collins, N. L., & Read, S. J. (1990). Adult attachment, working models and relationship quality in dating couples. *Journal of Personality and Social Psychology, 58*(4), 644–663.

Cotterell, J. L. (1992). The relation of attachments and supports to adolescent well-being and school adjustment. *Journal of Adolescent Research, 7*(1), 28–42.

Davila, J., & Bradbury, T. N. (2001). Attachment insecurity and the distinction between unhappy spouses who do and do not divorce. *Journal of Family Psychology, 15,* 371–393.

Davila, J., Karney, B. R., & Bradbury, T. N. (1999). Attachment change processes in the early years of marriage. *Journal of Personality and Social Psychology, 76*(5), 783–802.

Egeland, B., & Sroufe, L. A. (1981). Attachment and early maltreatment. *Child Development, 52,* 964–975.

Feeney, J. A. (1996). Attachment, caregiving, and marital satisfaction. *Personal Relationships, 3,* 401–416.

Fuller, T. L., & Fincham, F. D. (1995). Attachment style in married couples: Relation to current marital functioning, stability over time, and method of assessment. *Personal Relationships, 2,* 17–34.

Gottman, J. M., Notarius, C., Gonso, J., & Markman, H. J. (1976). *A couple's guide to communication.* Champaign, IL: Research Press.

Greenberg, J. S., & Johnson, S. M. (1988). *Emotionally focused therapy for couples.* New York: Guilford Press.

Hahlweg, K., Markman, H. J., Thurmaier, F., Engle, J., & Eckert, V. (1998). Prevention of marital distress: Results of a German prospective longitudinal study. *Journal of Family Psychology, 12*(4), 543–556.

Hamilton, C. E. (2000). Continuity and discontinuity of attachment from infancy through adolescence. *Child Development, 71* (3), 690–694.

Jacobson, N. S., & Addis, M. E. (1993). Research on couples and couple therapy: What do we know? Where are we going? *Journal of Consulting and Clinical Psychology, 61,* 85–93.

Jacobson, N. S. & Christensen, A. (1996). *Acceptance and change in couple therapy.* New York: Norton.

Jacobson, N. S., & Truax, P. (1991). Clinical significance: A statistical approach to defining meaningful change in psychotherapy research. *Journal of Consulting and Clinical Psychology, 48,* 696–703.

Johnson, S. M. (1996). *The practice of emotionally focused marital therapy: Creating connection.* New York: Brunner/Mazel.

Johnson, S. M., Hunsley, J., Greenberg, L., & Schindler, D. (1999). Emotionally focused couples therapy: Status and challenges. *Clinical Psychology: Science and Practice, 6,* 67–79.

Johnson, S. M., Makinen, J. A., & Millikin, J. W. (2001). Attachment injuries in couple relationships: A new perspective on impasses in couple therapy. *Journal of Marital and Family Therapy, 27*(2), 145–155.

Johnson, S. M., & Talitman, E. (1996). Predictors of success in emotionally focused marital therapy. *Journal of Marital and Family Therapy, 23*(2), 135–152.

Kirkpatrick, L. A., & Davis, K. E. (1994). Attachment style, gender, and relationship stability: A longitudinal analysis. *Journal of Personality and Social Psychology, 66*(3), 502–512.

Kirkpatrick, L. A., & Hazan, C. (1994). Attachment styles and close relationships: A four-year prospective study. *Personal Relationships, 1,* 123–142.

Kobak, R. R., & Hazan, C. (1991). Attachment in marriage: Effects of security and accuracy of working models. *Journal of Personality and Social Psychology, 60*(6), 861–869.

Kobak, R. R., Ruckdeschel, K., & Hazan, C. (1994). From symptom to signal: An attachment view of emotion in marital therapy. In S. M. Johnson & L. S. Greenberg (Eds.), *The heart of the matter: Perspective on emotion in marital therapy* (pp. 46–71). New York: Brunner/Mazel.

Lewis, M., Feiring, C., & Rosenthal, S. (2000). Attachment over time. *Child Development, 71(3),* 707–720.

Margolin, G., John, R. S., & O'Brien, M. (1989). Sequential affective patterns as a function of marital conflict style. *Journal of Social and Clinical Psychology, 8*(1), 45–61.

Markman, H. J., Floyd, F. J., Stanley, S. M., & Lewis, H. (1986). Prevention. In N. Jacobson & A. Gurman (Eds.), *Clinical handbook of marital therapy* (pp. 173–195). New York: Guilford Press.

Markman, H. J., Floyd, F. J., Stanley, S. M., & Storaasli, R. D. (1988). Prevention of marital distress: A longitudinal investigation. *Journal of Consulting and Clinical Psychology, 56,* 210–217.

Markman, H. J., Renick, M. J., Floyd, F. J., Stanley, S. M., & Clements, M. (1993). Preventing marital distress through communication and conflict management training: A 4- and 5-year follow-up. *Journal of Consulting and Clinical Psychology, 61*(1), 70–77.

McCullough, M. E., Worthington, E. L., Jr., & Rachal, K. C. (1997). Interpersonal forgiving in close relationships. *Journal of Personality and Social Psychology, 73,* 231–336.

Neidig, P. (1989). *The Stop Anger and Violence Escalation (SAVE) workbook.* Stony Brook, NY: Behavioral Science Associates.

Pasch, L. A., & Bradbury, T. N. (1998). Social support, conflict and the development of marital dysfunction. *Journal of Consulting and Clinical Psychology, 66*(2), 219–230.

Renick, M., Blumberg, S. L., & Markman, H. J. (1992). The Prevention and Relationship Enhancement Program (PREP): An empirically based preventive intervention program for couples. *Family Relations, 41,* 141–147.

Rogge, R., Cobb, R. J., Johnson, M., Lawrence, E., & Bradbury, T. N. (2002). Modifying pro-social behaviors to prevent adverse marital outcomes. In A. S. Gurman & N. Jacobson (Eds.), *Clinical handbook of couple therapy* (3rd ed., pp. 420–435). New York: Guilford Press.

Scharfe, E., & Bartholomew, K. (1994). Reliability and stability of adult attachment patterns. *Personal Relationships, 1,* 23–43.

Senchak, M., & Leonard, K. E. (1992). Attachment styles and marital adjustment among newlywed couples. *Journal of Social and Personal Relationships, 6,* 51–64.

Simpson, J. A. (1990). Influence of attachment styles on romantic relationships. *Journal of Personality and Social Psychology, 59,* 971–980.

Simpson, J. A., Rholes, W. S., & Nelligan, J. S. (1992). Support-seeking and support giving within couples in an anxiety-provoking situation: The role of attachment styles. *Journal of Personality and Social Psychology, 62*(3), 434–446.

Sroufe, L. A. (1988). The role of infant–caregiver attachment in development. In J. Belsky & T. Nezworski (Eds.), *Clinical implications of attachment* (pp. 136–174). Hillsdale, NJ: Erlbaum.

Stanley, S. M., Markman, H. J., St. Peters, M., & Leber, B. D. (1995). Strengthening marriages and preventing divorce: New directions in prevention research. *Family Relations, 44,* 392–401.

Sullivan, K. T., & Bradbury, T. N. (1997). Are prevention programs reaching couples at risk for marital dysfunction? *Journal of Consulting and Clinical Psychology, 65,* 24–30.

Thompson, R. A., Lamb, M. E., & Estes, D. (1982). Stability of infant–mother attachment and its relationship to changing life circumstances in an unselected middle-class sample. *Child Development, 53,* 144–148.

Vaughn, B., Egeland, B., Sroufe, L. A., & Waters, E. (1979). Individual differences in infant–mother attachment at twelve and eighteen months: Stability and change in families under stress. *Child Development, 50,* 971–975.

Waters, E. (1978). The reliability and stability of individual differences in infant–mother attachment. *Child Development, 48,* 1184–1199.

Waters, E., Merrick, S., Treboux, D., Crowell, J., & Albersheim, L. (2000). Attachment security in infancy and early adulthood: A twenty-year longitudinal study. *Child Development, 71(3),* 684–689.

Weinfield, N. S., Sroufe, L. A., & Egeland, B. (2000). Attachment from infancy to early adulthood in a high-risk sample: Continuity, discontinuity and their correlates. *Child Development, 71(3),* 695–702.

Whiffen, V. E., Kallos-Lilly, A. V., & MacDonald, B. J. (2001). Depression and attachment in couples. *Cognitive Therapy and Research, 25(5),* 577–590.

14

Attachment in Later Life

Implications for Intervention with Older Adults

J. MICHAEL BRADLEY
GAIL PALMER

In his seminal writings on attachment theory, John Bowlby repeatedly asserted that attachment representations are likely to exert influence "from the cradle to the grave" (Bowlby, 1979, p. 129). Indeed, it is likely that a major source of the appeal and durability of attachment theory is its utility as a conceptual framework for understanding close relationships at various points in the lifespan, from infant–caregiver bonds (e.g., Ainsworth, Blehar, Waters, & Wall, 1978) to adult romantic relationships (e.g., Hazan & Shaver, 1987). While theorists and researchers have been relatively slow to extend attachment theory to older adult populations, a growing body of research has begun to underscore the relevance of attachment issues in later life. Further, many approaches to couple and family therapy with older adults implicitly emphasize attachment themes as both sources of dysfunction and targets for intervention. This chapter presents attachment theory as a conceptual framework for informing couple and family interventions with older adults.

Theorists have long recognized the relevance of attachment themes in later life, given the range of aging-associated events likely to trigger a heightened sense of vulnerability and to raise the specter of distressing (and often permanent) separation and loss experiences. As time marches on, elders and their family members are likely to become increasingly sensitive to physical and/or cognitive limitations, the presence or threat of chronic illness, the loss of same-age peers or loved ones, and the realization that one's time on earth is limited. While these changes typically prove challenging for elders and their family members, individuals and families clearly differ in their ability to successfully adjust to and cope with the stresses of aging. Research examining attachment models and processes in later life suggests that attachment security is associated with "successful" aging across a variety of contexts (see Bradley & Cafferty, 2001, for a detailed review of literature applying attachment theory to older adults). For instance, in a study of elderly dementia patients, Magai and Cohen (1998) found that a secure premorbid attachment style predicted greater levels of positive emotional expression following the onset of illness, while an insecure style predicted negative emotional expression and dementia-related symptoms. Similarly, several authors have shown that attachment security is related to a lower subjective sense of burden and a greater commitment to provide care among adult children caring for chronically ill older parents (e.g., Cicirelli, 1993, 1995; Crispi, Schiaffino, & Berman, 1997). Attachment security has also been linked to greater adjustment following bereavement (Sable, 1989) and to general well-being among older adults (Webster, 1997; Wensauer & Grossmann, 1995).

Given the evidence suggestive of relationships between attachment security and positive adjustment to the stresses of aging, it seems reasonable to assume that attachment issues might prove especially relevant and useful in therapeutic work with older adults, particularly in the context of marital and family therapy. Much of the literature on couple and family interventions with older adults stresses the importance of attachment themes and issues without explicitly invoking attachment theory per se. For example, Qualls (1996, 1999) observes that as families age, older parents may be challenged to accommodate the increasing autonomy of their adult children and to view them as peers, while adult children may be challenged to come to terms with the increasing dependency or frailty of their older parents. While these changes are likely to be somewhat stressful or anxiety-provoking, successful adaptation is thought to be strongly linked to flexibility within interaction patterns, open communication, and mutual responsiveness and sensitivity among family members. Other authors underscore the importance of attachment themes in aging families, particularly the balance between dependence and autonomy. Many of these authors describe attachment in quantitative terms—for instance, along a continuum from detached to enmeshed (e.g., Greene, 1989) or from positive to negative (e.g., Shields, King, & Wynne, 1995). While a focus on the interdependence among elders and their families is certainly appropriate, attachment theory specifically addresses qualitative differences in attachment models and behaviors, and, as such, offers great promise for informing interventions with aging couples and families. (For a general review of literature on interventions with older adults, see Kennedy & Tanenbaum, 2000.)

Attachment theory may also prove to be a valuable complement to couple and family interventions in that attachment needs and their emotional and cognitive correlates provide a bridge between the psychological experience of individual members and the larger family context. Bowlby (1982) emphasized the idea that individuals' attachment systems are likely to be activated in times of distress related to vulnerability, separation, and loss (or the perception or expectation thereof). For clinicians working with older adults and their families, attachment theory provides a rich framework for understanding links between an individual's behavior in family relationships and his or her underlying fears, vulnerabilities, and needs. As such, attachment concepts may have clinical utility on several levels: (1) as templates to inform case conceptualization; (2) as the basis for techniques and strategies applied to couple and family interventions; and (3) as the theoretical foundation for attachment-based therapies such as emotionally focused therapy (EFT; Johnson, 1996).

ATTACHMENT THEORY AS A FRAMEWORK
FOR CASE CONCEPTUALIZATION

At the most basic level of application to psychotherapy, attachment theory holds much promise as a framework for case conceptualization and assessment. In an overview of applications of attachment theory to individual therapy with adults, Slade (1999) emphasizes that attachment patterns are likely to be related to individuals' ability and/or willingness to access certain kinds of thoughts, feelings, and memories. As such, the therapist as listener must be sensitive to the *function* of speech (and by implication, thought) patterns, particularly in terms of how verbal behavior relates to the regulation of emotion. For example, someone who has developed a preoccupied–anxious orientation with respect to attachment may show poorly regulated affect and may seem overwhelmed by emotion at times; in contrast, individuals with a dismissing–avoidant attachment orientation may appear rigid, constricted, or evasive, particularly when discussing emotionally charged subject matter. While avoidant individuals may use vague language and provide few details about attachment themes, preoccupied individuals may show disorganized, tangential speech and a tendency to "ramble on" about attachment themes (Main, 1991).

Among older adults, the therapist may be challenged to distinguish attachment-related patterns of emotion regulation from generational or cohort effects (e.g., the belief that it is inappropriate to share one's deepest feelings or to "complain" too much). Whereas some older adults may adhere to a general norm of emotional constraint, this behavior is likely to be most evident in casual or superficial conversation; by contrast, the tendency to restrict or suppress one's emotions characteristic of avoidant attachment is likely to be most evident when discussing events related to emotional vulnerability. The latter is evident in the following example, in which a man in his late 60s discusses how he coped with the death of his adult child:

THERAPIST: What is it like now, to talk about her?

CLIENT: Well, we remember the fun times. The memories, these are the strong memories. We don't remember the bad times. There wasn't, as I say, you don't . . . I can't think of times when . . . (*clears throat*) . . . only small . . . only happy anecdotes (*tearing up slightly, holding it back, not wiping his eyes*).

While the content of this man's speech might suggest a healthy optimism, the process of his speech suggests that he invests considerable effort in suppressing his emotions. This suppression is evident in his reluctance to acknowledge his sadness (and to call attention to his crying) and in the halting manner of his speech, particularly as he seems torn between acknowledging and denying the existence of "the bad times."

Attachment theory may prove particularly useful as a conceptual framework for therapists working with aging families. Byng-Hall (1991, 1999) describes the family system as the intersection point of family members' respective attachment models; collectively, individual models and family interaction patterns may represent a "shared working model," or "family script." Just as individual attachment systems are "goal-corrected," so is the family system, with each member attempting to find and maintain a "secure base" within the family. To the extent that the family system provides a network of supportive relationships, readily accessible by all family members, the shared working model will constitute a "secure family base." Under less-than-optimal circumstances, family members may learn to employ defensive strategies and develop insecure attachment models, which collectively will undermine the secure family base. For example, a child who experiences rejection, criticism, or negative affect when seeking support from a caregiver may develop a generalized expectation that support is unavailable; as such, the child may learn to avoid expressing attachment needs toward his or her caregivers. In turn, the caregiver may view the child as aloof, cold, or sullen, perhaps prompting continued criticism of or demands toward the child. Both the child's avoidance and the caregiver's criticism can be seen as attachment strategies, albeit defensive ones, in that their intent is to maintain a tenuous sense of security in the face of potential rejection or unresponsiveness.

A key element of Byng-Hall's model is the role of individual attachment models as distance regulators within the family system. For instance, a family member with a fear of rejection may engage in clingy, dependent, or critical behavior, which in turn may elicit negative responses (such as rejection or criticism) from family members. As such, the individual may experience an "approach–avoidance conflict" whenever the attachment system is activated; over time, the individual learns to change his or her strategy toward one of detachment or withdrawal in an attempt to avoid further rejection or criticism. This scenario seems particularly likely among older adults who have a history of conflict with or rejection by other family members; over time, these elders may learn not to turn to others to have their needs met, preferring to maintain a tenuous sense of security by conflict avoidance and compulsive self-reliance. This theme is suggested by a 65-year-old widow, who described learning not to express her opinions to her adult son after years of conflict, typically stemming from her son's perception of her as critical and overinvolved:

CLIENT: And I'd like for him to be able to spend more time with his children, and relatives, but right now it's pay the bills—both have to work to pay the bills for what they want, their lifestyle.

THERAPIST: So it sounds like you have these concerns, but at the same time you're letting him make his own decisions.

CLIENT: Oh yes, I don't make decisions anymore (*laughs*), I don't give many opinions either. . . . It's a good relationship, and even though I'm investigating long-term care, and what I'm going to do with myself when I'm no longer able to do for myself, I know my son would take me in, he would bend over backwards, but I don't want him to have to.

THERAPIST: Is this something that the two of you have discussed, or are you just looking forward?

CLIENT: We've discussed it before, and he's told me more than once, "Well, you can come live with us," my daughter-in-law too talks about my coming to stay with them, but I really don't want to stay with them—it would just be a problem.

While many older adults may be reluctant to "impose" on their adult children, several elements from the excerpt above suggest that attachment dynamics might be at work on a deeper level. For example, the woman hints at the history of conflict with her son by pointing out that she no longer expresses concerns to her son; then she spontaneously shifts to a discussion of her refusal to let her son care for her despite mentioning that he would "bend over backwards" for her. The discussion of the past conflict between this woman and her son seems to have elicited multiple examples of how she has shifted to a more avoidant stance with respect to her son in her later life. While this strategy may offer the advantage of avoiding future conflict and potential alienation of her son, this defensive stance prevents the use of potentially more adaptive strategies (e.g., accepting care from a willing caregiver, expressing her concerns openly to her son).

Byng-Hall (1999) discusses a number of possible scenarios in which individual models and family dynamics interact reciprocally in the context of caregiving families. While his discussion focuses on parents caring for infants or children, the issues involved seem readily applicable to families taking care of an aging family member. In families with a "secure family base," members collaborate in a manner that shows sensitivity to the needs of both the care recipient *and* the caregivers. Family members tend to work together to plan, delegate responsibility, and provide mutual support. In contrast, insecurity among one or more family members may be expressed in a variety of maladaptive ways. For instance, the threat posed by a chronically or terminally ill older member may lead to minimization or outright denial among the ill elder and/or family members, particularly those with avoidant attachment models. Alternately, anxious attachment models might lead to compulsive caregiving, power struggles among caregivers, or "competition for care" among care recipients. Regardless of how attachment models play out in the family context, a central task for clinicians working with aging families is to recognize that all of these manifestations represent strategies for obtaining and maintaining security in the face of threat and vulnerability—namely, the threat of separation and loss posed by the aging process in general and by illness in particular. Conceptualizing the aging family in terms of the individual attachment models that influence broader family dynamics provides a rich framework to structure interventions.

APPLYING ATTACHMENT CONCEPTS TO COUPLE AND FAMILY INTERVENTIONS

In addition to their utility in case formulation in assessment, techniques based on attachment concepts can be used as valuable therapeutic tools for clinicians working with older families and couples. Regardless of the specific therapeutic context or extent of application, clinicians would likely benefit from a thorough understanding of the relationship between symptoms of interpersonal or familial distress and underlying attachment signals. Central to this view is the notion that many problems in family contexts—such as excessive criticism or arguing, withdrawal and emotional detachment, and manipulative or controlling behaviors—are the result of distortions of "normal" attachment signals, such as fears of abandonment, the desire for closeness, and needs for security (Kobak, Ruckdeschel, & Hazan, 1994). Given the range of life transitions associated with older adulthood, it seems reasonable to assume that such attachment needs will take on greater prominence, thus increasing the potential for distress "symptoms" to play out in family contexts.

Application to Psychoeducational Interventions

One relatively common form of intervention with aging families involves the use of psychoeducational techniques to assist families caring for an older member. These approaches are typically geared toward families with an elder who is suffering from some type of age-related impairment, illness, or disability. Therapeutic aims may involve educating caregivers about the aging process, specific illnesses, or the health system; teaching caregivers coping skills; and providing support aimed at reducing caregivers' subjective sense of burden.

A common technique used to achieve these aims involves reframing or relabeling the ill elder's symptoms or "problem" behaviors. Zarit (1996) underscores the importance of helping caregiving family members to see ill elders' problematic behaviors as manifestations of their illness (and of their emotional needs related to the illness). Attachment theory offers a powerful tool for reframing in that it shifts focus away from care recipients' overt behaviors and symptoms and onto their underlying attachment needs (i.e., for comfort, reassurance, and security). As some theorists have observed, aging care recipients' needs for security are sometimes expressed indirectly, which may prove confusing or outright anxiety-provoking for caregivers. For example, Wright, Hickey, Buckwalter, and Clipp (1995) observe that some Alzheimer's sufferers are careful to avoid conflict or excessive requests for assistance (lest they alienate the caregiver), while in other cases care recipients may show clingy, dependent, or demanding behaviors (to ensure that their needs are met). In addition, some elders may display signs of rejection, hostility, or outright paranoia toward caregivers; these behaviors may indicate defensive attempts at self-reliance or a desire to appear "strong" in the face of a deeper sense of vulnerability. While overt behavior in these examples clearly differs across individuals, from an attachment perspective all of these behaviors reflect individual strategies aimed at ensuring security and proximity to the caregiver.

To the extent that therapists working with caregiving families can successfully reframe an aging family member's overt behavior in terms of his or her needs for security, caregivers may experience a shift from feelings of defensiveness, confusion, or resentment to a position of greater empathy, sensitivity, and responsiveness. For example, in the case of an adult son taking care of an older mother with terminal cancer who at times criticized her son's attempts to care for her and complained of his lack of involvement, the therapist might observe:

> "It sounds as though she's scared, like she's aware that she is dying and is feeling kind of desperate; and maybe she's trying to be strong and tough on the outside instead of expressing that fear directly. This could be her way of telling you she really needs you."

In this example, the therapist clearly connects the mother's behavior to her underlying vulnerability and need for security; in addition, her criticism is framed as an attempt to cope (by trying to appear strong), as opposed to a problem behavior or a sign of pathology. Ideally, an intervention of this sort shifts the focus away from assigning blame to an emphasis on empathic understanding of the care recipient's behavior in terms of her or his underlying attachment needs. When such understanding is attained, caregivers may experience less subjective burden as well as a heightened ability for sensitive, productive responding. Consider these comments made by a 68-year-old woman who recounted her experiences while caring for her terminally ill mother:

> "Sometimes me and her would have . . . not have words, but you know, she would say, 'I'm gonna get me some place else to go,' and I'd say, 'OK, when you do, let me know, so I can go with you,' and then she'd laugh and all. But it was hard for her to give up control to somebody else. It's hard, you know, I'm sure it's hard, after you've been your own person to be the child again."

Although the woman described her mother's behavior as "demanding" at times, her empathic understanding of her mother's increased sense of vulnerability and reduced autonomy allowed her to see her mother's behavior as an expression of her needs for security; as such, she was able to respond nondefensively, reassuring her mother that she was available.

Application to Couple and Family Therapy

While employing such reframing techniques in the context of psychoeducational interventions represents a relatively simple application, attachment concepts can also be extended to more intensive couple and family interventions. Employing an attachment perspective in interventions with aging families may be particularly useful in overcoming resistance or defensiveness at the outset of therapy. A number of authors underscore the potential for various forms of resistance in therapy contexts involving aging families. For instance, Qualls (1991) observes that elders are often "scapegoated" as the source of familial distress by family members who are having difficulty adapting to age-related changes in the elder's behavior. Conversely, family members may deny the scope or seriousness of aging relatives' difficulties and/or blame caregivers for not dealing with the elders appropriately. In all of these situations, a particular family member has been identified as the "patient," or the source of the problem, when the difficulties might be more appropriately conceptualized as the failure of the family system to adapt to changes related to the aging process (Qualls, 1999).

In cases involving defensiveness surrounding the assignment of blame and the identification of a specific family member as the "patient," an attachment perspective offers a framework for helping families take a broader, nondefensive stance while creating a sense of shared responsibility.

This end can be accomplished in the earlier stages of contact by framing distress symptoms as the frustrated expression of basic attachment needs such as closeness and security (Kobak et al., 1994). To the extent that the therapist validates each family member's individual perspective while reframing his or her feelings in a nonaccusatory fashion, the family is likely to be willing to accept greater shared responsibility in addressing the problems of concern.

In many circumstances in which an older relative is identified as the "patient," or primary source of difficulty, the elder may not even be included in the initial contact with the therapist. This pattern was illustrated by a woman in her early 60s who sought brief individual therapy to help cope with feelings of stress and burden related to caring for her elderly mother, who lived in a nearby residential facility. The woman reported feeling that her mother demanded a great deal of care and attention from her, often calling at all hours of the day to request assistance with various personal matters. In addition, the woman reported hearing from her brother (who lived several hundred miles away) that her mother occasionally complained to him about the care she was receiving. The woman reported that she had never brought these issues up with her mother, as she "didn't feel she could handle it," and went on to describe her mother as having had a troubled past and "low self-esteem." In this case, the therapist tactfully pointed out that the woman's reluctance to discuss these issues with her mother, as well as her view of her mother as needy, demanding, and weak, likely came across as thinly veiled resentment and a reluctance to emotionally support her mother. This shift in emphasis from the mother's difficult behavior to the interpersonal dynamic between mother and daughter opened the door for short-term family work, in which the mother was able to reveal her fears of abandonment by her daughter in the face of her imminent death, while the daughter was able to discuss her feelings of inadequacy or helplessness in meeting her mother's needs. For both parties, the experience of being able to directly express their attachment needs and fears, as well as to have them clearly heard and understood, helped them establish a warmer and more meaningful connection. The daughter reported that being able to see her mother in "a new light" helped her feel more sympathetic to her needs and more forgiving of her occasional complaints, while the mother began to express more gratitude for her daughter's efforts to care for her.

The shift from a defensive, blaming posture toward one of greater openness, sensitivity, and shared responsibility is often characterized as a "softening" (Johnson & Greenberg, 1995; Kobak et al., 1994). This phenomenon typically occurs when attachment-related emotions such as fear and sadness are identified and amplified in a safe therapeutic context. The experience of softening is particularly beneficial when participants experience this shift on an emotional level in the session and the therapist is successful in helping clients to process this experience and in facilitating greater engagement between partners (Johnson & Greenberg, 1988).

EMOTIONALLY FOCUSED THERAPY
WITH AGING COUPLES AND FAMILIES

While the attachment concepts described above may be incorporated into many forms of couple and family intervention with varying degrees of involvement and intensity, they may also be employed as a systematic basis for therapy. The most rigorous and thorough application of attachment theory concepts to clinical intervention with adults involves emotionally focused therapy (EFT; Johnson, 1996; Johnson & Greenberg, 1994, 1995). Although most of the EFT literature focuses on marital or romantic relationships, EFT principles may also be applied successfully at the family level (e.g., Johnson, Maddeaux, & Blouin, 1998). EFT is based on the assumption that the desire for attachment security motivates much behavior in close relationships (i.e., in couple and family settings). Events that affect the couple or family system—such as ongoing marital distress, illness of a family member, or even aging in general—may lead one or more members of the system to feel a sense of deterioration of the secure base (i.e., a sense that others have become less accessible and responsive). While individuals may attempt to cope with this vulnerability by using a variety of strategies, two of the more common approaches involve constellations of feelings, thoughts, and behaviors related to anxiety (e.g., protesting, clinging, demanding, criticizing, dependency) and to avoidance (e.g., withdrawal, affective "cutting off").

The practice of EFT involves two overriding goals: (1) accessing and identifying the primary emotions underlying individuals' attachment strategies; and (2) using the newly accessed emotions to help restructure couple and family interactions to promote a shared sense of security and engagement. While EFT shares some prominent features of behavioral, systemic, and narrative approaches (such as identifying and restructuring systemic patterns of interaction), EFT places primary emphasis on emotional engagement during the therapy session. Rather than having clients recount emotionally charged past events or discuss them in an abstract sense, the therapist closely follows the family's emotional experience in the session with the intent of accessing and enhancing the primary emotions underlying each member's interactional stance. Central to EFT is the notion that emotions serve as signals of underlying attachment needs as well as primary mechanisms of therapeutic change (Johnson & Greenberg, 1994). When family members successfully identify and express primary emotions in the session, these emotions serve as "signals" that guide other family members' responses toward a more caring, supportive stance. It should be emphasized that EFT does not simply involve indiscriminate "venting" of emotions; rather, the therapist helps family members express primary emotions in a manner that is likely to facilitate greater responsiveness and engagement among family members.

Case Example

George and Alice, ages 66 and 65, were seen for 10 sessions of EFT following a course of conjoint sessions with a mediator. George and Alice had been married for 41 years and had three grown children and six grandchildren. George had retired from a demanding job 1 year earlier, and as a result George and Alice were focused on how they would spend their retirement years together. They described their relationship as challenging from its inception, which they attributed to having very different backgrounds. A constant theme between the couple had been Alice feeling alone and responsible in the marriage and in the family and George feeling resentful and controlled. This dynamic played out in the early years of the marriage with George spending a lot of time outside of the home drinking with his family and friends and Alice at home alone raising the children. At this time the couple lived close to George's family, but Alice's unhappiness grew to the point that she eventually moved herself and the children back to her hometown. George followed her and the marriage improved in that George's drinking subsided; however, their interactional patterns remained unchanged. Alice continued to feel alone in taking care of the children and herself, although she resented her role as the "leader" in the family. In turn, George resented Alice's domination but typically responded with withdrawal and conflict avoidance.

George and Alice's decision to attend therapy began indirectly, with the inheritance of George's old family homestead, which presented a crisis in the marriage because of what it symbolized to the couple: Alice felt "haunted" by the house and the old wounds it represented, whereas for George it meant freedom and a chance to recapture his childhood. In the months prior to the beginning of therapy, the couple sought mediation to forge a separation, but through this process they were able to reach an agreement around the ownership of the homestead. This resolution prompted George and Alice to decide to work on their marriage, and they were subsequently referred for couple therapy.

Like George and Alice, for many older families the decision to seek professional help may be prompted by difficulty adjusting to a major transition, often brought on by the aging process. As many of these transitions (e.g., onset or worsening of a chronic illness, a change in residence or living arrangement, retirement) threaten to change or upset family and couple dynamics, individual attachment systems and their associated emotional reactions are likely to be highly activated among one or more of the family members seeking clinical help. Often these underlying attachment needs and fears may be masked or obscured by a focus on more specific issues related to the transition. It is important for clinicians to see the "objective" information regarding the family's current circumstances in light of the underlying attachment dynamics operating within and between family members. Even in cases where a relatively simple intervention is indicated—for instance, a brief psychoeducational intervention with caregivers of an infirm older family member—sensitivity to the needs and fears of family members from an attachment perspective can provide a basis for a more empathic understanding of the family's concerns and will allow the clinician to tailor the intervention to better fit the family.

The case of George and Alice also demonstrates another critical issue specific to work with older couples: as many older couples are likely to have relatively long histories of marital distress, conflict, withdrawal, or disengagement, one or both partners may feel a sense of resignation or hopelessness. Further, the couple may feel ashamed to be seeking treatment and may be skeptical about the potential for improving the relationship. Indeed, George and Alice came to therapy feeling discouraged and somewhat embarrassed to be seeking help at this late point in their marriage. They had sought counseling at other points in their life, and George had been in individual therapy for a number of years, which he stated "didn't fix me." As a result, both were consequently reserved in their expectations, wanting primarily to "get along peacefully." Alice was clear that she didn't trust George and had given up on feeling close to him years ago. Alice described feeling "sick and tired" of trying to make the marriage work, while George stated that he often felt "lost" and was unable to see how he could make a difference in the way his wife felt. The beginning of therapy was focused on building an alliance with each partner and validating their positions, as well as recognizing their courage in coming to sessions and their obvious commitment to one another, as evidenced through their marriage's longevity and their efforts to help both themselves and each other. The therapist congratulated George and Alice for their 40 years of marriage and praised their ingenuity in accessing services to help when faced with a problem. In addition, the therapist framed this stage in their marriage as an opportunity for growth as a couple and an optimal time to work on their relationship, as their children were grown and out of the home. An effort was made to create a therapeutic environment that acknowledged their struggle, reinforced their strengths, and suggested that changing their interaction patterns was indeed possible.

It is crucial that therapists working with older adults resist the temptation to view elders as "set in their ways" or unable to make meaningful life changes. Of course, therapists are not the only parties susceptible to such fatalistic assumptions; clients themselves may see their situation as hopeless or their problems as irreparable, particularly if they view their problems as the fault of other family members. In the example above, the therapist immediately attempted to establish an expectation that change was possible by reinforcing George and Alice's decision to work on their relationship and framing the longevity of their marriage as a further indication of their commitment to each other.

Therapists working with older couples can also foster more positive expectations for therapy by framing marital and family problems as the result of interaction patterns and dynamics, rather than as the result of individual flaws, personality features, or psychopathology. As the initial sessions of George and Alice's therapy were focused on accessing the emotions underlying the couple's negative interactional cycles, the therapist was careful to help George and Alice see their difficulties in systemic terms, rather than blaming each other or themselves. This emphasis allowed George and Alice to begin to discuss their interaction patterns in a relatively non-defensive fashion. During the early part of their marriage, the couple had been engaged in a pursue–withdraw cycle, with Alice doing the pursuing and George the withdrawing. In more recent years, the pattern changed to mutual withdrawal and disengagement, as Alice had experienced many years of feeling that George was unavailable to her. Currently there was very little closeness or trust experienced between the couple, and no physical intimacy. Alice talked about feeling alone and abandoned in the relationship, and she revealed her pain and hurt over George's lack of consideration of her needs. Historically, Alice reacted to her pain by attempting to control her environment and make demands and rules for the relationship. Alice managed all of the couple's decisions around money, recreation, and their children, while George remained quiet but resentful of what he termed the "boss–slave" relationship. Alice's complaints made George feel deficient and incompetent, and rather than fight or protest, he became emotionally withdrawn. George's withdrawal signaled to Alice that she was alone and that she needed to take care of herself rather than depending on George. The more Alice felt alone, the more she became self-reliant and managerial; the more George felt impotent and angry at himself and Alice, the more withdrawn he became. While George's compliance with Alice on one level appeared harmonious, on another level he was both resentful and depressed about his position in the marriage.

The dynamics of George and Alice's relationship over the course of their marriage underscore the idea that attachment is a dynamic system that adapts to changes in the (interpersonal) environment, rather than an immutable, trait-like variable. George and Alice's respective attachment systems seemed to adapt in response to external feedback at several points throughout their relationship. For instance, while George and Alice showed the familiar "attack–withdrawal" pattern in the earlier years of their relationship, Alice gradually shifted to a posture of withdrawal herself after years of unsuccessful attempts to "reach" George through criticism. Indeed, it seems likely that this pattern of mutual disengagement might be more common in older couples with histories of marital difficulty. While this pattern may offer a superficial sense of stability, it is important for the therapist and the family alike to realize that such "detachment" is not a normative aspect of the aging process, but a defensive attempt to maintain a sense of attachment security. As therapy progresses and this defensive stance is explored and questioned, one or both partners may feel threatened by the potential disruption of this stability and may fear the opening of old wounds. In these cases the therapist should remember that anxiety is a normal by-product of therapeutic change at *any* age or developmental stage; all the same, considerable tact and sensitivity to family members' anxiety (as well as to their desire to change) is essential.

In the case of George and Alice, the exploration of their interactional cycles in a safe therapeutic context allowed the couple to gradually reexperience disowned aspects of themselves and to express these directly to each other. Alice was able to talk about her past wounds and have them acknowledged and validated by George, who stated that he had a great deal of remorse around not being there for Alice and that he wished he had been more of a support to her over the years. Alice was increasingly able to let go of the past but was also uncertain that she could count on George to be there for her in the future, especially as she aged and felt more vulnerable. George also felt afraid about the future, remarking "I don't have a map." He described himself as always feeling like a "lone wolf" who didn't feel close to anyone and didn't accept help from anyone. For George, isolation felt safe; he added that "if someone said they loved me, I would freak out." George acknowledged that fear led him to avoid closeness with Alice, and pointed out that when the two shared a positive moment or Alice showed signs of appreciating him, he minimized these instances or pushed them out of awareness.

At this stage, therapy focused on helping George gradually explore his fears of closeness and his feelings of unworthiness and inadequacy. Some of these feelings were rooted in the injuries inflicted early in the marriage when George abandoned Alice by drinking and disappearing for days, behavior which made George feel shameful and self-critical. As George was able to feel more of his own grief around the past (and to be reassured that Alice heard and understood these feelings), George became more able to respond to Alice in a caring and loving fashion. In the middle of therapy, Alice became sick through the night and was able to rely on George; she mentioned that George responded to her like "my guardian angel." Processing this experience in therapy helped the couple consolidate a new pattern of responsive interaction, and they began to recognize and identify the gifts they were giving each other. George's ability to hear Alice's pain over past wounds and to express his own regrets allowed Alice to reexperience her longing for closeness with George. As George saw that Alice could accept his feelings of regret, he was able to acknowledge his fear and conflict over further disappointing her and to access his own pain and unmet needs for closeness. As Alice was able to see the softer side of her husband, she began to reflect more on her own behavior and apologize for criticizing him, which Alice found "had a big impact" on George. At the end of therapy, the couple reported that they were closer and were initiating physical affection; as such, they felt comfortable terminating sessions, knowing they could call again if needed.

Discussion

This case example illustrates the value in using attachment concepts as a systematic framework for therapy with older adult clients. Perhaps one of the most valuable aspects of an attachment framework is that it defines clients' presenting problems as manifestations of a universal human need, rather than as signs of weakness, frailty, or psychopathology. This shift in emphasis may be particularly important for older adults, who are often stigmatized as "difficult," "crotchety," or "senile." In addition, a focus on interpersonal patterns rather than individual symptoms may help reduce clients' initial defensiveness or "entrenchment." In the example above, conceptualizing George and Alice's difficulty in terms of an interaction cycle helped defuse any potential for assigning blame and "finger pointing." Reframing their behaviors in terms of their underlying vulnerabilities and emphasizing their strategies for maintaining a sense of security (albeit a tenuous one) implicitly shifted the focus of therapy toward their unmet needs for attachment and closeness. In this context, both partners found it relatively easy to acknowledge that they wanted to be close, although they hadn't known how to let down their guard and reach out to each other in the past.

Dankoski (2001) points out that EFT is a particularly useful treatment approach for couples and families whose distress is related to major life events that call for changes in the relationship system. Major life cycle transitions—including many normative later life events, such as retirement and the increased susceptibility to illness and death—may be particularly troublesome for families lacking a secure family base. In the present example, George's retirement and inheritance of his family's old homestead seemed to open up "old wounds," in that Alice seemed to perceive their returning to his family's home as a return to her frustrated past with George. In this sense, Alice's feelings of being "haunted" by the old home take on deeper significance. By zeroing in on the deeper fears triggered by the transitional event, the therapist was able to help George and Alice react to each other's needs for security with greater sensitivity and responsiveness.

It is particularly noteworthy that George and Alice were able to break their cycle of defensive withdrawal and to connect with each other in a relatively short period of therapy, despite their age and their long history of distance and avoidance. This outcome underscores an important aspect of attachment theory: while Bowlby conceptualized attachment models as remaining relatively stable over the lifespan, he also emphasized the "goal-corrected" nature of the attachment system in adapting to feedback from attachment figures (Bowlby, 1980). Contrary to the negative stereotype that older adults are rigid and "set in their ways," some elders—particularly in times of transition—may actually be more amenable to change in the later stages of life. Erikson (1982) observed that the developmental struggle between generativity and stagnation may continue from middle age to later life, particularly as aging adults strive to further define a meaningful sense of identity incorporating both past and future. The EFT model allows great sensitivity to both sides of this tension (i.e., the need for stability and security and the desire for growth and enhancement of meaning). Like narrative-based approaches to psychotherapy, EFT encourages therapists and clients to examine and actively construe their "life stories" in subjective, personalized terms. The therapist's skillful use of EFT may offer older couples and families a chance to jointly "write" a happy ending to their shared life story.

CONCLUSION

Increased attention to the mental health needs of elders and their families is strongly warranted, especially given the dramatic increase and projected further growth of the world's elderly population. While much of the current literature pertaining to interventions with older adults is highly sensitive to the importance of the family context, many of these treatment approaches lack a clear theoretical focus. Attachment theory has shown great promise both as a framework for guiding interventions (Johnson & Greenberg, 1994) and as a framework for understanding individual differences in adapting to lifespan transitions, including many developmental events associated with aging (Bradley & Cafferty, 2001). Further, the application of attachment concepts to interventions with older adults offers promise on many levels of integration, ranging from a framework for hypothesis formation or case conceptualization to the foundation of systematic approaches for working with couples and families. Perhaps most significantly, an attachment perspective respects the humanity and dignity of older adult clients, in that it views distress symptoms as manifestations of a basic, universal human need, rather than as signs of frailty, weakness, or decline. As such, the thoughtful use of attachment concepts in interventions with older couples and families offers the potential for continued growth and generativity, even in the later stages of life.

REFERENCES

Ainsworth, M. D. S., Blehar, M. C., Waters, E., & Wall, S. (1978). *Patterns of attachment: A psychological study of the Strange Situation.* Hillsdale, NJ: Erlbaum.

Bowlby, J. (1979). *The making and breaking of affectional bonds.* London: Tavistock.

Bowlby, J. (1980). *Attachment and loss: Vol, III. Loss: Sadness and depression.* London: Hogarth Press.

Bowlby, J. (1982). *Attachment and loss: Vol. I. Attachment* (2nd ed). New York: Basic Books. (First edition published in 1969)

Bradley, J. M., & Cafferty, T. P. (2001). Attachment among older adults: Current issues and directions for future research. *Attachment and Human Development, 3*(2), 200–221.

Byng-Hall, J. (1991). The application of attachment theory to understanding and treatment in family therapy. In C. M. Parkes, J. Stevenson-Hinde, & P. Marris (Eds.), *Attachment across the life cycle* (pp. 199–215). New York: Tavistock/ Routledge.

Byng-Hall, J. (1999). Family and couple therapy: Toward greater security. In J. Cassidy & P. R. Shaver (Eds.), *Handbook of attachment: Theory, research, and clinical applications* (pp. 625–645). New York: Guilford Press.

Cicirelli, V. G. (1993). Attachment and obligation as daughters' motives for caregiving behavior and subsequent effect on subjective burden. *Psychology and Aging, 8,* 144–155.

Cicirelli, V. G. (1995). A measure of caregiving daughters' attachment to elderly mothers. *Journal of Family Psychology, 9,* 89–94.

Cicirelli, V. G. (1996). Emotion and cognition in attachment. In C. Magai & S. H. McFadden (Eds.), *Handbook of emotion, adult development and aging* (pp. 119–132). San Diego, CA: Academic Press.

Crispi, E. L., Schiaffino, K., & Berman, W. H. (1997). The contribution of attachment to burden in adult children of institutionalized parents with dementia. *Educational Research, 37,* 52–60.

Dankowski, M. E. (2001). Pulling on the heart strings: An emotionally focused approach to family life cycle transitions. *Journal of Marital and Family Therapy, 27*(2), 177–187.

Erikson, E. H. (1982). *The life cycle completed: A review.* New York: Norton.

Greene, R. (1989). A life-systems approach to understanding parent–child relationships in aging families. *Journal of Psychotherapy and the Family, 5*(1–2), 57–69.

Hazan, C., & Shaver, P. R. (1987). Romantic love conceptualized as an attachment process. *Journal of Personality and Social Psychology, 52,* 511–524.

Johnson, S. M. (1996). *The practice of emotionally-focused marital therapy: Creating connection.* New York: Brunner/Mazel.

Johnson, S. M., & Greenberg, L. S. (1988). Relating process to outcome in marital therapy. *Journal of Marital and Family Therapy, 14*, 175–184.

Johnson, S. M., & Greenberg, L. S. (1994). Emotion in intimate relationships: Theory and implications for therapy. In S. M. Johnson & L. S. Greenberg (Eds.), *The heart of the matter: Perspectives on emotion in marital therapy* (pp. 3–22). New York: Brunner/Mazel.

Johnson, S. M., & Greenberg, L. S. (1995). The emotionally focused approach to problems in adult attachment. In N. S. Jacobson & A. S. Gurman (Eds.), *Clinical handbook of couple therapy* (pp. 121–141). New York: Guilford Press.

Johnson, S. M., Maddeaux, C., & Blouin, J. (1998). Emotionally focused family therapy for bulimia: Changing attachment patterns. *Psychotherapy, 35*(2), 238–247.

Kennedy, G. J., & Tanenbaum, S. (2000). Psychotherapy with older adults. *American Journal of Psychotherapy, 54*(3), 386–407.

Kobak, R., Ruckdeschel, K., & Hazan, C. (1994). From symptom to signal: An attachment view of emotion in marital therapy. In S. M. Johnson & L. S. Greenberg (Eds.), *The heart of the matter: Perspectives on emotion in marital therapy* (pp. 46–71). New York: Brunner/Mazel.

Magai, C., & Cohen, C. (1998). Attachment style and emotion regulation in dementia patients and their relation to caregiver burden. *Journals of Gerontology: Series B: Psychological Sciences and Social Sciences, 53B*, 147–154.

Main, M. (1991). Metacognitive knowledge, metacognitive monitoring, and singular (coherent) vs. multiple (incoherent) models of attachment: Findings and directions for future research. In C. M. Parkes, J. Stevenson-Hinde, & P. Marris (Eds.), *Attachment across the life cycle* (pp. 127–159). New York: Tavistock/Routledge.

Qualls, S. H. (1991). Resistance of older families to therapeutic intervention. *Clinical Gerontologist, 11*, 59–68.

Qualls, S. H. (1996). Family therapy with aging families. In S. H. Zarit & B. G. Knight (Eds.), *A guide to psychotherapy and aging: Effective clinical interventions in a life-stage context* (pp. 121–137). Washington, DC: American Psychological Association.

Qualls, S. H. (1999). Family therapy with older adult clients. *Journal of Clinical Psychology, 55*(8), 977–990.

Sable, P. (1989). Attachment, anxiety, and loss of a husband. *American Journal of Orthopsychiatry, 59*, 550–556.

Shields, C. G., King, D. A., & Wynne, L. C. (1995). Interventions with later life families. In R. H. Mikesell, D. D. Lusterman, & S. H. McDaniel (Eds.), *Integrating family therapy: Handbook of family psychology and systems theory* (pp. 141–158). Washington, DC: American Psychological Association.

Slade, A. (1999). Attachment theory and research: Implications for the theory and practice of individual psychotherapy with adults. In J. Cassidy & P. R. Shaver (Eds.), *Handbook of attachment: Theory, research, and clinical applications* (pp. 575–594). New York: Guilford Press.

Webster, J. D. (1997). Attachment style and well-being in elderly adults: A preliminary investigation. *Canadian Journal on Aging, 16*, 101–111.

Wensauer, M., & Grossmann, K. E. (1995). Quality of attachment representation, social integration, and use of network resources in old age. *Zeitschrift für Gerontologie und Geriatrie, 28*, 444–456.

Wright, L. K., Hickey, J. V., Buckwalter, K. C., & Clipp, E. C. (1995). Human development in the context of aging and chronic illness: The role of attachment in Alzheimer's disease and stroke. *International Journal of Aging and Human Development, 41*, 133–150.

Zarit, S. H. (1996). Interventions with family caregivers. In S. H. Zarit & B. G. Knight (Eds.), *A guide to psychotherapy and aging: Effective clinical interventions in a life-stage context* (pp. 139–159). Washington, DC: American Psychological Association.

15

Using an Attachment-Based Intervention with Same-Sex Couples

GORDON J. JOSEPHSON

Attachment theory offers a convincing explanation of romantic love. As described in Hazan and Shaver's (1987) seminal work, attachment theory accounts for the development of different relationship styles, including both functional and nonfunctional interactional patterns. Furthermore, the theory helps us understand the powerful negative and positive emotions that arise in close relationships and does so within an integrated conceptual framework. As demonstrated in the other chapters of this book, the conceptualization of romantic love as attachment has fostered a growing body of research that continues to inform our understanding of romantic relationships. It is not surprising, then, that attachment theory has been identified as one of the main theories used to guide couple interventions (Johnson & Lebow, 2000).

The application of attachment theory to same-sex romantic relationships can be characterized as new but rapidly expanding. As the research into same-sex relationships matures, there is a movement away from atheoretical descriptions toward the application of theories originally developed in the context of heterosexual relationships (Peplau, 1991; Mohr, 1999). Several authors have recently identified the importance of examining the use of empirically validated couple interventions with same-sex couples (Addis & Zamudio, 2001; Cochran, 2001; Greenan & Tunnell, 2003; Johnson & Lebow, 2000). The goal of this chapter is to explore the usefulness of an attachment-based intervention with same-sex couples. The intervention of interest here is emotionally focused therapy (EFT) as articulated by Johnson (1996). The chapter begins with a discussion of the applicability of attachment theory to same-sex couples. Following this, EFT is described and its usefulness in working with same-sex couples is explored.

THE APPLICABILITY OF ATTACHMENT
THEORY TO SAME-SEX COUPLES

A detailed description of attachment theory is beyond the scope of this chapter. For those requiring an introduction to this topic, several excellent resources exist (see, e.g., Hazan & Shaver, 1987; West & Shelden-Keller, 1994; Cassidy & Shaver, 1999; or McKinsey-Crittenden, 2000). In brief, attachment theory is based on two main principles: (1) there is a fundamental adaptive need for maintaining relatedness to others; and (2) one develops an attachment style (i.e., a habitual way of engaging significant others) through early childhood experiences with key caregivers (Bowlby, 1969). Attachment bonds are thought to differ from other social bonds in four ways: (1) the importance of proximity maintenance, (2) the presence of separation distress, and the role of the bond as both (3) a safe haven, and (4) a secure base (Hazan & Zeifman, 1999).

Adult attachment can best be construed as the product of two interacting dimensions, *anxiety* regarding intimate relationships and *avoidance* in such relationships (Brennan, Clark, & Shaver, 1998). These two dimensions have been used to define four categories of attachment style: secure (low in both anxiety and avoidance), anxious (high in anxiety, low in avoidance), avoidant (high in avoidance, low in anxiety), and fearful–avoidant or disorganized (high in both anxiety and avoidance) (Brennan et al., 1998). Attachment behaviors can also be conceptualized as self-protective strategies through which people protect themselves from danger and isolation (McKinsey-Crittenden, 2000). Such a conceptualization is useful in applying the theory to couple interventions as it is likely easier to help a client understand how he or she has become overly self-protective than to get the client to embrace the idea that he or she has an "insecure" attachment style. Regardless of the terminology used to define it, an attachment style is thought to affect the nature and stability of close relationships through influencing two types of behaviors: (1) support seeking and (2) protest at separation. For example, those with anxious or avoidant attachment styles are more likely than those with secure styles to express themselves by distancing, or by attempting to control, their partner. Distancing and control are strategies that contribute to relationship distress and separation (Feeney, 1999).

The discussion of the application of attachment theory to romantic relationships has referred almost exclusively to heterosexual unions, yet the principles involved in the theory appear transferable to any close bond. The applicability of attachment theory to same-sex couples is examined below by reviewing two areas of the literature: (1) the general differences between same-sex and heterosexual couples; and (2) the attachment styles of gay men and lesbians.

General Differences between Same-Sex and Heterosexual Couples

Several differences between heterosexual and same-sex couples are frequently presented in the literature. These proposed differences vary greatly in terms of the evidence on which they are based. Some differences are deduced from clinical observation, such as higher rates of childhood sexual, physical, and emotional abuse (Hardin & Hall, 2001); greater politicalization of same-sex relationships; lack of traditional sex roles; lack of role models; and both partners being socialized into the same gender role (Brown, 1995). Other, empirically derived, differences include less social support for the relationship (Meyer, 1990), higher frequency of sexual contact in male couples (Klinger, 1996), higher rates of substance use (Anderson, 1996), nonmonogamy in gay male relationships (Green, Bettinger, & Zacks, 1996), higher rates of fusion in lesbian relationships and of overdifferentiation of self among gay men (Krestan & Bepko, 1980), negative societal and internalized stigma toward lesbians and gay men and their relationships (J. Mohr, personal communication, July 2001), discrepancies between partners in the degree to which they are open about their orientation (Berger, 1990; Haas & Stafford, 1998), and elevated rates of acquired immune deficiency syndrome (AIDS) among gay men (MacDonald, 1998). However, for several of these characteristics (e.g., rates of substance use), the empirical findings are highly contradictory. Although some observed differences, such as the inability to legally wed, can be easily demonstrated (Ossana, 2000), the effect of such a difference on the couple's functioning remains unclear.

In summary, several articles discuss the potentially unique aspects of same-sex couples; however, the majority of these review the same limited studies. Indeed, two recent extensive reviews of this research both concluded that there is little substantive empirical work on gay and lesbian couples (Ossana, 2000; MacDonald, 1998). The research that does exist often lacks a detailed description of the differences and/or a discussion of their relevance. Factors that moderate or mediate the association between being gay or lesbian and these differences are rarely explored. Furthermore, the vast majority of studies are dated, having been conducted at a time when homosexuality was far less socially acceptable than it is today.

More recently, attempts have been made to clarify some of these inconsistencies. In contrast to samples in which gay men and lesbians are recruited at community centers or through social networks, epidemiological data now exist from random samples of the population in which sexual orientation is recorded. Such studies offer a more accurate account of differences between gay men and lesbians and heterosexual men and women than traditional samples. Epidemiological data indicate that gay men and lesbians are at elevated risk for stress-related disorders such as depression, and that lesbians may experience more difficulties with substance use (Cochran, 2001). Clarification of earlier research has also occurred through reinterpreting the concepts involved using a more informed understanding of lesbians' and gay men's development. For example, the idea that the gender role socialization of girls and boys makes lesbians prone to fusion and gay men prone to "overdifferentiation of self" has been reconsidered using a more detailed understanding of how the gender role socialization of lesbians and gay men may differ from that of heterosexuals (see, e.g., Green et al., 1996; Mackey, O'Brien, & Mackey, 1997; Igartua, 1998).

In summary, the literature on the differences between same-sex and heterosexual couples is characterized by many conjectures but a very limited number of empirically derived and consistent findings. In its present state, this research can only suggest general ideas to consider in clinical work with same-sex couples. Issues such as substance use, histories of abuse, frequency and quality of the couple's sexual contact, monogamy, social support, autonomy and intimacy, and conformity to traditional sex roles are important questions in working with any couple. Alternatively, the politicalization of the relationship, the client's feelings about the lack of legal and formal rituals proclaiming the union, how open each is about their orientation, and the experience of social and internalized stigma are aspects that clinicians may wish to specifically ask about when working with same-sex couples. Concerns regarding the AIDS epidemic could be of more interest in gay male couples than lesbian or heterosexual couples, depending on monogamy, HIV status entering the relationship, and the sexual practices they engage in.

In terms of the present analysis, none of these potential differences would appear to affect the applicability of attachment theory to same-sex relationships. Furthermore, some authors have suggested that attachment theory actually helps us to understand potential differences between same-sex and heterosexual couples. MacDonald (1998) recommended that what is often labeled "fusion" be reinterpreted as "anxious attachment," suggesting that such an attachment style might be a reflection of society's invalidation of lesbian relationships. He also noted that adult attachment theory has an established research base and that attachment style can be assessed using validated self-report questionnaires, whereas the concept of fusion is lacking in these areas.

In addition, evidence from studies comparing same-sex and heterosexual couples suggests that the basic bonds of love and intimacy, factors key to attachment, are the same in both types of couples (Klinger, 1996). A recent examination of long-term relationships concluded that patterns of roles, conflict and its management, decision making, and sexual and psychological intimacy were similar regardless of the sexual orientation of respondents (Mackey et al., 1997). Indeed, despite the potential differences discussed above, the majority of authors indicate that same-sex and heterosexual couples are more similar than they are different.

Attachment in Lesbians and Gay Relationships

Several authors suggest that it is important to explore attachment in same-sex relationships. Anti-gay prejudice and internalized negative views of same-sex attraction are thought to provide gay men and lesbians with unique challenges in forming intimate attachments with each other (Mohr, 1999). Ironically, threat, fear, shame, and anger from anti-gay stigma and hostility might both heighten the importance of a secure attachment and complicate its attainment. It may be that, as suspected for trauma survivors, adverse experience both heightens the need for attachment and renders achieving intimacy and trust more difficult (Johnson, 2002).

Very little has been published discussing the applicability of attachment theory to same-sex relationships. In his review of the literature, Mohr (1999) explored the role of attachment and fear systems in gay men's and lesbians' identity development and concluded that there was no reason to assume that same-sex romantic attachments operate differently than heterosexual ones. Only a few studies have actually measured gay men's and lesbians' attachment styles. Mohr and Fasinger (1997) found that the relationship between attachment style and relationship distress was similar in same-sex and heterosexual couples. They also found initial evidence that insecure attachment was associated with internalized homophobia. Ridge and Feeney (1998) found that the frequencies of the four attachment styles did not differ significantly between homosexual and heterosexual participants. Similarly, Gaines and Henderson (2002) found that the percentages of securely attached lesbians and gay men did not differ from those obtained in studies using heterosexual samples. Elizur and Mintzer (2001) did not obtain significant differences when they compared the rates of attachment styles for gay men in their study to previous research with heterosexual men. Kurdek (1997) found that attachment styles, conceptualized in terms of positive models of self and other, were related to commitment in same-sex couples. Based on these few studies, it appears that the attachment styles of gay men and lesbians can be measured using existing measures and that, as in heterosexual couples, they vary with relationship satisfaction and commitment. In contrast to Mohr's (1999) hypothesis that gay men and lesbians face unique challenges in forming intimate attachments, the research on gay men's and lesbians' attachment styles does not suggest higher frequencies of insecure styles. However, as with most studies about stigmatized minorities, it is difficult to make comparisons with rates in the majority population because the minority group samples are convenience samples that may be biased (i.e., insecurely attached gay and lesbian individuals may be less likely to identify their minority orientation and thus to participate in such a study).

Apart from the question of differences in the frequencies of insecure attachment styles, there remain many unexamined potential differences in the development and functioning of lesbians' and gay men's attachment styles. Variation in attachment style may, for example, be moderated by several factors specific to lesbians and gay men, including the age of coming out, the nature of the coming-out process, the presence of a family member or close friend with whom one could safely discuss sexuality, time spent in individual or group therapy addressing self-acceptance, and/or the experience of intimacy in heterosexual relationships prior to coming out. In the research measuring attachment discussed above, there are some indications that the factors determining attachment style in gay men and lesbians may differ from those in the heterosexual population. Specifically, an association between early parenting and attachment style, typically strong in heterosexual samples, was not found by Ridge and Feeney (1998). These authors called for further research on the predictors of attachment style in gay men and lesbians. In particular, they suggested peer relationships might be important. An initial examination of adult social support and attachment styles by Elizur and Mintzer (2001) suggests gay men's attachment styles may be more closely associated with support from friends than from parents. However, this study examined adult peer relations and, given the importance of experiences at a young age on attachment style (Bowlby, 1969), future studies may want to examine lesbians' and gay men's childhood peer relations.

Before leaving this topic, the following three observations are offered for consideration in future research. First, it appears to be important to distinguish more carefully between the effect of a same-sex orientation on attachment style and the effect of the minority status and stigma associated with that orientation. Second, the relationship between sexuality and attachment needs further clarification. Sexuality can be conceptualized as a component of romantic relationships distinct from attachment. For example, Shaver, Hazan, and Bradshaw (1988) suggested that attachment is one of three components of romantic relationships, with sexuality and caregiving being the other two. More recently, Hazan (Chapter 3, this volume) argued that sexual behavior between two adults promotes their attachment to each other. A more detailed understanding of the relationship between sexuality and attachment could benefit an appreciation of the similarities or differences of attachment in heterosexual and same-sex relationships. Third, concern was raised by Mohr (1999) that an explanation for attachment behaviors based on their evolutionary advantage in the raising of young might require an alternative explanation in someone who experiences same-sex desire. However, a same-sex orientation does not necessarily imply a lack of desire to procreate and/or to parent. In addition to the many gay men and lesbians who have children from earlier heterosexual unions, gay men and lesbians have always found, and continue to find, the means to become parents and to nurture attachment behaviors in their young. From this perspective, an evolutionary theory of the advantages of attachment behavior would be applicable to gay men and lesbians. More research is needed on gay men's and lesbians' parenting and attachment.

Overall, the investigation of attachment styles in lesbians and gay men is very limited. Existing studies have largely been published in only the past 5 years. Although the application of attachment theory to same-sex relationships is in its infancy, there is some evidence that, similar to heterosexual couples, attachment bonds exist and are associated with attraction, commitment, and relationship satisfaction. There is also some limited evidence that the development and operation of an attachment style may differ in some gay men and lesbians, specifically that it may be influenced more by peer than by parent relations and that it might be influenced by societal and internalized anti-gay stigma. Empirical research has not yet been published that examines how the potential differences between heterosexual and same-sex relationships discussed above might relate to attachment. Perhaps the cited differences, such as the lack of role models and public images, are most problematic when a couple does not feel safe enough to be themselves, state their desires, and negotiate with each other. An attachment-based couple therapy is one way in which to promote a safe haven and secure base from which couples can assert such needs.

USING AN ATTACHMENT-BASED
INTERVENTION WITH SAME-SEX COUPLES

From an attachment perspective, the underlying cause of marital distress is the lack of accessibility and responsiveness of at least one partner, and the problematic ways in which the partners deal with their insecurities when this occurs (Johnson, 1996). The goal of couple therapy is, therefore, to change the ways the couple deals with their insecurities and to establish a safe haven and secure base for each partner. The use of attachment-based interventions with same-sex couples is examined below in two steps: (1) existing interventions for same-sex couples are identified and their relationship to attachment theory are examined, and (2) the phases of EFT are examined from the perspective of therapy with a same-sex couple.

Interventions Specific to Same-Sex Couples and Their Relationship to Attachment Theory

Very little has been done in applying therapy interventions to same-sex couples. As recently as 1996, Cabaj and Klinger stated, "At this point, no formal treatment outcome studies on psychotherapy with gay male or lesbian couples have been completed" (p. 498). They speculated that the neglect of this area of study is probably a reflection of the low priority given to research about gay male and lesbian issues in couple therapy. The lack of studies could also be due to a lack of research on couple therapy in general and the complexity of outcome research.

In the review for this chapter, five descriptions of approaches to couple therapy specific to same-sex couples were identified. The five include an Adlerian approach (Fisher, 1993), a combination of psychodynamic and cognitive therapy (Gray & Isensee, 1996), a stage model (McWhirter & Mattison, 1982), a psychodynamic approach (Butler & Clarke, 1991), and a structural therapy approach (Greenan & Tunnell, 2003). None of these five approaches involves a clear theory of romantic relationships in their conceptualization. However, several have aspects that support the use of an approach based in attachment theory. These include attention to feelings and thoughts about self and other (Fisher, 1993), a concern with both interpersonal and intrapersonal dynamics and an acknowledgment of interactional cycles that promote distress and prevent closeness (Gray & Isensee, 1996), and efforts to understand oneself and one's relationship needs and to communicate this to one's partner, including expressing emotion to establish a secure base (Butler & Clarke, 1991). Although Greenan and Tunnell (2003) make explicit reference to attachment theory in their explanation of how some gay men learn to fear emotional bonds and value autonomy, they do not incorporate this into the description of their intervention.

Overall, there are relatively few descriptions of interventions specific to gay male couples and even fewer (only two of the five presented) for lesbian couples. In general, those that exist are not comprehensive approaches but instead offer suggestions for adding specific components to a general therapy model to address aspects of same-sex relationships. Several interventions appear to consist only of explaining concepts to clients, and yet research on the importance of emotional engagement in couple therapy suggests this may not be sufficient (Johnson, 1996). Those that do involve an exploration of the client's emotional experience do not include a clear guide for carrying out this exploration.

Emotionally Focused Therapy with Same-Sex Couples: Same Dance, Different Dance Club

EFT is an empirically validated couple intervention that is based on research on heterosexual romantic relationships (Johnson & Greenberg, 1985; Alexander, Holtzworth-Munroe, & Jameson, 1994; Johnson, Hunsley, Greenberg, & Schindler, 1999). Although EFT acknowledges that other factors, such as the socialization of gender roles, may play a role in the creation of relationship distress, EFT considers the most important factor to be attachment insecurity and how the couple deals with such insecurity (Johnson, 1996). In EFT, emotions are seen as the primary signaling system of attachment. The therapist helps distressed partners reprocess their emotional responses so that they can interact in new ways. By facilitating emotional engagement and responsiveness, the therapist helps the couple to overcome negative affect and to expand constricted interactions that are predictive of divorce (i.e., criticize–defend or pursue–withdraw) (Gottman, 1994).

There is as yet no empirical research on the application of EFT to same-sex couples, nor has any clinically based speculation been published. Johnson (1996) indicated that EFT is suited to couples with an emotional investment and a willingness to learn about how they contribute to the problems in the relationship. Based on these criteria, there is no reason to exclude same-sex couples.

As described above, the key therapeutic tasks of EFT can be summarized as accessing and reformulating emotional responses and shaping new interactions based on these responses. These tasks are carried out in a three-phase process: (1) assessment and deescalation of problematic interactional cycles, (2) the creation of specific change events where interactional positions shift and new bonding events occur, and (3) a consolidation and integration of these changes in the everyday life of the couple. The exploration of the application of EFT to same-sex couples, offered below, follows these three phases. In addition, therapy excerpts are used to demonstrate the existence, in a gay couple, of the four defining features of attachment bonds: (1) the importance of proximity maintenance, (2) the presence of separation distress, and the role of the bond as (3) a secure base, and (4) a safe haven (Hazan & Zeifman, 1999).

The couple discussed in the examples below will be identified as "Brad" and "David." The men were both in their 30s and had been together a year when they presented for therapy. They reported experiencing both a strong connection and mutually distressing conflicts. The couple moved in together after dating for 6 months. This was the first relationship for both of them involving cohabitation. From an attachment perspective, Brad presented as fearful–avoidant, intermittently expressing both desperation for connection and a desire to reject the relationship and its importance to him. David demonstrated an anxious attachment style, reporting that he monitored the relationship closely for signs that Brad's feelings for him were equal to his feelings for Brad.

In the first phase of EFT the following considerations seem important in working with same-sex couples. First, the alliance between therapist and couple is thought to be crucial for EFT, in part because the therapist leads the clients into uncharted emotional territory and asks them to express strong emotions to each other, in a real and authentic way, in the presence of the therapist. It is therefore important for the therapist to be comfortable with gay and lesbian people and with talking about their lives, love, and sexuality. Some familiarity with gay and lesbian culture, and with the local gay and lesbian community, would help in establishing this alliance. To foster a positive alliance, it is also important that clients perceive the tasks presented by the therapist as relevant to improving their relationship. Furthermore, the client's perception of the relevance of tasks affects their engagement in therapy, a factor that in the EFT model appears to be more important to therapy outcome than the initial severity of the couple's problems (Johnson & Talitman, 1997). Thus, it is important for both the alliance and the therapy outcome that the therapist be able to present the tasks involved in EFT clearly, and that they be confident about the relevance of these tasks and of an attachment-based therapy for same-sex couples.

In the first phase of EFT therapy, the therapist assesses the couple's problematic interaction cycle and attempts to deescalate their conflict. This is primarily done by helping the clients examine the unacknowledged attachment-related emotions underlying their interactional positions and how both partners are trapped in cycles that maintain attachment insecurity. With Brad and David, the therapist identified a complex negative interaction cycle in which David pursued Brad for closeness while Brad, at times threatened by closeness, would withdraw to protect himself. David would then give up and withdraw, which would cause Brad, fearful of losing the relationship, to switch to aggressively pursuing David for closeness and reassurance. Through helping the couple see this cycle and how it often left them both feeling alone and defeated, the therapist encouraged them to disrupt the cycle and stop their conflicts from escalating. An exploration of the emotions each experienced when caught in the negative interaction cycle helped them begin to understand themselves and each other better. It also assisted with their efforts to deescalate the frequency and intensity of their conflicts and encouraged them to achieve new levels of emotional engagement.

The attachment themes of proximity maintenance and separation distress were integral to the couple's negative interaction cycle. At the beginning of therapy, Brad was often unaware of, or uncomfortable with, the importance of proximity maintenance. For example, on Brad's return from a business trip, during which the two men did not speak for a week, he reacted to David's concerns about being unable to reach him as follows:

BRAD: He mentioned my not calling and I felt frustrated at that point.

THERAPIST: That's what happens to you, you feel frustrated?

BRAD: Yeah, cause I don't like the fact that . . . every time I need to go away . . . there is always some sort of issue with me going away and the fact that I didn't call. He made comments that I deliberately didn't give him my room number. It was ludicrous, I had things to do during the day. I did leave a message. In the evenings I had social gatherings with my colleagues but I was not avoiding him.

The therapist helped the men explore Brad's fears that he was being overly scrutinized and judged and David's concerns about being unable to reach Brad. As the therapist tracked David's experience and mirrored it back to him, he indicated that he withdrew instead of clearly voicing his worries because he feared that these worries indicated something was wrong with him. David believed that if Brad saw his anxieties he would either purposely reject him or be frightened away. David's tendency to not voice his worries also contributed to the couple's negative interaction cycle and a loss of proximity maintenance. For example, when Brad was away on business and David was distressed over Brad not calling, the following occurred:

DAVID: You know what? Something happened, he called me I guess, it was in the daytime. I saw "unknown name long distance" and I didn't answer it because I was angry. So he did try to call me but I didn't answer it . . . I knew it was Brad and I thought "too bad for him." I didn't want him thinking that I was sitting by the phone waiting for his call.

The therapist then helped David explore and express how hard it was to show Brad his need for comfort and reassurance.

This lack of accessibility and proximity maintenance evoked separation distress in both men. In the case of Brad not answering his cell phone or leaving a hotel number, David stated:

DAVID: I just feel alone. I'm supposed to have a partner that I can depend on, but I don't feel like he's there for me when I want him to be.

THERAPIST: What do you do with that feeling? (*silence*) . . . As you said, some of it goes to anger and . . .

DAVID: Um . . . I think about breaking up I guess, about running off and ending it.

On the occasions when David tired of pursuing Brad and withdrew, Brad's experience could also be conceptualized as separation anxiety. The therapist asked Brad what went on for him at this point in their cycle:

BRAD: At the moment he leaves I get desperate.

THERAPIST: What's that like, to be desperate?

BRAD: I don't know, I just, there is nothing I can do. . . . In my mind I am racing . . . what did I do? what is the big deal? why is he leaving? what did I say? Its hard to describe, the place I am standing doesn't feel like home anymore, I have lost any sense of attachment to anything.

Typically in their cycle, David would come home and go to sleep on the couch. Brad talked about what this was like for him:

BRAD: I need him. I need to feel that he is still there. If he doesn't come to me then I am alone. I am all alone in that lonely spot again.

Brad talked about how the feelings he had when David left were similar to those he had when he was a kid. He recalled not feeling heard by his father or older siblings and his response then was to have a temper tantrum that would get his mother's attention and comfort. Later, he described his feelings regarding David's withdrawal from him as follows:

BRAD: It's a loneliness, desperation, fear . . . I need to have David with me. Knowing he means so much to me and being scared of being alone, it's a dark place, scary, pitch black, dark.

The second phase of EFT, the shifting of interactional patterns and creation of new bonding events, involves a process of promoting identification with disowned attachment needs and aspects of self. As Johnson (1996, p. 171) notes, the conception of one's self as unlovable makes "self-disclosure and the communication of needs and desires seem extremely hazardous." EFT therefore involves an expansion, further differentiation, and validation of each partner's sense of self, thus increasing each partner's ability to be authentic and accessible (Johnson, 1996). This validation of self need not take place in separate individual therapy. The construct of self can be accessed in couple therapy through an examination of the interpersonal relationship. It is through an expansion of interpersonal cycles (e.g., from a withdrawn stance to an engaged stance) that the sense of self is able to also expand. For example, as Brad explored his concerns about being close and accessible to David, he spoke about how being teased as a child, and the death of his mother in his adolescence, had taught him to keep others at a distance. As he began to understand the roots of his conception of himself as a loner and as unlikeable, his self-perception gradually changed to "the kind of person that has a partner," someone who "can lean on someone and be leaned on."

It is possible that the goals of self-understanding and validation, inherent in EFT, could be fertile ground for gay men and lesbians. The literature on adolescent development and identity formation in gay men and lesbians suggests that the sense of self is constricted by a premature foreclosure on identity exploration due to an awareness of one's self as different from the norm (Martin, 1982; Maylon, 1981). This literature also suggests that attachment needs are often strongly disowned, and that many aspects of self are disregarded due to shame (Cass, 1979; Maylon, 1982). In "coming out" (i.e., accepting oneself as primarily attracted to the same sex and interested in pursuing a same-sex relationship), the individual reopens an exploration into the definition of self. However, it may not be at the time of coming out, but during the initial attempt to form an emotional connection to someone, that the real work of reintegrating the self and emotional experience begins. Couple therapy may therefore be a context that is particularly well suited to address the emotional aspects of the coming-out process. Perhaps, as Colgan (1987, p. 114) stated, it is "the safety of the relationship [that] provides the basis for redressing earlier developmental wounds." We can see this kind of development in Brad's reconsideration of his conclusion as an adolescent that he was in some way flawed and that he needed to hide himself from others. As therapy progressed, he spoke of how his connection with David made him feel joyful and how this caused him to worry less about what people thought of him.

This second phase of EFT, the shifting of interaction patterns and creation of new bonding events, appeared as follows in the intervention with Brad and David. In response to Brad's separation distress, the therapist attempted to facilitate emotional engagement in the couple by asking if Brad has ever felt like he could say "It hurts when you pull away" instead of getting angry. Brad responded as follows:

BRAD: It is not something I've ever thought about doing, it would be hard to say that as I have my hand on the "trigger"—I'm ready to point out David's shortcomings to cover up mine.

The therapist then asked Brad to turn to David and tell him, "When you leave I get confused, I don't understand, and I get scared." Brad did this and the therapist turned to David and asked:

THERAPIST: How do you feel when he says that?
DAVID: I feel good, I feel valued, but I also have doubts.

The therapist acknowledged and briefly explored David's doubts but turned again to Brad and supported him to further express the feelings that occurred before he experienced anger over David leaving. The therapist listened for and highlighted Brad's account of how his fear was related to David's importance to him. Again the therapist asked Brad to tell David directly about his fear and what losing David would mean to him. This time David responded that it "felt good to hear it, like he wants to be with me." Both men then looked at each other shyly and Brad took David's hand.

A further example of the shifting of interactional patterns and the creation of bonding events occurred during the exploration of David's worries that Brad cared for him much less than he cared for Brad, and that this put him in a vulnerable position. During this discussion David talked about how much Brad meant to him. The therapist supported David to tell Brad directly that his worry was a result of how much he wanted to be with Brad. When the therapist asked Brad how this made him feel, he indicated, "I definitely feel good about it, it makes me feel good, important." In these brief moments of profound connection, both David and Brad appeared to gain insight into what the relationship would feel like if it were a secure bond. Rather than becoming frustrated and leaving for several hours, David began to express his attachment needs clearly, and Brad, more aware of the importance of being accessible, became more engaged in the relationship.

The third phase of EFT consists of the creation of a narrative of how the couple first created a bond, how they got distressed, and how they repaired the relationship (Johnson, 2002). The construction of such a narrative may take more time in therapy with lesbian and gay couples as there are fewer role models for same-sex relationships. The third phase also involves a consolidation of the changes made. Societal stigma regarding same-sex relationships may slow down the couple's ability to integrate the changes made in the relative safety of the therapy office into their day-to-day life. The presence of social support for their relationship might be one factor that supports or threatens the changes the couple make.

As therapy continued, Brad and David increasingly resolved their conflicts outside of therapy in a manner that allowed them to experience the relationship as a safe haven and secure bond. For example, regarding the reoccurring conflict over Brad's business travel and David wanting him to call more, they described being able to talk about the conflict and cry about it together at home. As Brad stated, " I could sense that David was really hurt by my not calling more and that he wants this to work, I know that he loves me . . . and I went to David and we held each other."

With regards to the role of social support in consolidating a new interaction cycle, Brad and David both received acknowledgment and support of their relationship from their families and friends. Professionally, however, Brad worked in a conservative occupation and felt uncomfortable with his coworkers knowing that he was in a gay relationship. Brad therefore was reluctant to call David in the presence of colleagues. David interpreted this as Brad not caring about him or being embarrassed by him, and it remained a source of tension in their relationship. The couple terminated therapy after 13 sessions of EFT due to a job transfer to another city. At the time of their move, the level of distress in their relationship was greatly reduced and their ability to share secure moments had increased. They reported to the therapist that they valued the therapy experience.

CONCLUDING THOUGHTS

It is evident that much remains to be done in developing and testing couple therapy with same-sex couples. The study of same-sex couples is relatively new. McWirter and Mattison (1982) conducted their comparative studies in the early 1980s, only 20 years ago. In addition, there have been rapid changes in gay and lesbian communities in most North American cities. As social movements go, the speed with which society is changing with regard to attitudes toward gays and lesbians might mean research a decade old is questionable, and research with one generation is unlikely to be easily transferred to the next. Research with distressed same-sex couples in therapy is needed. Research is also needed that identifies factors that are associated with the different attachment styles of gay men and lesbians, and that further explores the specific nature of their relationship distress. Research is also needed on the commonalities between same-sex and heterosexual couples.

Attachment theory holds great promise for working with same-sex couples. The existing research on differences between same-sex and heterosexual couples and on the attachment styles of gay men and lesbians suggests the theory is applicable to same-sex romantic relationships. A review of the application of couples interventions to gay and lesbian couples indicates a lack of theory-based approaches for such couples. EFT is an empirically validated, attachment-based, couple intervention that offers a clearly delineated process that the present examination suggests could be very beneficial to same-sex couples. The goal of EFT is the establishment of a secure emotional bond. The formation of such a bond would likely allow for trust, flexibility, and an ability to be vulnerable that could play an important part in helping same-sex couples navigate the particular challenges they face, as outlined in the first half of this chapter. It is likely that issues such as legal recognition and the absence of rituals for legitimizing their bond, or the experience of social stigma, are less disruptive when the couple feels securely attached to each other.

REFERENCES

Addis, M. E., & Zamundio, A. (2001). Systemic and clinical considerations in psychosocial treatment dissemination: An example of empirically supported treatment for a gay couple. *Behavior Therapist, 24*, 151–154.

Alexander, J. F., Holtzworth-Munroe, A., & Jameson, P. (1994). The process and outcome of marital and family therapy: Research review and evaluation. In A. Bergin & S. Garfield (Eds.), *Handbook of psychotherapy and behavior change* (pp. 595–607). New York: Wiley.

Anderson, S. C. (1996). Addressing heterosexist bias in the treatment of lesbian couples with chemical dependency. In J. Laird & R. Green (Eds.), *Lesbians and gays in couples and families: A handbook for therapists* (pp. 316–340). San Francisco: Jossey-Bass.

Berger, R. M. (1990). Passing: Impact on the quality of same-sex couple relationships. *Social Work, 35*, 332–328.

Bowlby, J. (1969). *Attachment and loss: Vol. I. Attachment.* New York: Basic Books.

Brennan, K. A., Clark, C. L., & Shaver, P. R. (1998). Self-report measurement of adult attachment: An integrative overview. In J. A. Simpson & W. S. Rholes (Eds.), *Attachment theory and close relationships* (pp. 46–76). New York: Guilford Press.

Brown, L. S. (1995). Therapy with same sex couples: An introduction. In N. S. Jacobson & A. S. Gurman (Eds.), *Clinical handbook of couple therapy* (pp. 274–295). New York: Guilford Press.

Butler, M., & Clarke, J. (1991). Couple therapy with homosexual men. In D. Hooper & W. Dryden (Eds.), *Couple therapy: A handbook* (pp. 196–206). Philadelphia: Open University Press.

Cabaj, R. P., & Klinger, R. L. (1996). Psychotherapeutic interventions with lesbian and gay couples. In R. P. Cabaj & T. S. Stein (Eds.), *Textbook of homosexuality and mental health* (pp. 485–501). Washington, DC: American Psychiatric Press.

Cass, V. C. (1979). Homosexual identity formation: A theoretical model. *Journal of Homosexuality, 4*, 219–235.

Cassidy, J., & Shaver, P. R. (Eds.). (1999). *Handbook of attachment: Theory, research, and clinical applications.* New York: Guilford Press.

Cochran, S. (2001). Emerging issues in research on lesbians' and gay men's mental health: Does sexual orientation really matter? *American Psychologist, 56*, 931–947.

Colgan, P. (1987). Treatment of identity and intimacy issues in gay males. *Journal of Homosexuality, 14*, 101–123.

Elizur, Y., & Mintzer, A. (2001). A framework for the formation of gay male identity: Processes associated with adult attachment style and support from family and friends. *Archives of Sexual Behavior, 30*, 143–167.

Feeney, J. (1999). Adult romantic attachment and couple relationships. In J. Cassidy & P. R. Shaver (Eds.), *Handbook of attachment: Theory, research, and clinical applications* (pp. 355–378). New York: Guilford Press.

Fisher, S. K. (1993). A proposed Adlerian theoretical framework and intervention techniques for gay and lesbian couples. *Individual Psychology, 49*, 439–449.

Gaines, S. O., & Henderson, M. C. (2002). Impact of attachment style on responses to accommodative dilemmas among same-sex couples. *Personal Relationships, 9*, 89–93.

Gottman, J. M. (1994). An agenda for marital therapy. In S. M. Johnson & L. S. Greenberg (Eds.), *The heart of the matter: Perspectives on emotion in marital therapy* (pp. 256–293). New York: Brunner/Mazel.

Gray, D., & Isensee, R. (1996). Balancing autonomy and intimacy in lesbian and gay relationships. In C. J. Alexander (Ed.), *Gay and lesbian mental health: A sourcebook for practitioners* (pp. 95–114). New York: Harrington Park Press.

Green, R. J., Bettinger, M., & Zacks, E. (1996). Are lesbian couples fused and gay male couples disengaged?: Questioning gender straightjackets. In J. Laird & R. J. Green (Eds.), *Lesbian and gays in couples and families: A handbook for therapists* (pp. 185–230). San Francisco: Jossey-Bass.

Greenan, D. E., & Tunnell, G. (2003). *Couple therapy with gay men.* New York: Guilford Press.

Haas, S. M., & Stafford, L. (1998). An initial examination of maintenance behaviors in gay and lesbian relationships. *Journal of Social and Personal Relationships, 15,* 846–855.

Hardin, K., & Hall, M. (2001). *Queer blues: The lesbian and gay guide to overcoming depression.* Oakland, CA: New Harbinger.

Hazan, C., & Shaver, P. (1987). conceptualizing romantic love as an attachment process. *Journal of Personality and Social Psychology, 52,* 511–524.

Hazan, C., & Zeifman, D. (1999). Pair bonds as attachments: Evaluating the evidence. In J. Cassidy & P. R. Shaver (Eds.), *Handbook of attachment: Theory, research, and clinical applications* (pp. 336–354). New York: Guilford Press.

Igartua, K. J. (1998). Therapy with lesbian couples: The issues and the interventions. *Canadian Journal of Psychiatry, 43,* 391–396.

Johnson, S. M. (1996). *The practice of emotionally focused marital therapy: Creating connection.* New York: Brunner/Mazel.

Johnson, S. M. (2002). *Emotionally focused couple therapy with trauma survivors: Strengthening attachment bonds.* New York: Guilford Press.

Johnson, S. M., & Greenberg, L. (1985). The differential effects of experiential and problem solving interventions in resolving marital conflicts. *Journal of Consulting and Clinical Psychology, 53,* 175–184.

Johnson, S. M., Hunsley, J., Greenberg, L., & Schindler, D. (1999). Emotionally focussed couples therapy: Status and challenges. *Clinical Psychology: Science and Practice, 6,* 67–79.

Johnson, S., & Lebow, J. (2000). The "coming of age" of couple therapy: A decade review. *Journal of Marital and Family Therapy, 26,* 23–38.

Johnson, S. M., & Talitman, E. (1997). Predictors of success in emotionally focused marital therapy. *Journal of Marital and Family Therapy, 23,* 135–152.

Klinger, R. L. (1996). Lesbian couples. In R. P. Cabaj & T. S. Stein (Eds.), *Textbook of homosexuality and mental health* (pp. 339–352). Washington, DC: American Psychiatric Press.

Krestan, J., & Bepko, C. S. (1980). The problem of fusion in the lesbian relationship. *Family Process, 19,* 277–290.

Kurdek, L. A. (1997). The link between facets of neuroticism and dimensions of relationship commitment: Evidence from gay, lesbian, and heterosexual couples. *Journal of Family Psychology, 11,* 503–514.

MacDonald, B. J. (1998). Issues in therapy with gay and lesbian couples. *Journal of Sex and Marital Therapy, 24,* 165–190.

Mackey, R. A., O'Brien, B. A., & Mackey, E. F. (1997). *Gay and lesbian couples: Voices from lasting relationships.* Westport, CT: Praeger.

Malyon, A. K. (1981). The homosexual adolescent: Development issues and social bias. *Child Welfare, 55,* 321–330.

Malyon, A. K. (1982). Biphasic aspects of homosexual identity formation. *Psychotherapy, Theory, Research and Practice, 19,* 335–340.

Martin, A. D. (1982). Learning to hide: The socialization of the gay adolescent. *Adolescent Psychiatry, 10,* 52–65.

McKinsey-Crittenden, P. (2000). Introduction. In P. McKinsy-Crittenden & A. Hartl Claussen (Eds.), *The organization of attachment relationships* (pp. 1–10). Cambridge, UK: Cambridge University Press.

McWirter, D. P., & Mattison, A. M. (1982). Psychotherapy for gay male couples. *Journal of Homosexuality, 7,* 79–91.

Meyer, J. (1990). Guess who's coming to dinner this time?: A study of gay intimate relationships and the support for those relationships. *Marriage and Family Review, 14,* 59–82.

Mohr, J. (1999). Same-sex romantic attachment. In J. Cassidy & P. R. Shaver (Eds.), *Handbook of attachment: Theory, research, and clinical applications* (pp. 378–394). New York: Guilford Press.

Mohr, J., & Fassinger, R. (1997, August). Attachment, sexual identity and relationship functioning in same-sex couples. In K. M. O'Brien (Chair), *The role of attachment in psychological and vocational well-being.* Symposium conducted at the annual meeting of the American Psychological Association, Chicago.

Ossana, S. M. (2000). Relationship and couples counselling. In R. M. Perez, K. DeBord, & K. J. Bieschke (Eds.), *Handbook of counseling and psychotherapy with lesbian, gay, and bisexual clients* (pp. 275–302). Washington, DC: American Psychological Association.

Peplau, L. A. (1991). Lesbian and gay relationships. In J. C. Gonsiorek & J. D. Weinrich (Eds.), *Homosexuality: Research implications for public policy* (pp. 177–196). Thousand Oaks, CA: Sage.

Ridge, S. R., & Feeney, J. A. (1998). Relationship history and relationship attitudes in gay males and lesbians: Attachment style and gender differences. *Australian and New Zealand Journal of Psychiatry, 32,* 848–859.

Shaver, P., Hazan, C., & Bradshaw, D. (1988). Love as attachment. In R. J. Sternberg & M. L. Barnes (Eds.), *The psychology of love* (pp. 68–99). New Haven, CT: Yale University Press.

West, M. L., & Shelden-Keller, A. E. (1994). *Patterns of relating: An adult attachment perspective.* New York: Guilford Press.

PART IV

SPECIFIC ATTACHMENT INTERVENTIONS FOR PARTICULAR PROBLEMS

16

Looking Outward Together

Adult Attachment and Childbearing Depression

VALERIE E. WHIFFEN

Love does not consist in gazing at each other but in looking
outward together, in the same direction.
                                    —ANTOINE DE SAINT-EXUPÉRY

This chapter describes an attachment theory-based conceptualization of depression that occurs, for either men or women, in the context of childbearing. Initially, I challenge common assumptions about "postpartum depression" (PPD) with a brief review of the empirical literature. Next, I provide
an overview of the adult attachment literature, specifically as it applies to
the way couples cope with stress and distress. Then I present a model of
childbearing depression (CBD) that proposes that the birth of children can
threaten the attachment security of the couple and result in one or both
partners becoming depressed. Finally, I illustrate the model with a case example.

POSTPARTUM DEPRESSION

The Myths of Postpartum Depression

Many myths exist about depression that occurs after childbirth. PPD is
thought to be different from other kinds of depression and probably caused

by hormones. A related myth is that PPD episodes do not need to be treated because they dissipate as women's hormones return to normal levels. The third myth is that PPD occurs precipitously after the birth of the baby to women who are otherwise doing well. And the final myth is that only women become depressed. Collectively these myths perpetuate a conceptualization of PPD that is at best misleading and at worst a disincentive to the effective treatment of postpartum difficulties.

What Is Childbearing Depression?

Although childbirth is a normal life event, not all couples adjust smoothly to the birth of a new child. Among women, failure to adjust most often takes the form of depression, although some distressed women report symptoms of anxiety instead (Ballard, Davis, Handy, & Mohan, 1993). In part, the predominance of depression may reflect women's tendency to manifest their emotional distress in the form of depression (Nolen-Hoeksema, 1987). However, the fact that women become depressed also may be meaningful from an attachment theory perspective, a point to which I return later in this chapter.

The first myth I identified is the belief that PPD differs meaningfully from depression that occurs at other times, that it is caused by hormones, or that it does not feel the same as non-PPD. What is the empirical support for this belief? In 1992, I reviewed the literature to learn whether or not PPD is a distinct disorder, that is, whether or not it is different from depression occurring at other times. Supporting the distinctive position, women are more prone to depression during childbearing periods than at other times in their lives. Approximately 13% of recently delivered women experience depressive symptoms severe enough to warrant a diagnosis of depression, which is a significant increase over the rate normally found among women of childbearing age. However, a closer look at the data suggests a complex picture.

First, we have to distinguish between the *prevalence* of depression detected shortly after childbirth and the *incidence* of PPD. *Prevalence estimates* refer to the total number of cases identified in the postpartum period regardless of when episodes started, while *incidence estimates* refer only to those cases that began after delivery. This distinction is critical because the term *postpartum depression* implies that the depression started after delivery. However, as many as 40% of the cases that are present after delivery actually began *during* pregnancy (Whiffen, 1992). In recent years, PPD researchers have begun to realize that depression that is detected shortly after delivery could have begun at one of three conceptually different time points (Elliott, 2000). First, the episode could have started during pregnancy and be related to the meaning that the birth of this particular child has for the mother. Second, it could have started after childbirth and reflect either a failure to adjust to the birth of this particular child or a specific vulnerability to depression after childbirth. Some women seem to be uniquely susceptible to depression after childbirth, while others also experience episodes at other times (Cooper & Murray, 1995). Third, the depression could have begun before pregnancy and be unrelated to the child's birth. Unfortunately, these distinctions are rarely made by researchers. Therefore, we have no clear idea what proportion of the cases of "postpartum depression" would fall into each of the three categories.

In this chapter, I am concerned with cases of depression that began either during pregnancy or in the postpartum period, and that are related to the meaning of this child's birth for the depressed woman. If we adopt the perspective that depression could begin any time during the pregnancy and postpartum periods, then the term "postpartum depression" becomes a misnomer because of its implication that the depression is related etiologically to the "partum" event of having a baby. In recognition of the fact that the term "postpartum depression" is at best misleading, in this chapter I replace it with the more inclusive term "childbearing depression" (CBD).

Putting Childbearing Depression in Context

An additional caveat to the general statement that women are at increased risk for depression during childbearing periods is that most cases of CBD are of mild to moderate severity. Less than half of the cases meet DSM criteria for major depression, with the majority meeting RDC criteria for minor depression (Whiffen, 1992); the closest diagnosis in the DSM system would be "adjustment disorder with depressed mood." Depressive symptoms also are less severe among women with CBD than among women with nonchildbearing depression, with an average score in the mild to moderate range on the Beck Depression Inventory (Whiffen & Gotlib, 1993). Interestingly, when women with CBD and women with nonchildbearing depression are compared, there are few other differences between the groups (Whiffen & Gotlib, 1993). The types of symptoms they report, the courses of their episodes, and their scores on such psychosocial variables as coping are indistinguishable. Thus, CBD typically is mild but does not seem to differ qualitatively from depression that occurs at other times, at least on the variables assessed by researchers to date.

However, this does not imply that CBD is a trivial disorder about which clinicians do not need to be concerned. Our research showed that half of the episodes detected at 1 month postpartum were still present 5 months later; this recovery rate did not differ from that for the clinically depressed women in the nonchildbearing comparison group (Whiffen & Gotlib, 1993). Thus, there is no evidence that CBD remits quickly. In addition, women who experience CBD are at risk for subsequent depressive episodes, both after other pregnancies and at other times in their lives

(Bagedahl-Strindlund & Ruppert, 1998). Depending on the population sampled, between one-quarter and one-half of the women who experience a CBD will have another depressive episode after pregnancy (Cooper & Murray, 1995; Marks, Wieck, Checkley, & Kumar, 1996; Wisner et al., 2001). Thus, CBD may be one of the first episodes of depression in the life of a woman who is vulnerable to depression.

In addition, an episode of depression at this point in a woman's life can have enduring consequences. An episode of CBD has a clear, negative impact on the development of the infant and on the marriage. Research conducted with the 2-month-old infants of women with CBD found that these infants already showed cognitive and temperamental deficits compared with the infants of nondepressed women (Whiffen & Gotlib, 1989b). The infants of the women with CBD were developing more slowly, and they showed evidence of negative emotionality during testing. Similar findings have now been reported by several other research groups (see meta-analysis by Beck, 1998). Additionally, a recent meta-analysis showed that the infants of mothers with CBD were less likely than other infants to form secure attachments to their mothers (Atkinson et al., 2000). Thus, an episode of CBD puts the index infant at risk for social-emotional difficulties. Finally, women who experience CBD continue to report lower levels of marital satisfaction up to 5 years later (Nettelbladt, Uddenberg, & Englesson, 1985). Thus, an episode of CBD can have serious and long-lasting consequences for the woman involved as well as her family.

The implication that depression follows from a "partum" event, as well as the tendency to consider CBD a unique and/or a hormonal disorder, leads most researchers to overlook the data showing that new fathers also can experience emotional distress. Although little research has been done on this topic, fathers are clearly at elevated risk for depression and anxiety after the birth of a child; 3–9% meet criteria for an Axis I disorder, particularly depression and anxiety (Ballard, Davis, Cullen, Mohan, & Dean, 1994; Ballard et al., 1993). This rate is much higher than the point prevalence rate for men typically obtained in community samples (Regier et al., 1988). In samples of men whose wives have already been identified as depressed, one in four of the husbands also meets criteria for an Axis I disorder (Zelkowitz & Milet, 1996). Studies of nonclinical samples show that, while having a baby is disruptive for both partners, for fathers it is measurably worse. While women's levels of emotional distress and marital satisfaction return to their prepartum levels by a year after the birth of the child, fathers continue to be distressed (Vandell, Hyde, Plant, & Essex, 1997).

Collectively, the research suggests that the birth of a new child can be problematic for either partner. A depressed or anxious husband and father is likely to have a negative impact on his wife. Husbands' depression may exacerbate and amplify their wives' depression. When a husband is depressed, he tends to feel unhappy in his marriage. His marital distress tends to make his wife unhappy as well (Whiffen & Gotlib, 1989a), and her marital dissatisfaction is a strong predictor of her subsequently experiencing an episode of major depression (Whisman, 1999). In addition, the high rate of paternal diagnosis when mothers are depressed suggests that maternal depression may be a symptom of a distressed *system* rather than of a distressed *individual*. Thus, it is important to consider the system that provides the immediate interpersonal context for CBD.

Who Is at Risk for Childbearing Depression?

Two reviews of the literature concluded that the best predictors of a new episode of CBD are a history of depression and depression levels during pregnancy (O'Hara & Swain, 1996; Whiffen, 1992). Women who are at risk for depression typically have sought help for emotional problems in the past and report higher levels of emotional distress during pregnancy than women who do not develop CBD. Consistent with a diathesis–stress model of depression, women are more likely to become depressed when they experience significant stress during the childbearing period that may or may not be related to pregnancy or the baby (Swendsen & Mazure, 2000). Interestingly, these are the same variables that are implicated in the onset of nonchildbearing depression (O'Hara, Schlechte, Lewis & Varner, 1991). Thus, the women who experience CBD are those who have had emotional difficulties in the past, and who presently are experiencing significant life stress.

The interpersonal context in which a woman lives also is a significant determinant of whether or not she will develop CBD. The onset of new episodes is predicted by several interpersonal variables even after initial symptom levels are taken into account. First, women are vulnerable if they perceive their relations with their own mother before the age of 16 to have lacked warmth or to have been explicitly rejecting (Gotlib, Whiffen, Wallace, & Mount, 1991). In the developmental literature, difficult relations with parents are associated with the development of insecure attachment (Ainsworth, Blehar, Waters, & Wall, 1968). Thus, many women who become depressed during childbearing periods experienced attachment difficulties during childhood that may predispose them to insecurity in their adult attachment relationships.

Second, lack of social support, particularly concrete help provided by the spouse, also contributes to depression (Collins, Dunkel-Schetter, Lobel, & Scrimshaw, 1993; O'Hara & Swain, 1996), particularly under conditions of high stress (Cutrona & Troutman, 1986). Lack of husband support may be a manifestation of marital distress, which is another reliable predictor of CBD (O'Hara & Swain, 1996; Whiffen, 1992). Marital factors may be especially important among women who are at risk because they previously experienced an episode of CBD. In one study, the husbands of high-

risk women who went on to experience a second CBD were rated by inter-
viewers during pregnancy as showing more indifference toward their wives
(Marks et al., 1996). This finding is fascinating because the researchers
were really interested in "expressed emotion"; they hypothesized that
women whose husbands were explicitly *critical* of them would be at greater
risk for depression, consistent with episodes of nonchildbearing depression
(see review by Coiro & Gottesman, 1996). However, the women who went
on to become depressed were those whose husbands seemed *indifferent* to
them. In my clinical experience, husbands' indifference is typically construed by their wives as an indication of their lack of love. Thus, the empirical literature suggests that both attachment difficulties in relations with
parents and specific difficulties in the marriage that may be characterized as
"husband neglect" are implicated in the etiology of CBD among women.

Reassessing the Myths

Based on this brief review, we can conclude that most of the myths of CBD
are contradicted by the data. Overall, no evidence exists that CBD differs
etiologically or symptomatically from nonchildbearing depression (O'Hara
et al., 1991; Whiffen, 1992; Whiffen & Gotlib, 1993). While some women
have been identified who experience CBD as a result of thyroid problems
(Harris et al., 1989), only a subgroup of women who become depressed is
uniquely susceptible after the birth of a child (Cooper & Murray, 1995).
Most women who experience CBD either have a history of depression or
they go on to have nonchildbearing episodes. CBD does not dissipate more
rapidly than nonchildbearing depression. It also does not begin only after
childbirth. Thus, the stereotype of a thriving young mother suddenly struck
down by CBD is simply false. Finally, the research suggests that CBD occurs in an interpersonal context, the couple, in which both partners may be
feeling maritally dissatisfied and distressed.

ADULT ATTACHMENT

Theory and Research

Attachment theory proposes that early relationships between children and
their primary caregivers shape the development of children's "working
models" of self and others (Bowlby, 1969, 1973). *Working models* are relational schemas that form because of regularities in interactions with key attachment figures (Baldwin, 1995). These schemas contain information both
about the emotional responsiveness of attachment figures and about the
self as experienced in these relationships. For instance, children who experience warmth and consistency in their relations with attachment figures develop a working model of the self as lovable and a working model of others
as loving and reliable. In contrast, children who experience rejection or in-

consistency develop working models of themselves as unlovable and of others as hostile or untrustworthy.

Hazan and Shaver (1987) proposed that attachment processes, parallel to those observed in parent–child relationships, also operate in romantic relationships. They proposed that romantic partners and spouses are the primary attachment figures for adults. Subsequently, Bartholomew (1990) hypothesized that adult attachment varies as a function of individuals' models of self and others. Individuals with positive models of both self and others are *securely* attached. They believe that they are lovable and that significant others will be emotionally responsive to them. Individuals with a negative model of self and a positive model of others are *anxious*. They look to others for reassurance because they feel unlovable. Individuals who have negative working models of both self and others are *fearful*. They believe that they are unlovable and that eventually they will be rejected by attachment figures. Finally, *dismissing* individuals have a negative working model of others but a positive working model of self. They are thought to protect their self-esteem from rejection by attachment figures by denying that attachment relationships are important.

The construct validity of the underlying dimensions as well as the four attachment styles has been confirmed empirically (Bartholomew & Horowitz, 1991; Griffin & Bartholomew, 1994). Recent factor analyses of various dimensional measures of adult attachment consistently indicate that there are two bipolar dimensions underlying adult attachment: anxiety–security and comfort with closeness–avoidance of closeness (e.g., Brennan, Clark, & Shaver, 1998). The first dimension reflects fears that one is unlovable and that rejection or abandonment by attachment figures is likely. This dimension appears to map onto Bartholomew's model of self. The second dimension reflects the extent to which individuals feel comfortable being close to and depending upon others as opposed to maintaining their autonomy. This dimension maps onto Bartholomew's model of others. A comparison of the dimensional model of attachment with Bartholomew's four-category system showed convergence between the two approaches (Brennan et al., 1998), which enables us to collate research done with the two systems.

Adult attachment researchers make no claims about the links between childhood relations with parents and adult attachment security. While some investigators believe that adult attachment security has more to do with the quality of adult relationships than with relations with previous attachment figures (Kobak, 1994), others point out that, as schemas, working models should summarize past experience (Baldwin, 1995). Indirect evidence suggests that there is a tendency for attachments to parents and to romantic partners to be associated. For instance, individuals who report attachment security with their romantic partners describe warm relationships with their parents, while adult attachment insecurity is associated with perceptions of parents as rejecting and uncaring (Hazan & Shaver, 1987; Oliver

& Whiffen, in press). This research seems to support the contention that, while relations with adult attachment figures may help individuals to rewrite their working models and redress adverse childhood relations with parents, there also is a strong tendency for individuals with insecure attachment histories to become involved in romantic relationships that perpetuate attachment insecurities (Bowlby, 1980).

Adult attachment researchers assume that infants and adults use their attachment figures for similar purposes. Just as a frightened or distressed infant seeks reassurance and comfort from his mother, a stressed, frightened, vulnerable, or distressed adult seeks reassurance and comfort from his spouse. The research indicates that securely attached individuals trust their partners to be emotionally responsive to them and that they seek out their partner when stressed or distressed (see review by Johnson & Whiffen, 1999). Individuals who are anxious about the availability of their attachment figures, that is, those who fear rejection or abandonment by them, cope with stress and emotional distress differently, depending on the extent to which they are comfortable with closeness. An anxiously attached individual who is comfortable with closeness (*anxious*) tends to actively seek reassurance from the partner and to blame and criticize the partner if he or she is perceived to be insufficiently available and responsive. These individuals report high levels of conflict with their partners, particularly when discussing relationship problems or when their trust has been violated. In contrast, an anxiously attached individual who is avoidant of closeness (*fearful*) tends to withdraw from the partner both physically and emotionally, and to avoid conflict and discussing problems. Individuals who are not anxious about rejection or abandonment but who are avoidant of closeness (*dismissing*) tend to be cold and critical, and to provide low levels of care in their close relationships (Bartholomew & Horowitz, 1991). Because they tend not to experience emotional distress themselves and to lack empathy for others, they tend to lack sensitivity to their partners' distress and need for comfort.

To summarize, the three insecure attachment styles demonstrate distinctive interpersonal styles when stressed and distressed. Anxiously attached individuals tend to engage in conflict with their partners and to blame them for difficulties, while fearfully attached individuals withdraw physically and emotionally from their partners. Dismissing individuals tend to be unaware of others' emotional distress and are likely to respond to their partners' bids for support and reassurance with coldness and a lack of empathy or care.

Adult Attachment and Depression

Depression researchers have begun to use the framework of attachment theory to understand adult depression. Following from Bowlby's (1980) seminal work on adult depression after loss, these researchers propose that attachment insecurity is a vulnerability factor for depression, which becomes salient under adverse interpersonal circumstances, such as the loss of a significant relationship or a life transition like childbirth (Anderson, Beach, & Kaslow, 1999; Ingram, Miranda, & Segal, 1998; Whiffen & Johnson, 1998). Furthermore, Bowlby (1980) believed that depression is more likely to occur when the individual experienced insecurity in early attachment relationships that resulted in the development of insecure adult attachment relationships.

Research supports the basic aspects of Bowlby's model. Attachment insecurity is correlated with both depressive symptoms (e.g., Roberts, Gotlib, & Kassel, 1996) and clinical depression (Carnelley, Pietromonaco, & Jaffe, 1994; Whiffen, Kallos-Lilly, & MacDonald, 2001). Additionally, individuals do not "recover" from attachment insecurity once episodes of depression remit, which suggests that insecurity is not merely a facet of clinical depression like distorted cognitions (Haaga et al., 2002). Finally, consistent with the general model, the onset of new episodes can be predicted from the combination of attachment insecurity and interpersonal stress (Hammen et al., 1995).

Adult attachment theory may be especially useful as a framework for understanding the development of depression in married individuals because there is strong evidence that depression, attachment insecurity, and marital distress covary. How might they be linked? I propose that specific types of marital interactions convey the impression that the partner is emotionally unavailable, which subsequently erodes the attachment security of the spouse and puts the spouse at risk for depression. Spouses who are warm and emotionally engaged mirror an image of the partner as lovable and worthy, while spouses who are cold, hostile, critical, or disengaged reflect back a picture of their partners as unlovable, defective, or unworthy of care. I propose that the marital context is a strong determinant of how individuals perceive and feel about themselves (Whiffen & Aube, 1999), and that feedback that one is unlovable or unworthy of care is inherently depressing.

Consistent with this model, depression in married or cohabiting individuals is associated specifically with *fearful* attachment, both for women (Carnelley et al., 1994; Whiffen et al., 2001) and for men (Oliver & Whiffen, in press). That is, depression is associated with the fear that one is unlovable and will be rejected. Additionally, we have shown that the partner's attachment style influences his or her spouse's depression. In a sample of clinically depressed women, we showed that husbands' avoidance of closeness exacerbated their wives' depressive symptoms over a 6-month period (Whiffen et al., 2001). These men's avoidance of closeness may have confirmed their wives' fears about them as attachment figures. In a subsequent study, we showed that avoidant partners tend to be unresponsive when their partners express vulnerable emotions, which increases their spouses' attachment insecurity and depressive symptoms over time (Whiffen, Varshney, & MacDonald, 2002). Thus, collectively, the research on adult attachment and depression in couples suggests that attachment processes are implicated in the worsening of depressive symptoms over time, and that a spouse who is avoidant of closeness may provide the interpersonal context for depression through his or her unresponsiveness to vulnerability.

AN ATTACHMENT THEORY MODEL OF CHILDBEARING DEPRESSION

Bowlby (1973) suggested that attachment needs become particularly salient during life transitions, which are periods of uncertainty and change. The introduction of a new child into an existing system, whether that system is a couple or a family, is a transition that brings uncertainty and change (Whiffen & Johnson, 1998). New mothers may feel challenged by their capacity to cope with the infant, particularly if the infant is difficult temperamentally or has medical problems. Mothers, fathers, and siblings may feel uncertain or resentful about the changes that a new baby brings to their established roles and to their relationships with one another. The way that a couple handles the birth of their children is an important test of their capacity to provide a secure base for one another under stressful circumstances. More critically, the integration of a child into the couple system may be the first opportunity that the partners have to demonstrate that they can remain emotionally available and responsive to other another, under circumstances that specifically threaten attachment security.

The birth of a new child has special implications for attachment because it threatens the security of existing attachments, between the mother and her other children and between the parents. Part of the couple's task as the parents of a newborn is to form an attachment to the infant. However, they must do so without compromising their existing attachments. At the beginning of romantic relationships couples gaze at each other, both literally and figuratively, as they form an exclusive pair bond that ideally fulfills their attachment needs and promotes attachment security. However, with each additional child, the couple must increasingly "look outward together"—that is, they must allow their relationship to evolve from an exclusive romance to an inclusive partnership focused extensively on achieving common life goals, including the raising of children. This evolution is best accomplished in a context of attachment security within the couple. If the couple's attachment is insecure, for either or both partners, then the transition from gazing at each other to looking outward together may raise attachment alarms and create emotional distress.

When an individual is stressed and distressed, he or she normally turns to an attachment figure for reassurance and comfort. According to attachment theory, this is one of the primary purposes served by attachment figures. For most couples, particularly in Western societies where nuclear families predominate, this attachment figure is most likely to be the spouse. If a stressed person turns to his or her partner for reassurance and that person is unable or unwilling to provide emotional support, then an attachment crisis may be precipitated for the reassurance-seeking partner. Research indicates that women need and anticipate increased involvement from their husbands in housework and childcare after the birth of a new child (Ruble, Fleming, Hackel, & Stangor, 1988). Their need for this support increases as the level of stress associated with infant care increases, for instance, when the child is temperamentally difficult (Cutrona & Troutman, 1986). If a husband does not provide support and help, his wife may construe his lack of involvement as a statement about how much he loves her. In a parallel manner, fathers may be distressed by the reduced intimacy and increased conflict with their wives that is normative after the birth of a child (Fincham & Beach, 1999). These changes may threaten the security of their attachment to their wives, and, in extreme cases, husbands may fear that the infant is replacing them as their wives' primary attachment figure.

The extent to which the birth of a child triggers attachment alarms is a function of the couple's specific attachment history and each individual's general attachment history. Partners who have proven to one another in the past that they are emotionally available and responsive during periods of crisis should be relatively resilient, while couples who have failed previous tests of their emotional availability will encounter more difficulties. These failed tests may be "attachment injuries" (Johnson, Makinen, & Millikin, 2001) from a previous time in the relationship that have never been resolved. *Attachment injuries* occur in moments when the injured person feels extremely vulnerable and needy and sees the partner as unavailable. These injuries may resurface as attachment fears become salient. The birth of a new child also may trigger attachment fears in an individual who experienced unavailability earlier in life with other attachment figures. For instance, a woman who felt that her mother left her to fend for herself as a child may expect her husband to do the same now.

Partners who are *anxiously* attached to their spouses or who default to an anxious pattern in attachment-salient situations will seek reassurance in a conflict-enhancing and blaming fashion. This strategy is likely to exacerbate marital distress; marital distress is a strong predictor of depression (Whisman, 1999). Partners who are *fearfully* attached to their spouses or who default to a fearful pattern will likely withdraw from their partners. This interpersonal coping strategy may indicate that the individual is already on the road to depression; indeed, Bowlby (1980) considered giving up on the attachment figure as the first step in the development of depression. Individuals who are fearfully attached want to be loved and accepted by their attachment figures but they fear being rejected or abandoned. They resolve this dilemma by keeping their emotional distance from attachment figures (Bartholomew & Horowitz, 1991) and by withdrawing physically and emotionally from their partners when stressed (Simpson, Rholes, & Nelligan, 1992). This strategy has the potential to become a self-fulfilling prophesy. Their partners may fail to recognize their distress and therefore neglect to provide the needed support. Subsequently, the partner's failure to provide support could be seen as confirming the fearful individual's perception that the partner is unavailable. This perception contributes to feelings of depression. From this description, it is apparent why a spouse who is avoidant of closeness may be depressogenic: these individuals are likely to be unaware of their partners' distress and need for support and to respond insensitively to those bids for reassurance that they do recognize.

Earlier in this chapter, I observed that depression is the most common manifestation of distress during childbearing periods, particularly for women. Why depression? Bowlby (1980) linked sadness and depression specifically to loss and disappointment. The potential for loss and disappointment during childbearing periods is substantial despite cultural pressure to view the birth of a child as a joyful event that marks the beginning of a new life (Nicolson, 1998). While the event is a beginning for the infant, it may be an ending for the parents. The birth of the first child marks the end of the couple's life together as a childless romantic couple. The transition from romantic couple to working partnership may be unexpected or it may come too early in the relationship for one or both partners. Similarly, the child's birth may change the structure of the caregiver's life. The caregiver may stop working outside the home for the first time and have to give up not only the work role but also the social support and self-efficacy that work provides. Even a caregiver who previously stayed at home with one or two children may feel her life suddenly constrained by a baby who has medical problems or who is temperamentally difficult. Change always is accompanied to some degree by loss. As a clinician, it is important to keep the idea of loss in mind when working with childbearing individuals and couples because they may feel that they are not entitled to experience and express feelings of loss about the beginning of their child's life.

CLINICAL EXAMPLE

The following case illustrates the use of two attachment-theory based interventions with a woman who presented for treatment of CBD. Initially, the client was treated individually with interpersonal therapy (IPT; Frank & Spanier, 1995). IPT focuses on life transitions and interpersonal difficulties as sources of depression. The goal of the therapy is to identify the interpersonal antecedents of the current depressive episode and to work with the client to renegotiate problematic relationships. While current interpersonal relations are thought to be rooted in early development, the focus in therapy is on the client's current relationships rather than on analyzing and reconstructing past relationships. Outcome studies show that IPT is as effective as tricyclic antidepressants in the treatment of depression (Frank & Spanier, 1995). Subsequently, the client and her husband were treated with emotionally focused therapy for couples (EFT; Greenberg & Johnson, 1988; Johnson, 1996). EFT is discussed extensively elsewhere in this volume. Briefly, the goals of treatment are to identify the attachment needs and emotions underlying repetitive, negative interaction cycles; to de-escalate these cycles; to encourage the expression of attachment needs and their acceptance by both partners; and to strengthen the attachment bond. A meta-analysis showed that EFT is highly effective in the treatment of marital distress (Johnson, Hunsley, Greenberg, & Schindler, 1999).

Background

Annie was a woman in her 30s who had been married for about 18 months when she became pregnant. Her husband was a U.S. citizen who had difficulty obtaining a work permit in Canada, with the result that he had been unemployed for more than a year at Annie's intake. She supported them financially through her demanding work as a lawyer. Initially, she told me that their relationship was good (although she reported a lifelong absence of interest in sex), and she focused on the stress she was experiencing at work. Symptomatically, Annie's scores were slightly elevated. She met DSM criteria for an adjustment disorder with depressed mood because her depressed mood developed after she became pregnant. On questionnaires, Annie reported a tendency toward dismissing attachment in her close adult relationships.

Attachment History

Annie was the third in a family of five children. Her mother was a stay-at-home mom who developed a terminal illness and died when Annie was an adolescent. Her father was a high-achieving professional who was critical of his children. Annie reported a weak attachment to her mother, whom she perceived as overwhelmed by the demands of looking after five small children. She told me that her only strong attachment was to her grandfather, who died when she was a child. She experienced other attachments throughout her life as weak and quickly compromised by feelings of anger or disappointment. As an adult, Annie felt distant in her romantic relationships, saying that they were conducted "at arms' length." She admitted that she found men's emotional demands on her overwhelming and that she was afraid of being hurt by romantic partners. She told me that being married to her husband was "a relief" because he required very little emotional intimacy. Thus, Annie reported a fearful to dismissing attachment style and she described her husband as dismissing.

Interpersonal Therapy for Depression

Although Annie continually began sessions by telling me that her depressed mood was due to her stress at work, she also continually drifted into talking about her marriage. At the same time, she was defensive about exploring her feelings about her husband or linking them to her mood. This can be a challenging aspect of working with an avoidant client: these clients tend to generalize about their relationships in ways that are incongruent with the specific stories that they tell, and to be inattentive to their immediate emotional experience (Johnson & Whiffen, 1999).

When Annie was approximately 6 months pregnant, she and her husband went on a week-long canoeing trip with several other couples. On the second day, Annie fell and twisted her ankle. Her husband took her back to the base lodge, got her medical attention, bought her some novels, then announced that he was finishing the trip and would return in five days time. Annie was devastated by what she saw as his lack of investment in her pregnancy. She said that although she wanted him to stay at the lodge with her, she felt that she did not have the right to ask that he give up the trip and stay with her because he had been "ambivalent" about her becoming pregnant. This incident became an attachment injury for Annie.

In discussing the trip with me and exploring her emotional response to her husband's behavior, Annie realized that she wanted more from him now that she was pregnant. She wanted to feel like a family with him instead of feeling like "separate checks." She asked him to come for marital therapy with her but he declined, saying that their marriage was fine. On one occasion she tried to tell him how she felt about the canoeing trip. He heard her out but when she finished he walked away from her without replying. Her husband's disinclination to discuss their problems is common among dismissing individuals who literally do not feel distressed and have great difficulty recognizing the distress of others. When their baby was born, Annie's feeling that he was not invested in her or their child intensified because she perceived him "carrying on with his life as if nothing [had] changed." At this point, she decided that he was as available to her as he was capable of being, and she decided to terminate individual therapy despite continuing feelings of depression and irritability.

Two years later Rob contacted me to ask for couple therapy. I had an individual session with him in which he told me that, after unsuccessfully trying to get a work permit in Canada for 2 years, he returned to the United States to take a job. Annie and the baby were alone in Canada for several months before they were able to join him. During this separation he led "the life of a bachelor," which he enjoyed immensely. Although he did not report involvements with other women, he did indulge his love of sports and the outdoors. When Annie and the baby joined him, he felt constrained by being part of a family with a small child. Their marriage deteriorated rapidly, and Annie returned to Canada after a few months because she feared that she would "end up a single mother in a foreign country." He followed her back to Canada after a further separation.

Couple Sessions

In the initial couple session, Annie told me that she felt "deserted" by Rob. She felt that she and their son were unimportant to him, and that eventually he would leave them both. She was aware of "shoring up her defenses" in preparation for this loss. For instance, she would not let him help in any way with the care of their child. She told me that she was afraid that if she "put down part of [her] burden" and let Rob pick it up, it would be too heavy to pick up again when he inevitably left her. Her depression had worsened considerably and now met DSM-IV criteria for major depression.

I began the couple therapy by finding out about Rob's experience of Annie's pregnancy. He was unequivocal: he felt "bulldozed" by Annie into having a child. He did not want to have a child so soon into their marriage and he claimed that he told her this clearly in their single conversation about the decision. He told me that it was very difficult for him to feel enthusiasm for a choice that he had not made. Once the baby was born, he felt displaced. He felt that he had been a "sperm bank" for Annie and that he had been discarded once his purpose was served. Rob had no difficulty telling me how angry he was with Annie. However, he was initially reluctant when I tried to reframe his anger in terms of his unmet attachment need to feel that his opinion mattered to her and that his needs were important. By continually reframing his anger in these more vulnerable terms, he was eventually able to tell Annie that he feared she loved their son more than she loved him.

Annie was aware that he "disagreed" with the decision to get pregnant, but she told herself that he would enjoy being a father because he enjoyed playing with other people's children. Initially, she blamed him for not being assertive enough in his objections to having a baby and for being intimidated by her. She stated repeatedly that she went out of her way to ensure that Rob felt included in their decisions and that he did not feel guilty about his lack of earnings. Annie saw herself as a democratic person and she rebelled against what she perceived as his view of her as strong-willed and controlling. Two shifts on Rob's part enabled her to hear how he experienced her. First, Rob was able to take responsibility for his part in the decision about the baby. He admitted that he did not voice his concerns strongly or persistently. He told her that he felt that he had no right to have an opinion about their life together as long as Annie was paying their bills. Second, he was able to tell her that his perception of her as "scary" and intimidating was partly due to her self-sufficient interpersonal style and partly due to his own feelings of inadequacy because he was unemployed. Once Rob took responsibility in these ways, Annie was able to acknowledge that they were both responsible for making the decision in a way that left him feeling unacknowledged and resentful.

However, she was unable to let go of her attachment injury, the canoeing trip, which came up repeatedly in our sessions. She talked about how lonely she felt in the lodge even though she had encouraged him to go off with their friends. She wanted him to stay behind with her but only because he wanted to, not because he felt guilty or because she asked him to. While I empathized immediately with how hurt Annie felt by Rob's unavailability, the incident had an extra emotional kick for her: it was significant because the basis of their relationship was doing physical activities together. There was little emotional intimacy and few common interests; she feared that without the "glue" of shared outdoor activities he would eventually find someone who was "more fun to play with." This was an important realization for Annie. She told Rob that she had not felt loved by him since becoming pregnant. While she had to limit her physical activities, he continued to engage with other people in sports that were too strenuous for her. Instead of feeling that he was "with her" in her pregnancy, she felt that he had abandoned her to endure it alone. She told him that she felt rejected by him in the same way that the last kid to be chosen for a sports team feels rejected: it seemed that Rob would rather do any activity with any other person than spend time with her and the baby. She told him that living every day with this lack of love made her feel depressed.

Initially, Rob told Annie that he did not like doing things with her anymore because the activities they used to enjoy could not be done easily with a baby. He found the activities they did together as a family boring, but eventually he admitted that he was still bucking being a family with her. Between our sessions, Rob began to plan new activities for them to do together as a couple and as a family. He arranged for babysitting and chose activities, like going to a film, that he knew they would both enjoy. These behaviors greatly reassured Annie that he still wanted to "play" with her.

The final significant change occurred when Rob talked about why he decided to return to the United States. She believed that he left because he wanted to get away from her and the baby, but he told her that he did it because he could tell she was unhappy and he surmised that this was because he did not have a job. He said that he wanted to "fix" her unhappiness. He already felt displaced by the baby, so he did not think that Annie would miss him or the scant material support he provided. He not only felt like he was useless to her, he also felt like he was part of the burden that she had to carry. By leaving, he thought he was reducing her burden. Annie told him that she wanted to rely on him after the baby was born but that when he began talking about leaving Canada, she "jumped ship." This came as a revelation to Rob who could not recall a time in their relationship that she had asked for his help. Hearing that she needed his help, both emotionally and instrumentally, reassured Rob that he was useful and important to her.

Summary of the Case

Both Rob and Annie were avoidant in their attachment styles: Rob was dismissing–avoidant while Annie was fearful–avoidant. These styles were evident in the way that they managed their difficulties. Both tended not to verbalize their feelings, Annie because she feared being rejected and Rob because he was uncomfortable about expressing vulnerable emotions. Rob tended to denigrate the importance of relationships both for himself and for Annie. For instance, he genuinely believed that he could return to the United States and that Annie would not miss him. Working with avoidant individuals can be challenging because they are only dimly aware of their own and others' feelings, and because, at times, they show a breathtaking lack of insight into what makes people tick. Rob and Annie's avoidant styles were compatible as long as they could lead relatively independent lives. However, once they needed to become interdependent, to look outward together, both felt that they could not count on the other person to be available and responsive. Annie was not responsive to Rob's concerns about having children; Rob was not responsive to the changes Annie had to make to her life when she became pregnant. Thus, the decision to become pregnant and the resulting birth of their child destabilized their relationship. Once destabilized, the interpersonal coping strategies associated with their attachment styles exacerbated and maintained their marital and Annie's emotional distress.

Rob and Annie's experiences after the birth of their child are consistent with the model of childbearing depression outlined in this chapter. Annie felt unsupported and abandoned by Rob, even though she reported that his behavior did not change much before and after the baby's birth. In fact, it was the *lack* of change when change was normative and expected that led her to believe that he was not invested in her pregnancy and their child. In Bowlby's terms, Annie's depression was linked to her loss of Rob as a romantic partner and his failure to make the transition to parent with her. Like many fathers, Rob felt displaced by Annie's affection for their son. Annie's attachment to their child appeared to supplant her attachment to Rob. Although he did not report clinical levels of depression, he reported feelings that are associated with depression, such as low self-esteem and feelings of inadequacy. Depressive feelings and unexpressed attachment needs to be respected and important often underlie the apparent insouciance of dismissing men.

CLINICAL IMPLICATIONS

Whenever a clinician is working with a childbearing depressed woman or man, it is essential that she or he assess the marriage. If the depression is co-occurring with marital distress, couple therapy is the treatment of choice. However, couple therapy may not be acceptable to the nondepressed partner who may not see the relevance of the marriage to the partner's depression (Emanuels-Zuurveen & Emmelkamp, 1996). In these situations, an attachment theory framework for understanding the depression within the context of individual therapy can help the depressed person to understand how specific relationship difficulties may be fueling the depression.

To summarize, attachment theory and adult attachment research provide a useful framework for understanding and treating depression that occurs in a childbearing context, whether it is the mother or the father who is depressed. The birth of a child has the potential to threaten the security of the parents' attachment to each other, and to prime attachment insecurities from earlier in the relationship or from previous relationships. An attachment-based intervention at this time has the potential both to strengthen the couple's relationship and to attenuate the impact of emotional distress on subsequent child development and marital relations.

REFERENCES

Ainsworth, M., Blehar, M., Waters, E., & Wall, S. (1968). *Patterns of attachment: A psychological study of the Strange Situation*. Hillsdale, NJ: Erlbaum.

Anderson, P., Beach, S. R. H., & Kaslow, N. J. (1999). Marital discord and depression: The potential of attachment theory to guide integrative clinical intervention. In T. Joiner & J. Coyne (Eds.), *The interactional nature of depression* (pp. 271–298). Washington, DC: American Psychological Association.

Atkinson, L., Paglia, A., Coolbear, J., Niccols, A., Parker, K. C. H., & Guger, S. (2000). Attachment security: A meta-analysis of maternal mental health correlates. *Clinical Psychology Review, 20,* 1019–1040.

Bagedahl-Strindlund, M., & Ruppert, S. (1998). Parapartum mental illness: A long-term follow-up study. *Psychopathology, 31,* 250–259.

Baldwin, M. W. (1995). Relational schemas and cognition in close relationships. *Journal of Social and Personal Relationships, 12,* 547–552.

Ballard, C. G., Davis, R., Cullen, P. C., Mohan, R. N., & Dean, C. (1994). Prevalence of postnatal psychiatric morbidity in mothers and fathers. *British Journal of Psychiatry, 164,* 782–788.

Ballard, C. G., Davis, R., Handy, S., & Mohan, R. N. (1993). Postpartum anxiety in mothers and fathers. *European Journal of Psychiatry, 7,* 117–121.

Bartholomew, K. (1990). Avoidance of intimacy: An attachment perspective. *Journal of Personal and Social Relationships, 7,* 147–178.

Bartholomew, K., & Horowitz, L. (1991). Attachment styles among young adults: A test of a four-category model. *Journal of Personality and Social Psychology, 61,* 226–244.

Beck, C. T. (1998). The effects of PPD on child development: A meta-analysis. *Archives of Psychiatric Nursing, 12*, 12–20.

Bowlby, J. (1969). *Attachment and loss: Vol. I. Attachment.* New York: Basic Books.

Bowlby, J. (1973). *Attachment and loss: Vol. II. Separation: Anxiety and anger.* New York: Basic Books.

Bowlby, J. (1980). *Attachment and loss: Vol. III. Loss.* New York: Basic Books.

Brennan, K. A., Clark, C. C., & Shaver, P. R. (1998). Self report measurement of adult attachment. In J. A. Simpson & W. S. Rholes (Eds.), *Attachment theory and close relationships* (pp. 46–76). New York: Guilford Press.

Carnelley, K. B., Pietromonaco, P. R., & Jaffe, K. (1994). Depression, working models of others, and relationship functioning. *Journal of Personality and Social Psychology, 66*, 127–140.

Coiro, M. J., & Gottesman, I. I. (1996). The diathesis and/or stressor role of expressed emotion in affective illness. *Clinical Psychology: Science and Practice, 3*, 310–322.

Collins, N. L., Dunkel-Schetter, C., Lobel, M., & Scrimshaw, S. C. M. (1993). Social support in pregnancy: Psychosocial correlates of birth outcomes and postpartum depression. *Journal of Personality and Social Psychology, 65*, 1243–1258.

Cooper, P. J., & Murray, L. (1995). Course and recurrence of postnatal depression: Evidence for the specificity of the diagnostic concept. *British Journal of Psychiatry, 166*, 191–195.

Cutrona, C., & Troutman, B. (1986). Social support, infant temperament, and parenting self-efficacy: A mediational model of postpartum depression. *Child Development, 57*, 1507–1518.

Elliott, S. A. (2000). Report on the Satra Bruk Workshop on Classification of Postnatal Mental Disorders. *Archives of Women's Mental Health, 3*, 27–33.

Emanuels-Zuurveen, L., & Emmelkamp, P. M. G. (1996). Individual behavioural-cognitive therapy v. marital therapy for depression in maritally distressed couples. *British Journal of Psychiatry, 169*, 181–188.

Fincham, F. D., & Beach, S. R. H. (1999). Conflict in couples: Implications for working with couples. *Annual Review of Psychology, 50*, 47–77.

Frank, E., & Spanier, C. (1995). Interpersonal psychotherapy for depression: Overview, clinical efficacy, and future directions. *Clinical Psychology: Science and Practice, 2*, 349–369.

Gotlib, I. H., Whiffen, V. E., Wallace, P. M., & Mount, J. H. (1991). A prospective investigation of postpartum depression: Factors involved in onset and recovery. *Journal of Abnormal Psychology, 100*, 122–132.

Greenberg, L., & Johnson, S. M. (1988). *Emotionally focused therapy for couples.* New York: Guilford Press.

Griffin, D., & Bartholomew, K. (1994). Models of the self and other: Fundamental dimensions underlying measures of adult attachment. *Journal of Personality and Social Psychology, 67*, 430–445.

Haaga, D. A. F., Yarmus, M., Hubbard, S., Brody, C., Solomon, A., Kirk, L., & Chamberlain, J. (2002). Mood dependency of self-rated attachment style. *Cognitive Therapy and Research, 26*, 57–71.

Hammen, C. L., Burge, D., Daley, S. E., Davila, J., Paley, B., & Rudolph, K. D. (1995). Interpersonal attachment cognitions and prediction of symptomatic responses to interpersonal stress. *Journal of Abnormal Psychology, 104*, 436–463.

Harris, B., Fung, H., Johns, S., Kologlu, M., Bhatti, R., McGregor, A. M., Richards, C.

J., & Hall, R. (1989). Transient post-partum thyroid dysfunction and postnatal depression. *Journal of Affective Disorders, 17*, 243–249.

Hazan, C., & Shaver, P. (1987). Romantic love conceptualized as an attachment process. *Journal of Personality and Social Psychology, 52*, 511–524.

Ingram, R. E., Miranda, J., & Segal, Z. V. (1998). *Cognitive vulnerability to depression*. New York: Guilford Press.

Johnson, S. M. (1996). *The practice of emotionally focused marital therapy: Creating connection*. New York: Brunner/Mazel.

Johnson, S. M., Hunsley, J., Greenberg, L., & Schindler, D. (1999). Emotionally focused couples therapy: Status and challenges. *Clinical Psychology: Science and Practice, 6*, 67–79.

Johnson, S. M., Makinen, J. A., & Millikin, J. W. (2001). Attachment injuries in couples: A new perspective on impasses in couples therapy. *Journal of Marital and Family Therapy, 27*, 145–155.

Johnson, S. M., & Whiffen, V. E. (1999). Made to measure: Adapting emotionally focused couples therapy to partners' attachment styles. *Clinical Psychology: Science and Practice, 6*, 366–381.

Kobak, R. (1994). Adult attachment: A personality or relationship construct? *Psychological Inquiry, 5*, 42–44.

Kobak, R. R., & Hazan, C. (1991). Attachment in marriage: Effects of security and accuracy of working models. *Journal of Personality and Social Psychology, 60*, 861–869.

Marks, M., Wieck, A., Checkley, S., & Kumar, C. (1996). How does marriage protect women with histories of affective disorder from post-partum relapse? *British Journal of Medical Psychology, 69*, 329–342.

Neddelbladt, P., Uddenberg, N., & Englesson, I. (1985). Marital disharmony four and a half years postpartum. *Acta Psychiatrica Scandinavica, 71*, 392–401.

Nicolson, P. (1998). *Postnatal depression: Psychology, science and the transition to motherhood*. New York: Routledge.

Nolen-Hoeksema, S. (1987). Sex differences in unipolar depression: Evidence and theory. *Psychological Bulletin, 101*, 259–282.

O'Hara, M. W., Schlechte, J. A., Lewis, D. A., & Varner, M. W. (1991). Controlled prospective study of postpartum mood disorders: Psychological, environmental, and hormonal variables. *Journal of Abnormal Psychology, 100*, 1–11.

O'Hara, M. W., & Swain, A. M. (1996). Rates and risks of postpartum depression: A meta-analysis. *International Review of Psychiatry, 8*, 37–54.

Oliver, L., & Whiffen, V. E. (in press). Perceptions of parents and partners in men's depressive symptoms. *Journal of Social and Personal Relationships*.

Regier, D., Boyd, J., Burke, J., Rae, D., Myers, J., Kramer, M., Robins, L., George, L., Karno, M., & Locke, B. (1988). One month prevalence of mental disorders in the United States. *Archives of General Psychiatry, 45*, 977–986.

Roberts, J. E., Gotlib, I. H., & Kassel, J. D. (1996). Adult attachment security and symptoms of depression: The mediating roles of dysfunctional attitudes and low self-esteem. *Journal of Personality and Social Psychology, 70*, 310–320.

Ruble, D., Fleming, A., Hackel, L., & Stangor, C. (1988). Changes in the marital relationship during the transition to first time motherhood: Effects of violated expectations concerning the division of household labor. *Journal of Personality and Social Psychology, 55*, 78–87.

Simpson, J. A., Rholes, W. S., & Nelligan, J. S. (1992). Support seeking and support giving within couples in an anxiety-provoking situation: The role of attachment styles. *Journal of Personality and Social Psychology, 62,* 434–446.

Swendsen, J. D., & Mazure, C. M. (2000). Life stress as a risk factor for postpartum depression: Current research and methodological issues. *Clinical Psychology: Science and Practice, 7,* 17–31.

Vandell, D. L., Hyde, J. S., Plant, E. A., & Essex, M. J. (1997). Fathers and "others" as infant-care providers: Predictors of parents' emotional well-being and marital satisfaction. *Merrill–Palmer Quarterly, 43,* 361–385.

Whiffen, V. (1992). Is postpartum depression a distinct diagnosis? *Clinical Psychology Review, 12,* 485–508.

Whiffen, V. E., & Aube, J. A. (1999). Personality, interpersonal context, and depression in couples. *Journal of Social and Personal Relationships, 16,* 369–383.

Whiffen, V. E., & Gotlib, I. H. (1989a). Stress and coping in maritally distressed and nondistressed couples. *Journal of Social and Personal Relationships, 6,* 327–344.

Whiffen, V. E., & Gotlib, I. (1989b). Infants of postpartum depressed mothers: Temperament and cognitive status. *Journal of Abnormal Psychology, 98,* 274–279.

Whiffen, V. E., & Gotlib, I. (1993). Comparison of postpartum and non-postpartum depression: Clinical presentation, psychiatric history, and psycho-social functioning. *Journal of Consulting and Clinical Psychology, 61,* 485–494.

Whiffen, V. E., & Johnson, S. M. (1998). An attachment theory framework for the treatment of childbearing depression. *Clinical Psychology: Science and Practice, 5,* 478–493.

Whiffen, V. E., Kallos-Lilly, A. V., & MacDonald, B. J. (2001). Depression and attachment in couples. *Cognitive Therapy and Research, 25,* 421–434.

Whiffen, V. E., Varshney, N. M., & MacDonald, B. J. (2002). *Marital relations, attachment, and depression in couples.* Manuscript submitted for publication.

Whisman, M. (1999). Marital dissatisfaction and psychiatric disorders: Results from the National Comorbidity Study. *Journal of Abnormal Psychology, 108,* 701–706.

Wisner, K., Perel, J., Peindl, K., Hanusa, B., Findling, R., & Rapport, D. (2001). Prevention of recurrent postpartum depression: A randomized clinical trial. *Journal of Clinical Psychiatry, 62,* 82–86.

Zelkowitz, P., & Milet, T. (1996). Postpartum psychiatric disorders: Their relationship to psychological adjustment and marital satisfaction in the spouses. *Journal of Abnormal Psychology, 105,* 281–285.

17

Understanding the Effects of Child Sexual Abuse History on Current Couple Relationships

An Attachment Perspective

PAMELA C. ALEXANDER

Among the most significant and pervasive long-term effects of childhood sexual abuse are interpersonal problems (Davis & Petretic-Jackson, 2000). Even though this observation should direct our attention to the abuse survivor's interactions with his or her family of creation (i.e., his or her spouse and children), the victim's relationships within this realm have frequently been ignored. Given that abuse survivors, usually female, are more vulnerable to marital violence (Follette, Polusny, Bechtle, & Naugle, 1996), to increased child abuse potential (Alexander, Schaeffer, Young, & Kretz, 2001), to marrying someone who abuses their children (Oates, Tebbutt, Swanston, Lynch, & O'Toole, 1998), and to general difficulties in parenting (Banyard, 1997; Cohen, 1995), these particular long-term effects of sexual abuse deserve more attention. Conversely, given that a current supportive marital relationship can help to overcome the negative effects of an abuse history on both marital functioning (Cohn, Silver, Cowan, Cowan, & Pearson, 1992) and parenting (Egeland, Jacobvitz, & Sroufe, 1988), the marriage of the abuse survivor is not only a potential source of difficulty, but also a potential source of solace and healing. Therefore, it is the purpose of this chapter to explore the current marital relationship of the sexual abuse survivor, both as a focus in itself and also as an important context for parenting.

The framework for discussing this relationship is the intersection between attachment theory and family systems theory. While attachment theory, like family systems theory, deals with patterns of self-reinforcing interactions, its focus has typically been upon the dyad (either marital or parent–child) as opposed to the broader family context. Cowan (1997) makes the case that a family systems model may provide a more substantive and complex understanding of a child's attachment than a simple mother–child dyadic model. In particular, the marital relationship has a direct impact on the parenting relationship (Cowan, Cowan, Cohn, & Pearson, 1996). For its part, attachment theory provides a way for conceptualizing the internalization of family systems and its transmission to a subsequent generation. Although Bowlby emphasized the points of connection between these two perspectives (Marvin & Stewart, 1990), it is unfortunate that little research has actually focused on this intersection.

This chapter is organized as follows. First, an overview of attachment theory is provided, with an emphasis on disorganized attachment (and its adult counterpart, unresolved or fearful–avoidant attachment), since that attachment pattern predominates in a sexually abused population (Alexander et al., 1998; Carlson, Cicchetti, Barnett, & Braunwald, 1989). Second, attachment theory is applied to the typical problems faced by abuse survivors in their marriages. Two constellations of problems are considered: first, the dysthymia, marital dissatisfaction, and problems with intimacy that even well-functioning abuse survivors describe in their marriages; and second, the increased risk for violence, including subsequent revictimization by and victimization of one's partner. Third, attachment theory is applied to what is known about the typical parenting problems of abuse survivors, with attention to the marital context of the parent–child dyad. Fourth, the implications for treatment of sexual abuse survivors are explored from the perspective of attachment theory and family systems theory.

OVERVIEW OF ATTACHMENT THEORY

As articulated by John Bowlby (1982), attachment is assumed to be a biologically based bond that assures the child's proximity to the caregiver, particularly during periods of perceived danger and fear. What is essential to emphasize when talking about an abused population is that, according to this theory, a child cannot *not* be attached, no matter how traumatizing the child's treatment by the caregiver. Therefore, in the absence of another attachment figure, a child must develop a strategy to maintain access to the parent, even if that parent is abusive. The caveat that the presence or absence of another attachment figure determines how dependent a child will be upon the abusive parent argues for the importance of the larger family system in understanding the relationship of the abusive parent and the child.

As a function of the caregiver's responses, the child develops a set of "internal working models" of relationships—that is, the child internalizes both sides of the relationship and not simply the role that the child initially assumed (Sroufe & Fleeson, 1986), an observation with obvious implications for the intergenerational transmission of violence. Longitudinal research suggests that these internal working models are fairly stable across time, showing a correspondence of 72% between infant attachment classification and adult attachment (Waters, Merrick, Treboux, Crowell, & Albersheim, 2000). Attachment tends to be independent of birth order (Main, 2000) and relatively independent of temperament (Hesse & Main, 2000). Not only do these internal working models serve as cognitive templates for relationships, but they also create a basis for affect regulation in that they determine *how* information is processed and what is accessible to memory (Zeanah & Zeanah, 1989).

Specific attachment patterns were described by Mary Ainsworth (Ainsworth, Blehar, Waters, & Wall, 1978) who validated her classification of a child's behavior in a separation–reunion paradigm (the "Strange Situation") with extensive observations of the child's interactions with the parent in the home. Adult attachment has been investigated within two different but overlapping perspectives. Personality and social psychology researchers (see Bartholomew & Horowitz, 1991; Collins & Read, 1990; Hazan & Shaver, 1987) refer to "attachment styles" that are typically assessed with self-report questionnaires, and validated by peer report, concurrent self-report measures, and observation of individuals in interactions with significant others. Developmental psychologists refer to the adult's "state of mind with respect to attachment." While not directly comparable to the child's attachment pattern because it does not refer directly to any particular relationship (Main, 2000), the adult's attachment pattern is a reflection of the adult's current internal working model and is assessed by means of Main's Adult Attachment Interview (AAI; Main & Goldwyn, 1998). Its continuity with the child's behavior is demonstrated both through longitudinal research (see Waters et al., 2000) and through research suggesting that the parent's state of mind with respect to attachment (even prior to the birth of the child) predicts the child's later behavior in the Strange Situation (van IJzendoorn, 1995; Ward & Carlson, 1995). In the interest of space, both the child's and the adult's behavior will be described together. When the personality and developmental perspectives differ in their terminology for adult attachment, both will be mentioned.

Organized Attachment Patterns

Three organized attachment patterns were initially identified. They are called *organized* in that a consistent pattern of behavior allows the child to access the attachment figure fairly reliably when needed (Main, 2000). However, only one of these patterns is called *secure* in that the child is able to express needs easily and straightforwardly with the confidence that the parent will respond quickly and appropriately. As a function of the parent's responsiveness, the secure child is easily soothed and uses the parent as a secure base, from which the child returns rapidly to exploration and play. Follow-up research with the secure child suggests that he or she has good and easy peer relationships, a positive sense of self and others, and, in interactions with peers, is neither a victim nor a victimizer, but instead is competent in play quality and conflict resolution (Bohlin, Hagekull, & Rydell, 2000; Troy & Sroufe, 1987; Wartner, Grossmann, Fremmer-Bombik, & Suess, 1994). The adult counterpart to this secure attachment is characterized by a positive, confident, and trusting sense of self and others; by a coherent, collaborative narrative with an apparently objective access to both positive and negative memories; and by a valuing of attachment relationships (Bartholomew & Horowitz, 1991; Main, 2000).

Two organized patterns of insecure attachment in children include avoidant attachment and anxious–ambivalent attachment. In *avoidant* attachment, the parent tends to be cold and rejecting precisely *when* the child is needy (Izard & Kobak, 1991). Therefore, the child's organized strategy for maintaining contact with the attachment figure is to suppress the negative affect that appears to drive the parent away and to deactivate his or her attachment needs. Unfortunately, this inattention to one's own distress is achieved at the expense of learning to recognize one's own negative affect. As a consequence, the avoidant child is frequently characterized by compulsive self-reliance, exhibiting both externalizing and internalizing behaviors (Lyons-Ruth, Easterbrooks, & Cibelli, 1997; Moss et al., 1999). Even though the avoidant child appears to express little distress, he or she experiences marked physiological arousal in a situation of stress (Spangler & Grossmann, 1993), and, if anything, becomes more fearful over time (Kochanska, 2001).

The adult counterpart to avoidant attachment is called *dismissing* attachment. In self-report measures (Bartholomew & Horowitz, 1991), it is characterized by a positive description of the self and a negative description of the other as well as by an avowed lack of need for intimate relationships. It is characterized in the AAI by idealization or derogation of the parent (as opposed to a realistic assessment of the parent), a fundamental reticence to broach topics of attachment, and inconsistencies and contradictions when forced to discuss attachment relationships (Main & Goldwyn, 1998). Like the avoidant child, the dismissing adult presents as "more normal than normal" (Crittenden, Partridge, & Claussen, 1991), exhibits increased physiological arousal when asked about parental rejection and separation (Dozier & Kobak, 1992), and is likely to be described as hostile by peers (Kobak & Sceery, 1988).

The *anxious–ambivalent* child maintains access to his or her inconsistent parent by heightening negative affect in order to get a reaction. Consequently, this child is clingy, fussy, dependent, coy, angry, and demanding (Crittenden, 1997; Moran & Pederson, 1998), not easily soothed because of the difficulty in relying upon the parent's response (Main, 2000), and therefore unable to use the parent effectively as a secure base. In relationships with peers and teachers, this child hyperactivates attachment needs, has low self-efficacy, is babied but disliked by teachers, and has shown a tendency to fall into the role of victim with aggressive playmates (Main, 2000; Troy & Sroufe, 1987). The adult counterpart of this attachment pattern (*preoccupied*) is characterized by a similar passive or angry preoccupation with the attachment figure, exhibiting superfluous, confusing, and irrelevant information when discussing the attachment figure (Bartholomew & Horowitz, 1991; Main & Goldwyn, 1998). Follow-up research suggests that preoccupied adults tend to experience more distress, distrust, intrusive psychological symptoms, difficulty in seeking help, and loneliness (Gittleman, Klein, Smider, & Essex, 1998; Kemp & Neimeyer, 1999; Larose & Bernier, 2001). They also tend to view conflict as a strategy for attaining intimacy (Fishtein, Pietromonaco, & Barrett, 1999).

Disorganized Attachment

In addition to the three organized attachment patterns, there is a fourth *disorganized* pattern. The high rates of this disorganized–disoriented attachment in maltreated samples (82% vs. 19% in a demographically matched sample; Carlson et al., 1989) suggest that it is clearly related to the experience of abuse. In the Strange Situation, disorganized attachment is characterized by contradictory approach–avoidant behavior on the part of the child in the presence of the caregiver. This disorganized behavior may include conflicting behavioral tendencies (such as either simultaneously or sequentially exhibiting approach and avoidant behaviors toward the parent), apprehension when the parent returns to the room after a separation, actual freezing or stilling, or a dazed disoriented expression on the face of the child in the presence of the parent (Main & Solomon, 1990).

The underlying dynamics of this rather unusual parent–child interaction was described in a model developed by Liotti (1992) which incorporates many of the observations of others. Namely, the parent of the disorganized child often has a history of abuse or unresolved loss (Ainsworth & Eichberg, 1991; Heller & Zeanah, 1999). The parent responds to this unresolved loss or trauma by relying inappropriately upon the child to reduce the parent's own anxiety. Not only does this role reversal signal to the child that the parent is not in control, but the parent of the disorganized child may either overtly frighten the child (as in the case of an abusive parent) or, in the case of a parent unresolved with respect to her or his own trauma or loss, may appear to be frightened by the child or in the presence of the child (Hesse & Main, 2000). However, given that the response of any child in a situation of threat or fear is to turn to the attachment figure, the disorganized child attempts to seek comfort from the very parent who is causing the fear in the first place. Thus, in the face of this dilemma of experiencing "fright without solution" (Main, 1995), the disorganized child develops multiple incompatible models of self, seeing the self as victim of the frightening parent, as persecutor of the frightened or out-of-control parent, and as rescuer of the vulnerable parent (Liotti, 1999). Liotti (1992, 1999) presents this scenario as a basis for the development of dissociative disorders, especially if this attachment dynamic is also accompanied by actual abuse. In fact, Ogawa, Sroufe, Weinfield, Carlson, and Egeland (1997) have found that the most significant predictor of dissociation at age 19 is the presence of disorganized attachment at age 2, even controlling for intervening trauma.

By age 6, the disorganized child is characterized by either punitive controlling or caregiving controlling behavior toward the parent (Main & Cassidy, 1988). Moreover, Jacobvitz and Hazen (1999) have noted that the punitive controlling behavior exhibited by the disorganized child appears to be reinforced by the marital conflict of the parents and the cross-generational alliance of the child with the other parent. The disorganized child's controlling behavior is also manifested in high rates of internalizing behavior and externalizing behavior with peers (Lyons-Ruth et al., 1997; Moss et al., 1999). In fact, Lyons-Ruth, Alpern, and Repacholi (1993) noted that disorganized attachment status was the strongest single predictor of hostile behavior toward peers in the classroom, with 71% of hostile preschoolers classified during infancy as disorganized. Moreover, in a longitudinal study, Kochanska (2001) found that disorganized children became more angry over time. Clearly, the disorganized child demonstrates significant difficulties with both affect regulation and cognition.

The concept of role reversal is, of course, familiar to family systems theorists, and is particularly prevalent among families characterized by sexual abuse (Alexander, in press; Burkett, 1991; Sroufe, Jacobvitz, Mangelsdorf, DeAngelo, & Ward, 1985). However, as would also be expected by a family systems theorist, this dynamic of the parent's reliance upon the child and the child's approach–avoidant behavior toward the parent occurs within a wider family or marital context. If a child has an alternate attachment figure, there would be no need to approach the problematic parent. Indeed, Anderson and Alexander (1996) found that their sample of eight severely dissociative incest survivors not only experienced more severe abuse than the larger sample of nondissociative incest survivors, but were also more likely to describe their abusive fathers as their primary attachment figures and their mothers as neglectful and rejecting. For example, Marianne reported being raped by her father at age 4. She described him as "Ted Bundyish" in that he would frequently sneak up behind her and grab her legs in order to dislocate her kneecaps. Moreover, she reported that, while her father was away on business trips, her mother would leave her at a young age alone with her two younger siblings for days at a time. She stated that her mother forced her and her sibs to eat rotting moldy food from the refrigerator, and tortured their pets in order to punish the children. Therefore, in spite of her father's sadistic abuse, Marianne described herself as closer to him than to her mother ("At least he was better than her"). Thus, the stage was set for needing to turn for comfort to the very person who was causing so much distress. Marianne's diagnosis of dissociative identity disorder is thus understandable when considering both the specific disorganized attachment dynamic and the wider family context (i.e., her inability to turn to a soothing other).

The adult counterpart to disorganized attachment in a child is referred to as *fearful* attachment in the personality literature and is suggestive of an avoidance of intimate relationships as well as a negative view of self and others (Bartholomew & Horowitz, 1991). The developmental literature refers to the adult counterpart of disorganized attachment in childhood as *unresolved*, and refers to a lack of resolution specifically with respect to abuse or loss. On the AAI, adults are classified as unresolved when they display lapses in reasoning or dissociated ideas or memories precisely when they are asked to speak about any experiences of trauma or loss (Main & Goldwyn, 1998). Research suggests not only that unresolved parents are more likely to have children who are disorganized in their interactions with that particular parent (Ainsworth & Eichberg, 1991; Heller & Zeanah, 1999; Main & Hesse, 1990), but are also more likely to be characterized by psychiatric disorders, including borderline personality disorder (Fonagy et al., 1996) and dissociation (Alexander et al., 1998). Unresolved attachment has been found to predominate in samples of male batterers (Holtzworth-Munroe, Stuart, & Hutchinson, 1997). Finally, both the developmental and the personality literature find that the unresolved or fearful individual is characterized by a fundamental sense of badness or shame (Bartholomew & Horowitz, 1991; Main & Hesse, 1992). Thus, the relevance of this attachment classification to the sexual abuse survivor is obvious.

ATTACHMENT THEORY AND THE MARITAL INTERACTIONS OF SEXUAL ABUSE SURVIVORS

While sexual abuse has a negative impact no matter what the attachment status of the individual, the long-term effects of the abuse appear to be determined more by the nature of the initial attachment relationship than by the characteristics of the abuse itself (Alexander, 1993). Furthermore, even specific posttraumatic reactions to the abuse are moderated by the amount and type of soothing the child received from attachment figures (Lyons-Ruth, Bronfman, & Atwood, 1999). Thus, it should not be surprising that abuse survivors bring both abuse effects and attachment effects and expectations to their relationship with their marital partner. Conversely, their marriage may either exacerbate these early effects or counteract them. Therefore, the following discussion is organized with respect to two constellations of these effects: (1) dysthymia, marital dissatisfaction, and problems with intimacy; and (2) increased risk for violence in the current attachment relationship. Both of these constellations of effects are important to consider in working with abuse survivors and their partners.

Dysthymia, Marital Dissatisfaction, and Problems with Intimacy

At a minimum, the intimate relationships of sexual abuse survivors are frequently characterized by mistrust, interpersonal sensitivity, and feelings of isolation (Davis & Petretic-Jackson, 2000; Harter, Alexander, & Neimeyer, 1988). For example, DiLillo and Long (1999) observed less relationship satisfaction, poorer communication, and lower levels of trust in their partners among sexual abuse survivors. Similarly, in an Army sample of young mothers, Alexander, Schaeffer, et al. (2001) found that sexual abuse history was uniquely predictive of marital dissatisfaction, low family cohesion, and high family conflict (even controlling for history of physical abuse, neglect, witnessing domestic violence, emotional abuse, and growing up with alcoholic parents). Waltz (1994) compared the coded interactions of heterosexual abuse survivors and their male partners with the marital interactions of nonabused women. Survivors and their partners in this sample were more dissatisfied with their marriages and exhibited more sadness and dampened emotional expressivity. Needless to say, a sample of women who are able to convince their spouses to participate in a study of marital interactions is undoubtedly functioning at the higher end of the continuum, at least with respect to their marriage. Therefore, the fact that they nonetheless exhibited blunted affect and dysthymia in their interactions with their partners points to the pervasiveness of the long-term effects of abuse on intimacy.

So what can attachment theory add to the understanding of this scenario? First, the negative self-construal associated with many individuals' experience of abuse appears to mediate many of the long-term effects (Coffey, Leitenberg, Henning, Turner, & Bennett, 1996; Harter, 2000). Research suggests that this fundamental feeling of shame and badness characteristic of unresolved or fearful attachment (Main & Hesse, 1992) is also clearly related to concerns about attachment. The self is considered unlovable and unentitled, making it very difficult to either express needs or to accept the nurturing of others. Loos and Alexander (2001), for example, found that core negative self-descriptors in a sample of highly dissociative individuals predicted attachment-related anxiety (but not general anxiety) in an emotional Stroop task. Therefore, attachment theory tells us that the depression and shame observed in abuse survivors will necessarily interfere with the establishment of intimate attachment relationships in adulthood.

The depression of the abuse survivor can also be understood as an effect of disrupted attachment on affect regulation. Evidence suggests that both the disorganized child and the abused child are seriously vulnerable to dysregulation of affect in dealing with later stressors, as a function of both an early experience of severe stress and the lack of adequate caregiving (Lyons-Ruth et al., 1999). Disorganized toddlers are significantly more likely to exhibit dysregulation of the hypothalamic–pituitary-adrenocorticol axis and higher cortisol concentrations than are nondisorganized toddlers (Hertsgaard, Gunnar, Erickson, & Nachmias, 1995), as are sexual abuse survivors (Weiss, Longhurst, & Mazure, 1999). These elevated cortisol levels are associated with helplessness and vulnerability in response to subsequent stressors (Spangler & Grossmann, 1993; Weiss et al., 1999). In fact, females (both humans and animals) may be even more vulnerable to this effect than males, thereby accounting in part for their increased vulnerability to depression in adulthood (Weiss et al., 1999). Thus, the affect dysregulation associated both with disorganized attachment and with the experience of sexual abuse may explain, from a physiological perspective, later vulnerabilities in coping with stress.

Although the distorted internal working models and disrupted affect regulation of the insecure, and especially disorganized, child can explain the dysthymia of the abuse survivor, the effect of early attachment relationships on current depression is moderated by the effect of current attachment relationships. For example, Whiffen, Judd, and Aube (1999) emphasized that support by a partner has an important impact on the functioning of the abuse survivor. Sexual abuse survivors were both better protected from depression than nonabused women when they described their relationships as of high quality and more vulnerable to depression when they did not. Alexander, Grelling, and Anderson (1995) similarly observed that secure incest survivors were more likely to have partners who were actively engaged with them and who thus counteracted their own tendency to shut down (as observed by Waltz, 1994). The following case example illustrates the positive impact of a supportive marital relationship on an abuse survivor, the continuing vulnerability of the woman even within the context of this supportive marriage, and the challenge to her partner in attempting to maintain this level of support in light of her continued depression.

Joanne was sexually abused by her father who was an FBI agent and a lay minister. He sodomized her when she was 9; when she was 11, on the way home from a Sunday evening church service, he took her with him to a motel where several other men were present. He stripped her, bound her hands and feet, inserted his gun into her vagina, and took pictures. She reported being so afraid that she passed out. He later said nothing of the event. She reported that the last abuse event occurred when she was 12, when her father sodomized her in the bathroom and she yelled loudly. Joanne described her mother as unavailable (probably depressed over the death of an older child when Joanne was 1.5 years old) and more like a sibling than a parent. She stated that her father found her interesting intellectually and that she allied herself with her father. Joanne's mother's experience of traumatic loss within 2 years of Joanne's birth (cf. Liotti, 1999), as well as her own report that she regarded her very sadistic father as her primary attachment figure, are consistent with her attachment classification of unresolved.

Joanne's second husband, Joe, is the son of a domestically violent father. He and Joanne have been married for 10 years and have been in marital therapy off and on for several years. Joe was classified as "secure" on an attachment interview. Although he describes himself as feeling secure in his relationship with Joanne, confident of her support, and able to come to new solutions, he has also learned how specific behaviors (e.g., standing in a doorway) may trigger anxiety attacks in her. He notes that she becomes frightened of him easily if he loses his temper. His description of his wife is poignant: "Joanne's a pretty great person, but there's a sadness to her that will never go away."

This case example represents an ideal of partner support and understanding in the face of continued distress and trauma in the incest survivor. However, even the supportive partner is not immune from the effects of his wife's dysthymia and history of trauma. Indeed, it is quite common for partners to experience secondary traumatization from their relationship with the survivor. Maltas and Shay (1995) described the phenomenon of *trauma contagion* in which the partner of the abuse survivor comes to develop a number of reactions secondary to his interaction with his wife, including shattered assumptions regarding his normal expectations of sexuality in an intimate relationship. For example, one incest survivor explained quite articulately how she was no longer able to remain with her husband because he expected that sex be part of their relationship. Trauma contagion for the partner may also result from the chronic stress of living with someone who is having flashbacks. As Maltas and Shay (1995) point out, the partner may have the experience of being on an emotional roller coaster. To the extent that the partner himself may be a trigger for the woman's flashbacks, he may find himself becoming hypervigilant and constantly worried about being misinterpreted. Ironically, many of these types of vicarious traumatization may be experienced most acutely by the supportive partner who is sensitive to his wife's anxiety and dysthymia. Both he and his partner may also be so focused on her history of abuse that even normal marital conflicts may be attributed to her past, thus obviating the fact that they are not exempt from normal conflicts within the marriage. Thus, even in the ideal scenario of the supportive partner of the dysthymic but functioning survivor, the effect of the abuse history on the marriage is palpable and may contribute to a vicarious experience of trauma for the partner. In conclusion, the negative self-construal and problems with affect regulation make it harder for incest survivors and their spouses to create and maintain a secure bond.

Increased Risk for Violence and Reenactment of the Original Attachment Relationship

In addition to general relationship dissatisfaction, sexual abuse survivors tend to be at increased risk for victimization in an adult intimate relationship (Follette et al., 1996; Messman & Long, 1996). In a comparison of low-income women with and without a history of sexual abuse, DiLillo, Giuffre, Tremblay, and Peterson (2001) found not only more marital violence in sexual abuse survivors, but also more woman-to-man aggression. Moreover, in a sample of 293 pairs of mothers and fathers participating in the Army's New Parent Support Program, mothers who were child sexual abuse survivors were significantly more likely to be in marriages characterized by mutual marital violence and dual-parent risk for child abuse, as well as in marriages in which only the mother was at risk for child abuse (Alexander, Kretz, Schaeffer, & Young, 2001). This apparent reenactment of the original family experience may be a result of assortative mating since unresolved individuals are more often married to each other than would be expected by chance (van IJzendoorn & Bakermans-Kranenburg, 1996). Alternatively, this increased risk for violence may simply be the result of newly established patterns of interactions within the marriage. In either case, a history of child sexual abuse appears to increase a woman's risk for subsequent family violence, including both unilateral and mutual marital violence.

Attachment theory can be useful in its ability to explain this increased risk for violence from several different perspectives, namely, the effect of disorganized attachment on (1) internal working models, (2) mentalizing, and (3) subsequent aggressive behavior. Each of these short-term effects has important implications for unresolved attachment in adulthood. First, as Sroufe and Fleeson (1986) have pointed out, the internal working model consists not of learned or observed roles, but instead the internalization of the whole attachment relationship. As such, individuals unconsciously have access to *both* aspects of the relationship—not only to their previously experienced victim role, but also to their perpetrator's victimizer role. For the child who is faced with the contradictory and unintegrated internal working models presented by the abusive unresolved parent, either pole of this dichotomy is a behavioral possibility and may be actualized either in different relationships (e.g., an abusive parent and a battered spouse) or even within the same relationship (Lyons-Ruth et al., 1999).

Second, Fonagy's concept of "mentalizing" also can be used to account for sexual abuse survivors' increased vulnerability to subsequent involvement in a violent relationship. According to Fonagy (Fonagy, Target, & Gergely, 2000), *mentalizing* refers to the child's ability to see another individual as an intentional thinking person. A deficit in mentalizing or reflective function is common among maltreated children and also among disorganized children. According to Fonagy, the parent of the disorganized and severely abused child fails to view the child as a distinct individual with his or her own subjective state. Instead, all behaviors of the child are interpreted vis-à-vis the parent's projections and needs. Moreover, the parents' denial or distortion of his or her abusive behavior, general family dysfunction, and the child's need to deny the hatred implied by the parent's abusive behavior all interfere with the child's ability to develop a reflective function (Fonagy et al., 2000). As a consequence of not being experienced as an independent person by one's parent, the child similarly fails to develop the ability to view him- or herself and others as individuals with intentional mental states. Instead, the child views self and others as physical transitional objects, with no sense of personal agency. An example of the long-term effect of this lack of agency was recounted by Herman (1981). She described an incest survivor who was raped as an adult by a stranger. This woman subsequently married her rapist 2 weeks later because that was *his* desire, with no sense of awareness that what *she* wanted should also enter into this decision.

Fonagy also points out that a fear of abandonment triggers nonmentalizing in disorganized children as the parent withdraws from the child in either anxiety or rage. Thus, the child equates his or her own arousal with the dangerous withdrawal or rage of the parent. In this way, disorganized attachment leads to a disorganized self (Fonagy et al., 2000) that feels unsafe, vulnerable, and in danger of disappearing unless certain unacceptable parts of the self can be externalized on to relationships. Evidence suggests, of course, that these characteristics implied by borderline personality disorder are indeed closely associated both with a history of sexual abuse (Gladstone, Parker, Wilhelm, Mitchell, & Austin, 1999) and with unresolved attachment (Alexander et al., 1998; Stalker & Davies, 1995).

A final way of thinking about the relationship between sexual abuse history, disorganized attachment, and subsequent vulnerability to relationship violence is suggested by follow-up research with disorganized children. Comparisons with other attachment categories and with other abused populations suggest that anger is particularly prominent in disorganized and sexually abused samples (Elhai, Frueh, Gold, Gold, & Hamner, 2000; Kochanska, 2001). As mentioned previously, disorganized latency-age children exhibit controlling behavior, both with their parents and with their peers (Lyons-Ruth, 1996; van IJzendoorn, Schuengel, & Bakermans-Kranenburg, 1999). Unresolved attachment in adulthood is similarly associated with violent behavior and has been found to predominate among samples of male batterers (Dutton, 1999; Holtzworth-Munroe et al., 1997). Moreover, research suggests that the other pertinent aspects of the disorganized relationship as described by Liotti (i.e., role reversal, dissociation, and shame) are also associated with a greater risk for violence (Alexander & Warner, 2003). For example, the role-reversing behavior observed in disorganized children (Main & Cassidy, 1988) is not dissimilar from the boundary intrusive behavior observed in couples exhibiting possessiveness, jealousy, and marital violence (Goodman & Fallon, 1995; Green & Werner, 1996). Furthermore, dissociation has been found to predict both internalized and externalized aggression (Putnam et al., 1996; Simoneti, Scott, & Murphy, 2000). Finally, shame has been found to predict both revictimization among sexual abuse survivors (Kessler & Bieschke, 1999) and self-reported anger and abusive behavior (Dutton, van Ginkel, & Starzomski, 1995). Therefore, follow-up research suggests that the dynamics of disorganized and unresolved attachment are intricately linked to subsequent vulnerability to violence.

In conclusion, attachment theory contributes to an understanding of the ubiquitous symptoms of depression and dissatisfaction of the sexual abuse survivor, and, at times, the same symptoms of her spouse. It also emphasizes the power of the current attachment figure (i.e., the spouse) in moderating the effects of either the abuse or early attachment experiences. Similarly, attachment theory helps to explain why many sexual abuse survivors are at an increased risk for violence in their current relationships. Namely, the long-term effects of disorganized attachment include distorted internal working models, problems with mentalizing, and variants of controlling behavior. These mechanisms as well as the choice of a partner with similar concerns can account for the increased risk for violence. On the other hand, a supportive, stable, and secure spouse can greatly reduce this risk for violence and conflict.

MARRIAGE AS THE CONTEXT
FOR THE ABUSE SURVIVOR'S PARENTING

Sexual abuse survivors are clearly at risk for problems with regard to parenting (Alexander, Schaeffer, et al., 2001), including inadequate sensitivity, lack of support, and role reversal (Alexander, Teti, & Anderson, 2000; Burkett, 1991; Cohen, 1995; Zuravin & DiBlasio, 1992). Indeed, the research previously reviewed that describes the family-of-origin experience of the disorganized child is equally applicable to describing the parenting of the unresolved sexual abuse survivor, thus explaining the risk for the inter-generational transmission of violence (Alexander & Warner, 2003). More-over, Crittenden et al.'s (1991) research on assortative mating, based on only the three organized attachment categories, suggests that certain types of partnerships (i.e., a dismissing individual married to a preoccupied indi-vidual) were at greatest risk for marital violence, child abuse, and neglect. One can only imagine that the assortative mating of two unresolved indi-viduals (van IJzendoorn & Bakermans-Kranenburg, 1996) would prove even more problematic for parenting. On the other hand, research also sug-gests that a supportive marriage can overcome the negative effects of a his-tory of abuse on parenting (Cohn, Cowan, Cowan, & Pearson, 1992). For example, mothers with a history of abuse are less likely to abuse their own children or to even engage in a role-reversing behavior to the degree that they are in a supportive relationship (Alexander et al., 2000; Egeland et al., 1988). Moreover, the positive impact of marital adjustment on parenting is especially important for mothers who are insecure, as would be characteris-tic of many abuse survivors (Eiden, Teti, & Corns, 1995).

Unfortunately, much of the recent research on attachment theory tends to ignore the importance of the marriage when evaluating parenting. For example, mothers with a history of trauma who do *not* typically exhibit the frightened/frightening behavior thought to elicit disorganized behavior in the child (Jacobvitz, Hazen, & Riggs, 1997) appear instead to exhibit an *in-hibition* of behavior with respect to their child (Schuengel, Bakermans-Kranenburg, & van IJzendoorn, 1999). While this behavioral inhibition and withdrawal on the part of the mother certainly seems to protect the child from either disorganized attachment (Schuengel et al., 1999) or inse-cure attachment (Lyons-Ruth et al., 1999), the larger effect of the mother's withdrawal on the child may be dependent upon the father's relationship with the child.

Consider the example of Betty, who is a 39-year-old incest survivor who described physical abuse and neglect by her mother and severe sadistic physical and sexual abuse by her father, who was undoubtedly dissociative. Betty reported that, as a result of many years of individual therapy, she has recognized the need to withdraw from her two young daughters in situa-tions that tend to elicit her anger. For example, she stated, "At the dinner table, I become my father—just a ball of rage." Consequently, she reported that for the past year, she has made her children their dinner, and then has gone off to eat by herself, whether or not her husband is at home. She simi-larly described refusing to give her daughters baths because of the negative association with bathtime in her family of origin. Any benefit to her daugh-ters from Betty's withdrawal from them obviously is dependent upon her husband or others providing a responsible alternative to her parenting. Otherwise, her daughters may be as vulnerable as she was as a child. While there was no evidence to the contrary in this particular case, the inference that behavioral inhibition on the part of an unresolved mother is beneficial to the child must be considered within the larger context of the family environment. Therefore, a focus solely on the parent–child interactions of the abuse survivor may fail to consider other sources of risk for the child.

IMPLICATIONS FOR THERAPY WITH THE ABUSE SURVIVOR, HER PARTNER, AND HER CHILDREN

There are a number of implications of attachment theory for intervening with the sexual abuse survivor. First, even before discussing interventions with the survivor and her family of creation (i.e., her husband and her children), it is important to remember that individual therapy does have an important role in working with someone who has been severely traumatized. The therapist may need to initially serve as the primary secure base for the survivor when her partner cannot or will not. For a survivor confronted with body trauma memories, threat is excessively high precisely because information processing is occurring at the midbrain or limbic system level, where only minimal contextual learning or cortical involvement is involved (Crittenden, 1997). Therefore, an individual therapist's involvement may be absolutely essential. Attachment theory can provide specific suggestions for individual therapy with the abuse survivor (see Alexander & Anderson, 1994).

On the other hand, there is a risk to the abuse survivor of only participating in individual or group therapy without attention to her family of creation. Follette, Alexander, and Follette (1991) found that being married predicted relatively poorer outcome for incest survivors participating in group therapy. It was inferred that participating in a group (or individual therapy) focusing on incest increased attachment-related anxiety within one's marriage. Without another venue to address these attachment issues in one's family of creation, progress in the group therapy was hampered. Therefore, any therapist working with abuse survivors individually or in groups must consider the potentially iatrogenic effect of the therapy itself on the abuse survivor's marriage and relationship with her children.

So what does attachment theory offer marital and family therapy with the abuse survivor? First, no matter what the goal for therapy, behavior change must proceed from a secure base (Alexander & Anderson, 1994). As mentioned previously, this is one reason that particularly traumatized women may need to rely initially upon an individual therapist. Eventually, of course, many marital therapies strive to enhance the healthy use of the marriage as a secure base for the partners (Cowan & Cowan, 2001). However, the abuse survivor's experience of betrayal and powerlessness in an early attachment relationship will necessarily interfere with her ability to explore her fears and vulnerabilities with her spouse, no matter how supportive he may be. Furthermore, his experience of vicarious traumatization in their relationship may make him cautious and mistrustful of requests for self-disclosure. Therefore, the marital therapist of the abuse survivor may initially need to play a much more central role as a secure base for both partners than is usually required in working with couples.

Second, attachment theory describes the process of affect dysregulation and suggests how subsequent attachment relationships become triggers for this dysregulation. Visual images and tactile stimuli may elicit a sudden anxiety or rage. For example, one woman who was sexually abused over a period of many years by her mother reported the beginning of flashbacks only when she reached the age at which her mother began abusing her and her own reflection in the mirror brought back images of the abuse. Physical similarities of one's partner to the abuser or one's children to oneself may similarly trigger reactions. Thus, an explicit focus on the process of affect regulation is essential with marital therapy with the abuse survivor. One of the most pertinent perspectives for dealing with the affect is emotionally focused couple therapy (Johnson, 1996). Johnson (2002) describes its use with abuse survivors and their partners as well as its emphasis on accessing and reprocessing affect, the development of strategies to tolerate and manage negative affect, and eventually the integration of new emotional experiences into a new sense of self.

A third contribution of attachment theory to the process of marital therapy comes from its emphasis on the internal working model. The internal working model of the unresolved adult was established preverbally and is unquestionably confused, contradictory, and unintegrated. Consequently, the distorted and dissociated components of the abuse survivor's internal working model is not going to be readily available for examination and discussion. Depending upon the insight and the observing ego of the partner, the marital therapist will need to attend closely to the interactions of the couple in the session; at least initially, self-report may be highly unreliable. In fact, videotaping may prove useful in slowing down and dissecting a particular interaction as well as the unstated internal working models underlying it. In addition to bringing working models to conscious awareness, it is important for the therapist to remember that the whole multifaceted relationship with the abuser will have been internalized and that the abuse survivor may be subtly reenacting different components of this early attachment relationship. Longitudinal research with disorganized children and retrospective research with unresolved adults suggest that abuse survivors are vulnerable to revictimization by and/or abuse of their own partners or their children, but may also have little insight into how their behavior may be abusive. Therefore, the therapist will need to be especially alert to the risk for victimization of either the woman, her partner, or their child. Ultimately, the goal is to help couples begin to recognize links between their parents and their current marriage, between their experience as children in their family of origin and their current experience and behavior as parents, and between their current marriage and their parenting (Cowan & Cowan, 2001).

Fourth, according to Main (1991), the most essential characteristic of a secure individual is the coherence of his or her narrative. The lack of a coherent narrative is the sine qua non of insecure attachment, and, by definition, a lack of coherence specifically with respect to one's trauma history is characteristic of the unresolved or fearful individual (Main & Goldwyn, 1998). Fonagy et al.'s (2000) concept of mentalizing or reflective function—that is, the ability to view one's own and one's partner's thoughts and perspectives objectively and as subject to change—is similar. This acceptance of one's own and one's partner's perspective is obviously the basis for both self-forgiveness and tolerance and acceptance of the other. While this is certainly the goal of many types of therapies, it is particularly central to narrative therapy (White & Epston, 1989). Developing a coherent narrative of one's current and past experience is frequently the goal of individual therapy. However, the opportunity to have one's story heard and witnessed by an intimate partner (in other words, by one's attachment figure) in addition to one's therapist is especially powerful in helping an individual understand, modify, and integrate her own story within her memory (Freedman & Combs, 2000). Explicitly, attachment theory implies that this process of telling one's story should be part of couple therapy.

Finally, it may be necessary to directly observe an abuse survivor's and her partner's interactions with their children. For example, attachment theory, like family systems theory, alerts the family therapist to attend to any particular indications of role reversal or emotional overdependence upon the child. Moreover, although the resolution of marital difficulties will help to protect both partners from problematic parenting, the specific emotional triggers of the child will undoubtedly be quite different than the triggers that define the partners for each other. It is especially important to monitor whether a woman's decision to withdraw from her child in certain situations of stress leaves the child vulnerable to abuse either by the other parent or by someone from outside the home. The distinction between a parent's behavioral inhibition and a parent's neglect is important, but not necessarily always apparent to a child. Therefore, the abuse survivor may need, with the help of her partner, to discover ways to structure her interactions with her children with respect to certain specific situations that trigger a negative reaction from her.

CONCLUSION

In conclusion, attachment theory has much to tell us about the experience of the sexual abuse survivor, especially the woman who remains fearful or unresolved about her abuse. In particular, attachment theory's recent focus on disorganized attachment helps to explain the significant problems with affect regulation, distorted internal working models, problems engaging in perspective taking, the fundamental sense of shame, and the anger and aggression observed in children who have been sexually abused. However, the dyadic parent–child interaction cannot be understood meaningfully without attention to the larger family context. So also, the abuse survivor's internal working model will be revealed most richly in her interactions with her partner and with her children. Therefore, these attachment relationships in the family of creation not only warrant attention in and of themselves, but also provide the most pertinent avenue for intervening with the survivor of childhood abuse. As such, they are of special interest to the marital and family therapist.

REFERENCES

Ainsworth, M. D. S., Blehar, M., Waters, E., & Wall, S. (1978). *Patterns of attachment*. Hillsdale, NJ: Erlbaum.

Ainsworth, M. D. S., & Eichberg, C. G. (1991). Effects on infant–mother attachment of mother's unresolved loss of an attachment figure or other traumatic experience. In P. Marris, J. Stevenson-Hinde, & C. Parkes (Eds.), *Attachment across the life cycle* (pp. 160–183). New York: Routledge.

Alexander, P. C. (1992). Application of attachment theory to the study of sexual abuse. *Journal of Consulting and Clinical Psychology, 60*, 185–195.

Alexander, P. C. (1993). The differential effects of abuse characteristics and attachment in the prediction of long-term effects of sexual abuse. *Journal of Interpersonal Violence, 8*, 346–362.

Alexander, P. C. (in press). Parent–child role reversal: Development of a measure and test of an attachment theory model. *Journal of Systemic Therapies*.

Alexander, P. C., & Anderson, C. L. (1994). An attachment approach to psychotherapy with the incest survivor. *Psychotherapy, 31*, 665–675.

Alexander, P. C., Anderson, C. L., Brand, B., Schaeffer, C. M., Grelling, B. Z., & Kretz, L. (1998). Adult attachment and longterm effects in survivors of incest. *Child Abuse and Neglect, 22*, 45–81.

Alexander, P. C., Grelling, B. Z., & Anderson, C. L. (1995, July). *Adult attachment as a predictor of the marital interactions of incest survivors*. Paper presented at the fourth International Family Violence Research Conference, Durham, NH.

Alexander, P. C., Kretz, L., Schaeffer, C. M., & Young, V. (2001). *Contrasting dual-parent, mother-only and father-only risk for child abuse: A typology of at-risk families*. Unpublished manuscript.

Alexander, P. C., Schaeffer, C., Young, V., & Kretz, L. (2001). *Trauma history and the prediction of child abuse potential*. Unpublished manuscript.

Alexander, P. C., Teti, L., & Anderson, C. L. (2000). Child sexual abuse history and role reversal in parenting. *Child Abuse and Neglect, 24*, 829–838.

Alexander, P. C., & Warner, S. (2003). Attachment theory and family systems theory as frameworks for understanding the intergenerational transmission of family violence. In P. Erdman & T. Caffery (Eds.), *Attachment and family systems: Conceptual, empirical, and therapeutic relatedness* (pp. 241–257). New York: Brunner/Routledge.

Anderson, C., & Alexander, P. C. (1996). The relationship between attachment and dissociation in adult survivors of incest. *Psychiatry, 59,* 240–254.

Banyard, V. L. (1997). The impact of childhood sexual abuse and family functioning on four dimensions of women's later parenting. *Child Abuse and Neglect, 21,* 1095–1107.

Bartholomew, K., & Horowitz, L. M. (1991). Attachment styles among young adults: A test of a four-category model. *Journal of Personality and Social Psychology, 61,* 226–244.

Bohlin, G., Hagekull, B., & Rydell, A. (2000). Attachment and social functioning: A longitudinal study from infancy to middle childhood. *Social Development, 9,* 24–39.

Bowlby, J. (1982). *Attachment and loss: Vol. I. Attachment.* New York: Basic Books. (First edition published in 1969)

Burkett, L. P. (1991). Parenting behaviors of women who were sexually abused as children in their families of origin. *Family Process, 30,* 421–434.

Carlson, V., Cicchetti, D., Barnett, D., & Braunwald, K. G. (1989). Finding order in disorganization. In D. Cicchetti & V. Carlson (Eds.), *Child maltreatment: Theory and research on the causes and consequences of child abuse and neglect* (pp. 484–528). New York: Cambridge University Press.

Coffey, P., Leitenberg, H., Henning, K., Turner, T., & Bennett, R. T. (1996). Mediators of the long-term impact of child sexual abuse: Perceived stigma, betrayal, powerlessness, and self-blame. *Child Abuse and Neglect, 20,* 447–455.

Cohen, T. (1995). Motherhood among incest survivors. *Child Abuse and Neglect, 19,* 1423–1429.

Cohn, D. A., Cowan, C. P., Cowan, P. A., & Pearson, J. (1992). Mothers' and fathers' working models of childhood attachment relationships, parenting styles, and child behavior. *Development and Psychopathology, 4,* 417–431.

Cohn, D. A., Silver, D. H., Cowan, C. P., Cowan, P. A., & Pearson, J. (1992). Working models of childhood attachment and couple relationships. *Journal of Family Issues, 13,* 432–449.

Collins, N. L., & Read, S. J. (1990). Adult attachment, working models, and relationship quality in dating couples. *Journal of Personality and Social Psychology, 58,* 644–663.

Cowan, P. A. (1997). Beyond meta-analysis: A plea for a family systems view of attachment. *Child Development, 68,* 601–603.

Cowan, P., & Cowan, C. P. (2001). A couple perspective on the transmission of attachment patterns. In C. Clulow (Ed.), *Adult attachment and couple psychotherapy* (pp. 62–82). Philadelphia, PA: Taylor & Francis.

Cowan, P. A., Cowan, C. P., Cohn, D. A., & Pearson, J. L. (1996). Parents' attachment histories and children's externalizing and internalizing behaviors: Exploring family systems models of linkage. *Journal of Consulting and Clinical Psychology, 64,* 53–63.

Crittenden, P. M. (1997). Toward an integrative theory of trauma: A dynamic-maturation approach. In D. Cicchetti & S. L. Toth (Eds.), *Rochester Symposium on Developmental Psychopathology: Vol. 8. Developmental perspectives on trau-

ma: Theory, research, and intervention (pp. 33–84). Rochester, NY: University of Rochester Press.

Crittenden, P. M., Partridge, M. F., & Claussen, A. H. (1991). Family patterns of relationship in normative and dysfunctional families. *Development and Psychopathology, 3*, 491–512.

Davis, J. L., & Petretic-Jackson, P. A. (2000). The impact of child sexual abuse on adult interpersonal functioning: A review and synthesis of the empirical literature. *Aggression and Violent Behavior, 5*, 291–328.

DiLillo, D., & Long, P. J. (1999). Perceptions of couple functioning among female survivors of child sexual abuse. *Journal of Child Sexual Abuse, 7*, 59–76.

DiLillo, D., Giuffre, D., Tremblay, G. C., & Peterson, L. (2001). A closer look at the nature of intimate partner violence reported by women with a history of child sexual abuse. *Journal of Interpersonal Violence, 16*, 116–132.

Dozier, M., & Kobak, R. (1992). Psychophysiology in attachment interviews: Converging evidence for deactivating strategies. *Child Development, 63*, 1473–1480.

Dutton, D. G. (1999). Traumatic origins of intimate rage. *Aggression and Violent Behavior, 4*, 431–447.

Dutton, D. G., van Ginkel, C., & Starzomski, A. (1995). The role of shame and guilt in the intergenerational transmission of abusiveness. *Violence and Victims, 10*, 121–131.

Egeland, B., Jacobvitz, D., & Sroufe, L. A. (1988). Breaking the cycle of abuse. *Child Development, 59*, 1080–1088.

Eiden, R. D., Teti, D. M., & Corns, K. M. (1995). Maternal working models of attachment, marital adjustment, and the parent–child relationship. *Child Development, 66*, 1504–1518.

Elhai, J. D., Frueh, B. C., Gold, P. B., Gold, S. N., & Hamner, M. B. (2000). Clinical presentations of posttraumatic stress disorder across trauma populations: A comparison of MMPI-2 profiles of combat veterans and adult survivors of child sexual abuse. *Journal of Nervous and Mental Disease, 188*, 708–713.

Fishtein, J., Pietromonaco, P. R., & Barrett, L. F. (1999). The contribution of attachment style and relationship conflict to the complexity of relationship knowledge. *Social Cognition, 17*, 228–244.

Follette, V. M., Alexander, P. C., & Follette, W. (1991). Individual predictors of outcome in group treatment for incest survivors. *Journal of Consulting and Clinical Psychology, 59*, 150–155.

Follette, V. M., Polusny, M. A., Bechtle, A. E., & Naugle, A. E. (1996). Cumulative trauma: The impact of child sexual abuse, adult sexual assault, and spouse abuse. *Journal of Traumatic Stress, 9*, 25–35.

Fonagy, P., Leigh, T., Steele, M., Steele, H., Kennedy, R., Mattoon, G., Target, M., & Gerber, A. (1996). The relation of attachment status, psychiatric classification, and response to psychotherapy. *Journal of Consulting and Clinical Psychology, 64*, 22–31.

Fonagy, P., Target, M., & Gergely, G. (2000). Attachment and borderline personality disorder: A theory and some evidence. *Psychiatric Clinics of North America, 23*, 103–122.

Freedman, J. H., & Combs, G. (2000). Narrative therapy with couples. In L. J. Bevilacqua (Ed.), *Comparative treatments for relationships dysfunction* (pp. 342–361). New York: Springer.

Gittleman, M. G., Klein, M. H., Smider, N. A., & Essex, M. J. (1998). Recollections of parental behaviour, adult attachment and mental health: Mediating and moderating effects. *Psychological Medicine, 28*, 1443–1455.

Gladstone, G., Parker, G., Wilhelm, K., Mitchell, P., & Austin, M-P. (1999). Characteristics of depressed patients who report childhood sexual abuse. *American Journal of Psychiatry, 156*, 431–437.

Goodman, M. S., & Fallon, B. C. (1995). *Pattern changing for abused women: An educational program.* Thousand Oaks, CA: Sage.

Green, R.-J., & Werner, P. D. (1996). Intrusiveness and closeness-caregiving: Rethinking the concept of family "enmeshment." *Family Process, 35*, 115–136.

Harter, S. L. (2000). Quantitative measures of construing in child abuse survivors. *Journal of Constructivist Psychology, 13*, 103–116.

Harter, S. L., Alexander, P. C., & Neimeyer, R. A. (1988). Longterm effects of incestuous child abuse in college women: Social adjustment, social cognition, and family characteristics. *Journal of Consulting and Clinical Psychology, 56*, 5–8.

Hazan, C., & Shaver, P. (1987). Romantic love conceptualized as an attachment process. *Journal of Personality and Social Psychology, 52*, 511–524.

Heller, S. S., & Zeanah, C. H. (1999). Attachment disturbances in infants born subsequent to perinatal loss: A pilot study. *Infant Mental Health Journal, 20*, 188–199.

Herman, J. L. (1981). *Father–daughter incest.* Cambridge, MA: Harvard University Press.

Hertsgaard, L., Gunnar, M., Erickson, M. F., & Nachmias, M. (1995). Adrenocortical responses to the Strange Situation in infants with disorganized/disoriented attachment relationships. *Child Development, 66*, 1100–1106.

Hesse, E., & Main, M. (2000). Disorganized infant, child, and adult attachment: Collapse in behavioral and attentional strategies. *Journal of the American Psychoanalytic Association, 48*, 1097–1127.

Holtzworth-Munroe, A., Stuart, G. L., & Hutchinson, G. (1997). Violent versus nonviolent husbands: Differences in attachment patterns, dependency, and jealousy. *Journal of Family Psychology, 11*, 314–331.

Izard, C., & Kobak, R. (1991). Emotion system functioning and emotion regulation In J. Garber & K. Dodge (Eds.), *The development of affect regulation* (pp. 303–321). Cambridge, UK: Cambridge University Press.

Jacobvitz, D., & Hazen, N. (1999). Developmental pathways from infant disorganization to childhood peer relationships. In J. Solomon & C. George (Eds.), *Attachment disorganization* (pp. 127–159). New York: Guilford Press.

Jacobvitz, D., Hazen, N., & Riggs, S. (1997, April). Disorganized mental processes in mothers, frightening/frightened caregiving, and disoriented/disorganized behavior in infancy. In D. Jacobvitz (Chair), *Caregiving correlates and longitudinal outcomes of disorganized attachments in infants.* Symposium conducted at the biennial meeting of the Society for Research in Child Development, Washington, DC.

Johnson, S. M. (1996). *The practice of emotionally focused marital therapy: Creating connection.* New York: Brunner/Mazel.

Johnson, S. M. (2002). *Emotionally focused couple therapy with trauma survivors: Strengthening attachment bonds.* New York: Guilford Press.

Kemp, M. A., & Neimeyer, G. J. (1999). Interpersonal attachment: Experiencing, expressing, and coping with stress. *Journal of Counseling Psychology, 46*, 388–394.

Kessler, B. L., & Bieschke, K. J. (1999). A retrospective analysis of shame, dissociation, and adult victimization in survivors of childhood sexual abuse. *Journal of Counseling Psychology, 46*, 335–341.

Kobak, R., & Sceery, A. (1988). Attachment in late adolescence: Working models, affect regulation, and representations of self and others. *Child Development, 59*, 396–399.

Kochanska, G. (2001). Emotional development in children with different attachment histories: The first three years. *Child Development, 72*, 474–490.

Larose, S., & Bernier, A. (2001). Social support processes: Mediators of attachment state of mind and adjustment in late adolescence. *Attachment and Human Development, 3*, 96–120.

Liotti, G. (1992). Disorganized/disoriented attachment in the etiology of the dissociative disorders. *Dissociation, 5*, 196–204.

Liotti, G. (1999). Disorganization of attachment as a model for understanding dissociative psychopathology. In J. Solomon & C. George (Eds.), *Attachment disorganization* (pp. 291–317). New York: Guilford Press.

Loos, M. E., & Alexander, P. C. (2001). Dissociation and the processing of threat related information: An attachment-theoretical perspective on maintenance factors in dissociative pathology. *Maltrattamento e abuso all'infanzia, 3*, 61–83.

Lyons-Ruth, K. (1996). Attachment relationships among children with aggressive behavior problems: The role of disorganized early attachment patterns. *Journal of Consulting and Clinical Psychology, 64*, 64–73.

Lyons-Ruth, K., Alpern, L., & Repacholi, B. (1993). Disorganized infant attachment classification and maternal psychosocial problems as predictors of hostile-aggressive behavior in the preschool classroom. *Child Development, 64*, 572–585.

Lyons-Ruth, K., Bronfman, E., & Atwood, G. (1999). A relational diathesis model of hostile–helpless states of mind: Expressions in mother–infant interaction. In J. Solomon & C. George (Eds.), *Attachment disorganization* (pp. 33–70). New York: Guilford Press.

Lyons-Ruth, K., Easterbrooks, M. A., & Cibelli, C. D. (1997). Infant attachment strategies, infant mental lag, and maternal depressive symptoms: Predictors of internalizing and externalizing problems at age 7. *Developmental Psychology, 33*, 681–692.

Main, M. (1991). Metacognitive knowledge, metacognitive monitoring, and singular (coherent) vs. multiple (incoherent) models of attachment. In C. M. Parkes, J. Stevenson-Hinde, & P. Marris (Eds.), *Attachment across the life-cycle* (pp. 127–159). London: Routledge.

Main, M. (1995). Recent studies in attachment: Overview, with selected implications for clinical work. In S. Goldberg, R. Muir, & J. Kerr (Eds.), *Attachment theory: Social, developmental and clinical perspectives* (pp. 407–474). Hillsdale, NJ: Analytic Press.

Main. M. (2000). The organized categories of infant, child, and adult attachment: Flexible vs. inflexible attention under attachment-related stress. *Journal of the American Psychoanalytic Association, 48*, 1055–1096.

Main, M., & Cassidy, J. (1988). Categories of response to reunion with the parent at age 6: Predictable from infant attachment classifications and stable over a 1–month period. *Developmental Psychology, 24,* 415–426.

Main, M., & Goldwyn, R. (1998). *Adult attachment scoring and classification system.* Unpublished manuscript, Department of Psychology, University of California at Berkeley.

Main, M., & Hesse, E. (1990). Parents' unresolved traumatic experiences are related to infant disorganized attachment status: Is frightened and/or frightening parental behavior the linking mechanism? In M. T. Greenberg, D. Cicchetti, & E. M. Cummings (Eds.), *Attachment in the preschool years* (pp. 161–182). Chicago: University of Chicago Press.

Main, M., & Hesse, E. (1992). Disorganized/disoriented infant behavior in the Strange Situation, lapses in the monitoring of reasoning and discourse during the parent's Adult Attachment interview, and dissociative states. In M. Ammaniti & D. Stern (Eds.), *Attachment and psychoanalysis* (pp. 86–140). Rome: Gius, Laterza and Figli.

Main, M., & Solomon, J. (1990). Procedures for identifying infants as disorganized/disoriented during the Ainsworth Strange Situation. In M. T. Greenberg, D. Cicchetti, & E. M. Cummings (Eds.), *Attachment in the preschool years* (pp. 121–160). Chicago: University of Chicago Press.

Maltas, C., & Shay, J. (1995). Trauma contagion in partners of survivors of childhood sexual abuse. *American Journal of Orthopsychiatry, 65,* 529–539.

Marvin, R. S., & Stewart, R. B. (1990). A family systems framework for the study of attachment. In M. T. Greenberg, D. Cicchetti, & E. M. Cummings (Eds.), *Attachment in the preschool years: Theory, research, and intervention* (pp. 51–86). Chicago: University of Chicago Press.

Messman, T. L., & Long, P. J. (1996). Child sexual abuse and its relationship to revictimization in adult women: A review. *Clinical Psychology Review, 16,* 397–420.

Moran, G., & Pederson, D. R. (1998). Proneness to distress and ambivalent relationships. *Infant Behavior and Development, 21,* 493–503.

Moss, E., St.-Laurent, D., Rousseau, D., Parent, S., Gosselin, C., & Saintonge, J. (1999). L'attachement à l'âge scolaire et le développement des troubles de comportement. *Canadian Journal of Behavioural Science, 31,* 107–118.

Oates, R. K., Tebbutt, J., Swanston, H., Lynch, D. L., & O'Toole, B. I. (1998). Prior childhood sexual abuse in mothers of sexually abused children. *Child Abuse and Neglect, 22,* 1113–1118.

Ogawa, J. R., Sroufe, L. A., Weinfield, N. A., Carlson, E. A., & Egeland, B. (1997). Development and the fragmented self: Longitudinal study of dissociative symptomatology in a nonclinical sample. *Development and Psychopathology, 9,* 855–879.

Putnam, F. W., Carlson, E. B., Ross, C. A., Anderson, G., Clark, P., Torem, M., Bowman, E. S., Coons, P. M., Chu, J. A., Dill, D. L., Loewenstein, R. J., & Braun, B. G. (1996). Patterns of dissociation in clinical and nonclinical samples. *Journal of Nervous and Mental Disease, 184,* 673–679.

Schuengel, C., Bakermans-Kranenburg, M., & van IJzendoorn, M. (1999). Frightening maternal behavior linking unresolved loss and disorganized infant attachment. *Journal of Consulting and Clinical Psychology, 67,* 54–63.

Simoneti, S., Scott, E. C., & Murphy, C. M. (2000). Dissociative experiences in partner assaultive men. *Journal of Interpersonal Violence, 15,* 1262–1283.

Spangler, G., & Grossmann, K. E. (1993). Biobehavioral organization in securely and insecurely attached infants. *Child Development, 64,* 1439–1450.

Sroufe, L. A., & Fleeson, J. (1986). Attachment and the construction of relationships. In W. Hartup & Z. Rubin (Eds.), *Relationship and development* (pp. 51–71). Hillsdale, NJ: Erlbaum.

Sroufe, L. A., Jacobvitz, D., Mangelsdorf, S., DeAngelo, E., & Ward, M. J. (1985). Generational boundary dissolution between mothers and their preschool children: A relationships systems approach. *Child Development, 56,* 317–325.

Stalker, C. A., & Davies, F. (1995). Attachment organization and adaptation in sexually-abused women. *Canadian Journal of Psychiatry, 40,* 234–240.

Troy, M., & Sroufe, L. A. (1987). Victimization among preschoolers: Role of attachment relationship history. *Journal of the American Academy of Child Psychiatry, 26,* 166–172.

van IJzendoorn, M. (1995). Adult attachment representations, parental responsiveness, and infant attachment: A meta-analysis on the predictive utility of the Adult Attachment Interview. *Psychological Bulletin, 117,* 387–403.

van IJzendoorn, M. H., & Bakermans-Kranenburg, M. J. (1996). Attachment representations in mothers, fathers, adolescents, and clinical groups: A meta-analytic search for normative data. *Journal of Consulting and Clinical Psychology, 64,* 8–21.

van IJzendoorn, M., Schuengel, C., & Bakermans-Kranenburg, M. J. (1999). Disorganized attachment in early childhood: Meta-analysis of precursors, concomitants, and sequelae. *Development and Psychopathology, 11,* 225–249.

Waltz, J. (1994). The long-term effects of childhood sexual abuse on women's relationships with partners. *Dissertation Abstracts International: Section B: The Sciences and Engineering, 55*(2-B), 609.

Ward, M. J., & Carlson, E. A. (1995). Associations among adult attachment representations, maternal sensitivity, and infant–mother attachment in a sample of adolescent mothers. *Child Development, 66,* 69–79.

Wartner, U. G., Grossmann, K., Fremmer-Bombik, E., & Suess, G. (1994). Attachment patterns at age six in south Germany: Predictability from infancy and implications for preschool behavior. *Child Development, 65,* 1014–1027.

Waters, E., Merrick, S., Treboux, D., Crowell, J., & Albersheim, L. (2000). Attachment security in infancy and early adulthood: A twenty-year longitudinal study. *Child Development, 71,* 684–689.

Weiss, E. L., Longhurst, J. G., & Mazure, C. M. (1999). Childhood sexual abuse as a risk factor for depression in women: Psychosocial and neurobiological correlates. *American Journal of Psychiatry, 156,* 816–828.

Whiffen, V. E., Judd, M. E., & Aube, J. A. (1999). Intimate relationships moderate the association between childhood sexual abuse and depression. *Journal of Interpersonal Violence, 14,* 940–954.

White, M., & Epston, D. (1989). *Literate means to therapeutic ends.* Adelaide, SA, Australia: Dulwich Centre Publications.

Zeanah, C. H., & Zeanah, P. D. (1989). Intergenerational transmission of maltreatment: Insights from attachment theory and research. *Psychiatry, 52,* 177–196.

Zuravin, S. J., & DiBlasio, F. A. (1992). Child-neglecting adolescent mothers: How do they differ from their nonmaltreating counterparts? *Journal of Interpersonal Violence, 7,* 471–489.

18

Attachment and the Experience of Chronic Pain

A Couples Perspective

SAMUEL F. MIKAIL

The research on the relationship between attachment styles and adjustment to illness/disability is sparse. This is surprising considering the origins of attachment theory. Bowlby's early formulations on attachment theory emerged from observations of children subjected to prolonged separation from their parents as a result of hospitalization (see Ainsworth and Bowlby, 1991, for a review). In the 1940s Bowlby began to make systematic observations of hospitalized and institutionalized children. This work eventually led to the influential film, *A Two-Year-Old Goes to Hospital* (Robertson, 1952). The foundation of attachment theory was based on the juxtaposition of two critical experiences: separation from significant figures (attachment figures) and coping with illness.

The following chapter draws on the tenets of attachment theory to explore the experience of chronic pain as one form of ill health. Chronic pain is discussed as an interpersonal phenomenon that affects an individual as well as his or her social network. I begin with a definition of chronic pain and an overview of the way it has been understood. This is followed by a review of research that has examined the impact of chronic pain on dyadic and family adjustment. Attachment theory is briefly summarized in an effort to present an interpersonally based model of chronic pain and its emerging empirical support. A case description is interspersed throughout the discussion in order to elaborate the theoretical and empirical review and highlight treatment themes.[1]

THE NATURE OF CHRONIC PAIN

Chronic pain is pain that persists beyond the expected time of healing, with 3 months taken as the most convenient point of division between acute and chronic pain (International Association for the Study of Pain, Subcommittee on Taxonomy, 1986). Our initial understanding of pain was based on *specificity theory*, which proposed that a specific pain system was responsible for the transmission of pain signals. Pain intensity was considered to be directly proportional to the intensity of the stimulus or the degree of tissue injury (see Melzack & Wall, 1982, for a review). But specificity theory failed to account for much of the observed clinical phenomena. For example, in some instances relatively small degrees of tissue damage, or even an absence of tissue damage, led to intense and intractable pain. In other situations severe injury, such as that experienced by soldiers in battle, was accompanied by unexpectedly minimal complaints of pain (Beecher, 1946). Melzack and Wall (1965) proposed the *gate control theory* of pain in an attempt to reconcile clinical observation and contemporary knowledge of neurophysiology, neuroanatomy, and cognitive science. A critical feature of gate control theory was the proposition that there exists in the nervous system a mechanism referred to as the "central control trigger," or "gate," that activates and incorporates cognitive processes that exert control over sensory input. These processes include memory, past experience with pain, appraisal of contextual variables, and so on. Psychological theories of pain management have been based largely on this premise, and have proven essential in the treatment of chronic pain. The evolution of these theories paralleled the evolution of pain theories more generally. For example, the operant theories of pain were somewhat limited in their emphasis on reward, punishment, stimulus, and response. Cognitive behavioral theories expanded this focus considerably by stressing the importance of appraisal, core beliefs, and cognitive distortion. Most recently, biopsychosocial theories emphasize the integration of biological, intrapsychic, and interpersonal/social factors in the management of pain.

THE INTERPERSONAL IMPACT OF CHRONIC PAIN: MARITAL AND FAMILY FUNCTIONING

Chronic pain is associated with high levels of psychosocial impairment including depression (Sullivan, Reesor, Mikail, & Fisher, 1992), unemploy-

---

[1] All identifying data have been altered in order to protect the patient's privacy.

ment (Taylor & Curran, 1985), physical deconditioning and disability (Fordyce, 1990), and emotional maladjustment (Polatin, Kinney, Gatchel, Lillo, & Mayer, 1993). An extensive body of literature has also examined the interpersonal concomitants of chronic pain. In particular, numerous investigations have revealed that chronic pain negatively impacts marital and family functioning (Romano, Turner, & Jensen, 1997; Schwartz & Ehde, 2000).

Mohamad, Weisz, and Waring (1978) were among the first to examine the relationship between depression and the marital adjustment of chronic pain patients. They reported that depressed pain patients had a significantly higher prevalence of marital discord than depressed patients without pain. Similarly, chronic pain has been found to have a deleterious effect on the emotional and dyadic adjustment of partners of chronic pain patients (Flor, Turk, & Scholz, 1987).

The above findings led researchers and clinicians to begin viewing chronic pain as a systemic phenomenon that impacts the individual and his or her social system. Some investigators wondered if there was a temporal relationship between the onset and progression of chronic pain and marital distress. Using retrospective ratings of dyadic adjustment, Flor et al. (1987) found that as many as 66% of patients indicated that their relationships had been negatively affected by chronic pain.

Others investigations have identified specific dimensions of dyadic adjustment impacted by chronic pain. These have included decreased sexual functioning (Maruta, Osborne, Swanson, & Halling, 1981), decreased cohesion, and higher levels of interpersonal control (Romano et al., 1997). Romano et al. (1997) found spouse marital satisfaction to be negatively correlated with patient depression and the spouse's ratings of the patient's level of disability and pain behavior. Flor et al. (1987) found dyadic adjustment of patients to be related to patients' pain levels and physical dysfunction and spouses' levels of solicitousness. Other dimensions of the pain experience found to be associated with poor martial adjustment include pain chronicity (Block & Boyer, 1984), functional impairment (Ahern & Follick, 1985), and depression (Kerns & Turk, 1984).

A small body of literature points to possible gender differences in marital and family adjustment of chronic pain patients and their partners. Comparisons of women's and men's marital adjustment and mood have shown that women are negatively impacted by a partner's chronic pain to a greater extent than men (Romano, Turner, & Clancy, 1989).

Other investigators have extended this body of research by focusing on the broad construct of family functioning as rated by patients and their partners (Dura & Beck, 1988; Mikail & von Baeyer, 1990). Several studies found that chronic pain patients report decreased levels of family activity and recreation (Dura & Beck, 1988; Nicassio & Radojevic, 1993), increased family conflict (Romano et al., 1997; Feuerstein, Sult, & Houle,

1985), decreased family cohesion (Romano et al., 1997; Nicassio & Radojevic, 1993), and lower expressiveness (Romano et al., 1997; Mikail & von Baeyer, 1990).

Most of this research has been based either on an operant or on cognitive-behavioral models of pain. Within the operant tradition the clinical focus targets pain behavior, with no attention given to the patient's or the partner's subjective experience. Behavioral techniques are applied in an effort to extinguish illness behavior. For example, within the context of a dyadic relationship, pain behavior might be viewed as a means of avoiding certain responsibilities while seeking nurturance. Treatment would focus on increasing activity level by reinforcing efforts to assume more instrumental tasks. At the same time solicitous behavior in response to displays of pain would be extinguished.

The cognitive-behavioral perspective focuses on pain beliefs, perceptions, and cognitively based coping mechanisms. A patient's perception of spousal responses to pain, the spouse's beliefs about pain and illness, and the couple's associated behaviors become the targets of clinical intervention. For example, patients and partners would be taught that increased activity does not lead to further disability and injury.

ATTACHMENT THEORY AND ATTACHMENT STYLES: AN OVERVIEW

Attachment theory complements both models through its emphasis on the primacy of emotional attachment in understanding human adaptation and the role of relationship as a source of security. Bowlby (1988) defined *attachment behavior* as "any form of behavior that results in a person attaining or maintaining proximity to some other clearly defined individual who is conceived as better able to cope with the world. It is most obvious whenever a person is frightened, fatigued, or sick, and is assuaged by comforting and caregiving" (pp. 26–27). Bowlby's definition stresses the adaptive nature of attachment behavior. Attachment behaviors function to protect the organism and return the individual to a state of physical and psychological homeostasis. Johnson and Whiffen (1999) describe *attachment* as "a behavioral control system that has as its goal the maintenance of a safe, predictable environment so that physiological homeostasis is possible. . . . Contact with a supportive other . . . makes the individual less reactive to perceived stress" (p. 372). Bowlby emphasized that attachment behaviors are enduring and can be observed throughout the life cycle. He also specified that attachment behaviors emerge or are expressed whenever the individual is experiencing a sense of threat or distress. Individuals living with chronic pain often experience such distress on an ongoing basis.

Mikail, Henderson, and Tasca (1994) proposed a model of chronic pain syndrome based on the tenets of attachment theory. Research has established that pain arising out of biological alteration such as injury, degenerative processes, or disease evokes stress and impacts other areas of functioning such as sleep, appetite, concentration, and mood. Mikail et al. (1994) suggested that if pain persists, the resulting disruption in biological, emotional, and social homeostasis evokes a sense of threat and triggers attachment behaviors. Bowlby (1988) noted that the first stage in the initiation of attachment behavior is the appraisal of perceived threat. When pain persists, the appraisal process typically includes informing one's partner and eventually consulting appropriate health care professionals. However, research has demonstrated that considerable variability exists among individuals in their willingness to seek the support of partners and professionals. Within the proposed model these differences are conceptualized as reflecting features of individual attachment style and the associated internal working model. Specifically, the authors proposed that insecurely attached individuals delay seeking support and/or have partners who are unresponsive to their expressions of distress. An individual experiencing pain and having an insecure attachment style would respond by avoiding activity and guarding the affected site, thereby giving rise to a gradual and rapid process of physical deconditioning. A negative cycle ensues, with further deteriorations in physical, emotional, and interpersonal function; increased disability; and an erosion of intimate relationships. Within this model the progression of chronic pain is considered an interpersonal process involving the identified patient, the partner, and their respective social networks. Mikail et al. (1994) made specific predictions regarding ways in which individuals with specific attachment styles adjust to the onset of pain. These are outlined below following a brief description of attachment styles.

ATTACHMENT STYLES AND INTERNAL WORKING MODELS

Ainsworth (1979) was the first to distinguish specific attachment styles and their associated behaviors in children. She identified three styles of attachment that she termed "secure," "anxious–avoidant," and "anxious–resistant." Ainsworth's observations revealed that securely attached children responded to threat by seeking contact with their mothers in order to be comforted. Once comforted, these children resumed play and exploration. In contrast, when anxious–avoidant children experienced stress or separation from their mothers, they responded with hostility and/or avoided them. In fact, Bowlby (1988) noted that these children were friendlier with strangers than with their own mothers. Anxious–resistant children responded to heightened stress by vacillating between seeking proximity and contact with their mothers and rejecting them. These children exhibited either anger or passivity in interactions with their mothers.

Ainsworth proposed that attachment styles become stable and enduring by age 2. Research has demonstrated that adults exhibit similar patterns of attachment in the context of intimate relationships (Collins & Reed, 1990; Bartholomew & Horowitz, 1991). Bartholomew and Horowitz (1991) modified Ainsworth's categorization of attachment styles by partitioning the anxious–avoidant group into two distinct groups, which they termed *dismissing* and *fearful*. Their proposed system was derived from Bowlby's contention that attachment styles stem from two underlying dimensions: anxiety and avoidance. The anxiety dimension reflects the individual's sense of self-worth and beliefs about the extent to which the self is accepted or rejected by others. Avoidance refers to the individual's tolerance of intimacy and interdependence. In a recent investigation Collins and Feeney (2000) provided empirical support for these two dimensions and the ways in which they impact support seeking and caregiving among adult couples.

Griffin and Bartholomew (1994) emphasized that the four styles are prototypes, with most people exhibiting features of several styles. Contemporary writings on attachment posit that attachment styles "are linked more and more to specific relationships rather than being seen as global tendencies that are formed in childhood and then become self-reinforcing" (Johnson & Best, 2002). Increasingly, attachment styles are being seen as more malleable than originally thought.

Bartholomew and Horowitz (1991) suggested that secure individuals have a positive view of self and their intimate others. Within a relational context, they exhibit low levels of anxiety and avoidance and appear to be comfortable with intimacy and interdependence. Generally, their early relationships were characterized by exposure to caretakers who were empathically attuned to and responsive to their needs. Through such mirroring they learned to identify and express internal emotional states. Mikail et al. (1994) hypothesize that securely attached individuals experiencing pain can offer descriptions of their symptoms and concerns that aid clinicians in reaching an accurate diagnosis. This is an expression of the confidence they feel in the responsiveness of caretakers, be they intimate partners or health care professionals. At the same time they also posses the internal resources to self-soothe when distressed. Mikail et al. (1994) suggested that securely attached individuals are unlikely to delay seeking consultation when ill or in need of health care.

Preoccupied individuals harbor a negative view of self and a positive view of intimate partners (Griffin & Bartholomew, 1994). They display a high degree of anxiety and low levels of avoidance. Their anxiety is born out of a strong desire for closeness (i.e., low avoidance) coupled with a fear of rejection (i.e., a firm belief that the self is unacceptable). Preoccupied individuals have experienced attachment figures as inconsistent in their availability and responsiveness. Out of this relational history emerges a view of the self as unworthy of care. They vacillate between requesting the support of attachment figures and withdrawing out of fear of rejection. Mikail et al. proposed that preoccupied individuals are likely to exhibit high levels of distress, life disruption, and symptom reporting. Their interactions with partners would be characterized by ambivalent dependence and submissiveness. Consistent with these predictions, Pianta, Egeland, and Adam (1996) found that preoccupied individuals had the highest indices of psychiatric symptoms indicative of self-reported distress and relationship problems.

Dismissing individuals have a positive self-image and view others negatively (Griffin & Bartholomew, 1994). Overtly, they display low levels of attachment-related anxiety, yet they tend to avoid intimacy and interdependence. Their pattern of avoidance is built on an expectation that others cannot be relied on. Their positive self-concept is maintained by viewing others as being incapable of responding adequately to their expressed needs. Mikail et al. (1994) suggest that on the surface dismissing individuals with chronic pain might present in a manner that is similar to those classified as securely attached. The strong conviction that the self is worthy and valuable equips these individuals with the capacity to be aware of their instrumental needs, though perhaps not their emotional needs. However, a history of experiencing others as incapable or unresponsive results in a propensity to silence the expression of emotional vulnerability and to dismiss the possibility that their emotional needs would be recognized or taken seriously. Thus, this group of individuals is likely to underreport symptoms, downplay distress, and present as coping effectively. Their interactions with intimate partners is apt to be characterized by hostility and emotional detachment. Pianta et al. (1996) found that the MMPI-2 profiles of dismissing individuals were characterized by relatively little emotional distress. They reported a sense of independence and exhibited the lowest levels of self-reported anxiety.

Fearful individuals have a negative view of self and intimate others. They exhibit high levels of attachment anxiety and avoidance (Griffin & Bartholomew, 1994). Even though they desire close relationships, their avoidance of intimacy is driven by a fear of rejection and abandonment. Fearful individuals view themselves as unworthy of caring and concern and believe that they have little intrinsic value to others. Attachment figures are seen as unlikely to be available or interested, or alternatively as incapable of offering the needed help. This constellation of beliefs contributes to a chronic state of fear and anxiety. Their ongoing devaluing of themselves results in an inability to identify and recognize basic needs. Thus, in the face of distress, needs are likely to be experienced as unspecified, generalized anxiety. The expectation that attachment figures are unavailable and unresponsive further exacerbates this situation, resulting in a silencing of what vague concerns these individuals may be aware of. Mikail et al. (1994) predicted that fearfully attached individuals would report the highest levels of distress and life disruption. The authors argued that the tendency of these individuals to delay seeking help is apt to contribute to a more marked progression of disability.

Partial support for the model proposed by Mikail et al. was offered in a recent empirical investigation (McWilliams, Cox, & Enns, 2000). These investigators employed data from the National Comorbidity Survey and compiled a sample of 381 individuals diagnosed with arthritis or related conditions. They found that ratings of insecure attachment were positively correlated with pain intensity and level of disability. Furthermore, multiple regression analyses revealed that pain severity and ratings of anxious attachment accounted for over 20% of the variance in predictions of disability level.

A body of emerging evidence points to a relationship between attachment styles and health behaviors (Cooper, Shaver, & Collins, 1998; Feeney, 1995). Feeney and Ryan (1994) found that, in a sample of college students, those exhibiting an avoidant attachment style (i.e., Griffin and Bartholomew's [1994] dismissing attachment style) were the least likely to seek medical care in response to illness. Feeney (1995) found that subjective ratings of poor health were correlated with anxious–ambivalent attachment (Griffin and Bartholomew's [1994] preoccupied attachment style).

Further support for the model comes from investigations examining the relationship between attachment style and affect regulation. Simpson, Rholes, and Nelligan (1992) found that under conditions of heightened anxiety securely attached women had no difficulty seeking comfort and reassurance from their partners. In contrast, women classified as avoidant (dismissing or fearful attachment styles in Griffin and Bartholomew's [1994] system) responded to heightened anxiety through avoidance of their attachment figures. They became silent in the presence of an intimate partner when exposed to a stressor in the laboratory. Finally, women classified as preoccupied verbalized their anxiety more extensively than their secure or avoidant counterparts but were less calmed in response to their partners' supportive gestures

CHRONIC PAIN AS A TRIGGER FOR ATTACHMENT BEHAVIORS

Chronic pain patients tend to seek multiple consultations from a variety of traditional and nontraditional health care providers (Holzman & Turk, 1986). Their persistence in seeking an answer to an unresolved health condition can contribute to an escalation of frustration and fear for both patient and partner. Many of these patients live with uncertainty about their health and future. They report feeling physically and emotionally fatigued by their pain and by treading through a complex and often unsympathetic health care system. Emotional and financial strains contribute to a heightened sense of vulnerability. They fear that they have overwhelmed members of their support network and express guilt that they have not been equal partners in their relationships. At times the anger toward one's body and the pain is directed toward others, particularly the partner, with a firm belief that the partner is resentful and exasperated.

This is the emotional and interpersonal backdrop to the initial consultation. Many chronic pain patients experience a mix of resentment and magical hope when meeting a new clinician. In Bowlby's terms, the clinician "is conceived as better able to cope with the world" (Bowlby, 1988, p. 27), or at the very least the world of ill health. This context contains the essential components necessary for the expression of the patient's attachment behaviors. The individual is frightened, fatigued, and seeking the aid of someone who is viewed as more capable. The story of Joanna P., a patient assessed in a multidisciplinary pain clinic, is particularly instructive.

JOANNA P.:
PSYCHOLOGICAL CONSULTATION IN THE PAIN CLINIC

Joanna was a 40-year-old clerk. She reported low back, neck, and right leg pain that had begun 2 years prior to her marriage. At the time she was treated surgically and reported marked improvement, although she continued to experience mild intermittent pain. Her pain became much more severe and persistent following childbirth several years after the surgery. For the next 10 years Joanna was treated in a variety of ways that included bed rest, mild exercise, and several trials of physiotherapy. She reported that following one trial of physiotherapy she was unable to move and the pain became intractable. She was placed on long-term disability a few months following this incident.

Joanna was seen in a multidisciplinary pain clinic 4 years after being placed on disability. She reported that at times her pain was so severe that it caused her to forget what she had been doing. Joanne was physically deconditioned, depressed, and anxious. She was overweight and described herself as a compulsive overeater. Joanna was reluctant to attend social events due to the unpredictability of her pain. She feared that her pain had negatively impacted her teenage daughter, who was unsure about how to respond to her mother's disability and had expressed considerable disappointment with her mother's unavailability and reluctance to engage in various family activities. Psychometric testing revealed that Joanna was interpersonally distressed—she felt an absence of support in her relationships and her marital adjustment was low. Specifically, she noted that there was little affection expressed between her and her husband. The couple frequently disagreed, and Joanna felt as if she was letting her husband down because of her inability to contribute financially or to maintain their home as she once had done. With considerable frustration and sadness Joanna said that prior to the onset of her pain she kept her house spotless, usually mopping the floors and vacuuming daily. Joanna was quite angry and self-critical due to her inability to maintain this standard of cleanliness.

ATTACHMENT STYLES AND INTERPERSONAL BEHAVIOR

Mikail et al. (1994) hypothesized that each adult attachment style would be associated with a characteristic relational or interpersonal pattern. In a pilot study aimed at identifying these patterns Mikail and Frank (1996) asked 86 individuals attending a chronic pain assessment clinic to complete a measure of adult attachment style (Relationship Questionnaire; Bartholomew & Horowitz, 1991) and the Inventory of Interpersonal Problems (IIP), a measure that classifies difficulties reported by respondents along the interpersonal circumplex (Horowitz, Rosenberg, Baer, Ureno, & Vallasenor, 1988; Alden, Wiggins, & Pincus, 1990). Results revealed that individuals falling into each of the attachment groups reported a unique set of interpersonal problems and associated patterns of engagement. Specifically, chronic pain patients classified as dismissing reported a pattern of interpersonal difficulties reflecting an autocratic and attacking relational stance (Mikail & Frank, 1996). From the perspective of interpersonal theory, these individuals fell within the dominant-hostile octant of the interpersonal circumplex (see Kiesler, 1996, for a detailed description of the circumplex). Kiesler (1996) pointed out that hostile responses evoke hostility in others. Mikail and Frank (1996) note that within a clinical context the hostility of this patient group may lead others to view them as uncooperative and attacking. Extrapolating from their findings, they suggest that the marriages of dismissing individuals are apt to be characterized by the type of negative affectivity associated with high degrees of marital distress, namely, contemptuous, critical, and detached engagement (Gottman, 1994). This style of engagement and its associated responses confirms these patients' expectations that caretakers will remain unavailable.

The IIP profile of preoccupied individuals emerged as subassertive and expressive (Mikail & Frank, 1996). Interpersonally, these patients appeared friendly and submissive, an interpersonal posture that "pulls" for others to take charge. Preoccupied individuals are adept at expressing their distress and making known their needs. Therefore these patients have a high likelihood of being referred for further treatment following initial evaluation. However, preoccupied individuals are apt to have an ambivalent attitude toward treatment. This stems from a negative self-concept coupled with a limited sense of self-efficacy. On the one hand, these individuals have a desire to please the clinician in order to gain approval and affirmation. On the other hand, they feel that they are unworthy of attention. One of the primary means by which they protect themselves from the pain of rejection or criticism is to retreat within relationships prior to being hurt emotionally. This ambivalence can evoke within the clinician a feeling of frustration and a desire to disengage. If this response is indeed forthcoming, these patients conclude that they do not deserve the care of others.

Fearfully attached individuals demonstrated a pattern of interpersonal behaviors characterized by a subassertive, introverted, and exploitable stance (Mikail & Frank, 1996). They assumed a position of rigid submissiveness. Kiesler (1996) suggests that this interpersonal posture will "pull" for others to be dominant and in control. Our data suggested that they were interpersonally distressed, reported high levels of pain severity, and exhibited elevations on measures of depressive symptoms. Within the rehabilitation context such a presentation is likely to lead to recommendations for psychopharmacological treatments—a treatment approach that is consistent with the belief held by fearful individuals regarding the nonresponsiveness of caretakers. The case of Joanna is consistent with a number of these findings.

Joanna exhibited a fearful attachment style. Psychometric testing revealed her level of disability and pain intensity to be more than one standard deviation above the mean compared to other patients with chronic pain. Over the course of her condition, she repeatedly delayed seeking treatment because she expected health care professionals to be unresponsive. Joanna was unable to work and felt ineffective as a partner and as a mother. She reported receiving minimal support from her family and felt that she was a disappointment to them. She vacillated between guilt and anger in her primary relationships. During the initial assessment and throughout the early stage of treatment she remained guarded and skeptical.

Joanna felt that she had little worth and viewed herself as a burden to her family and friends. Her inability to return to work or to maintain the household in the manner that she had been accustomed to made her feel unworthy of her husband's respect or love. She firmly believed that if she suddenly left her home her husband and daughter would not miss her. Feelings of low self-worth, coupled with a near constant anger toward her husband, neutralized her sexual desire. On the rare occasions that Joanna's husband approached her sexually she rebuffed him, and the anger and distance between the two escalated. Both Joanna and her husband felt deeply hurt and isolated. Her husband sought refuge in his relationship with his daughter. He would take her out to various sporting events or the movies—the unpredictability and intensity of Joanna's back pain made it difficult for her to engage in such activities. She became jealous of their relationship and felt inadequate as a mother.

Joanna discharged her anger by pushing herself physically to do more housework or to complete projects at home. Invariably, this led to an exacerbation of pain that necessitated days of bed rest and physical withdrawal.

This cycle was repeated countless times and served to deepen Joanna's feelings of inadequacy and hopelessness. The persistence of her pain made her feel that health care professionals had failed her. She was caught between desperately wanting help, yet expecting to be disappointed by others. She viewed herself as a "screwed-up person" who is likely to fail and burden those around her. As treatment unfolded, it became evident that these beliefs reflected the ways in which Joanna had been treated as a child.

The initial assessment was challenging; Joanna's anxiety, distress, anger, and hostility were palpable. Her description of her distress was understated because she feared that her concerns would be either dismissed or pathologized. Her defensive self-reliance and stoicism led several clinicians to underestimate the urgency of her clinical needs, thereby confirming her belief that caregivers are indifferent and unresponsive. Her expectation that her concerns would be pathologized was quite realistic. In several instances health care professionals who tried to offer assistance were met with hostility, agitation, and Joanna's exceedingly high standards. Unfortunately, this interpersonal stance was "louder" than her need for help. She was referred to the psychologist and offered nothing in the way of rehabilitation.

THE TREATMENT PROCESS

Chronic pain is a complex condition that impacts all aspects of the individual's functioning. Effective treatment requires a multidisciplinary approach that includes physiotherapy, occupational therapy, medicine, and psychology. Typically, physiotherapy targets physical deconditioning, chronic muscle tension, and compromised physical endurance. Occupational therapy focuses on work hardening, energy conservation, and teaching strategies for pacing activity level. Medical management addresses medication dependence or the inappropriate use of multiple medications, and may also involve use of antidepressants and/or time-limited use of narcotics or anti-inflammatories. Psychological treatment typically begins with cognitive-behavioral group therapy. Emphasis is placed on teaching various pain management strategies, including relaxation; proper sleep hygiene; reinforcing the importance of pacing, planning, and prioritizing; addressing the impact of cognitive distortions and catastrophizing; and so on. In many instances, individuals experiencing chronic pain are unable to return to previous forms and/or levels of employment. This has a profound impact on the individual's sense of identity. Psychological treatment may include a component that addresses changes in one's sense of self and the associated life adjustment. A detailed description of these various treatment modalities is beyond the scope of this chapter. For excellent summaries the interested reader is referred to Turk, Meichenbaum, and Genest (1983) and Holzman and Turk (1986).

Couple therapy is an important component of treatment and can vary slightly in focus and approach depending on the gender of the identified patient.[2] Many pain clinics require patients and partners to attend the initial assessment together in order to identify issues that are impacting the relationship. At the same time the couple can be given valuable information regarding the nature of chronic pain and the rehabilitation process. Frequently, couples harbor a false hope that the pain will resolve entirely. One of the most valuable outcomes of the assessment is in helping couples understand that although chronic pain persists indefinitely it does not signal the presence of active organic pathology. Many patients fear a worsening of their condition that may ultimately necessitate the use of a wheelchair. Couples can be reassured that they can continue to lead active and productive lives.

It is at this point that clinicians can address the ways in which chronic pain impacts a couple's relationship. For example, the profound fatigue associated with chronic sleep disturbance contributes to marked alterations in mood and decreased libido. Decreased physical endurance and deconditioning are associated with significant reductions in activity level, including paid employment, household chores, and childcare. Depression, anxiety, or symptoms of posttraumatic stress lead to social withdrawal and a reluctance to engage in recreational activities.

At the end of assessment a comprehensive and progressive treatment is outlined for the couple. The various components of treatment are described and the partner is asked to attend several "family" sessions that are part of a pain management group. Pain management groups combine cognitive behavioral and psychoeducational interventions and focus on many of the above themes. Group discussion is encouraged as a means of creating a sense of universality, with shared experiences being highlighted in order to normalize partners' experiences.

Joanna was offered individual therapy following her involvement in the pain management group. It was evident that she was still in a great deal of distress and that further intervention was needed. Her interpersonal or attachment history was explored in greater detail and she was asked to write a brief autobiographical sketch. The following is an excerpt from her story.

> "When I was born I was my mother's fifth child and my father's first. My parents weren't married at the time, and for some reason I was given my mother's first husband's name. I only learned this when I was 17 and I wanted to obtain a copy of my birth certificate. I still recall the utter

---

[2]A discussion of these gender differences is beyond the scope of this chapter. Here the discussion has been limited to issues and themes common to both male and female patients.

confusion and shock that I felt. All of a sudden I felt unsure as to who my real father was. I rushed home and spoke to my older sister, who told me that when I was brought home from the hospital after my birth she didn't know which father I belonged to. My mother's explanation of this was confused. She was reluctant to discuss it and was rather dismissive. I was filled with anger. The fact that my parents didn't bother to straighten these papers out made me feel that my identity wasn't important to them. . . .

". . . Throughout my childhood my mother worked outside the home. She often worked evening and night shifts and I recall being afraid whenever she wasn't there at night. I felt that it wasn't safe to be in the house without her. I would be angry with her for this but I never said anything because I knew that I would either be ridiculed or punished for complaining. My mother's moods were very unpredictable; I never knew when she would fly off the handle next and beat me for something I did or didn't do. I put a lot of my energy into trying to be good in order to avoid her anger, but it didn't seem to matter. My grandparents lived downstairs from us. I remember them as being very caring and kind. I envied my older brother who lived with them. I wasn't allowed to have much of a relationship with them because my father wouldn't permit it. He didn't want me having any private conversations with them or visiting them and he always badmouthed them. . . .

". . . One of my first memories is from about age 2. I remember being in the crib and shouting to get out, but nobody came and I don't know what I was yelling and crying about. When I was older I recall hiding in the bathroom at home, especially when mom was working, but I'm not sure why."

Initially Joanna was very cautious and mistrustful, making it a challenge to establish a therapeutic alliance. Her autobiographical account reflected an attachment history characterized by parental neglect and abuse. Treatment began with a focus on symptom relief and an acknowledgment of the legitimacy of Joanna's pain complaints. The psychologist worked closely with the physiotherapist in an effort to address and accommodate Joanna's fear of touch. Members of the treatment team were attentive to the importance of stability and consistency of contact. For example, changes to scheduled appointments were avoided if at all possible and a treatment routine was established and adhered to. She was given a rationale for the various recommendations and interventions. The psychologist and the occupational therapist collaborated on addressing Joanna's unrealistically high expectations regarding the management of household chores. This was a laborious process in which the occupational therapist focused on teaching Joanna various pacing and energy conservation strategies, while the psychologist addressed themes of self-worth and the associated cognitive distortions. Joanna tried to compensate for feeling broken by spending more time on manageable tasks such as light housekeeping. Gradually, these activities took precedence over her relationships, and although this lessened her feelings of inadequacy temporarily, Joanna's inability to work with her previous vigor fed her self-criticism and perpetuated a vicious cycle.

Following individual treatment, Joanna was referred to a process-oriented psychotherapy group comprised of individuals with various physical disabilities. The objectives were to lessen her isolation and to offer interpersonal support. The group members challenged her avoidance of intimacy and her fear of relationships. Other members affirmed her resilience and strength and offered feedback that stood in stark contrast to her silent self-derogation and negative self-concept. During this time Joanna's mother became ill and died. Joanna struggled with her ambivalence toward her mother and the group facilitated her efforts to come to terms with what her mother had failed to offer her. This was a critical juncture in her treatment. The group's support and empathy initiated a shift in Joanna's expectation that others will fail to respond to her emotional needs.

Following the death of her mother Joanna revealed to the psychologist that her father had sexually abused her during childhood and requested that she be seen in individual therapy. Her willingness to share this aspect of her past reflected her evolving trust in the responsiveness of others. This phase of treatment lasted approximately 2 years. During this time Joanna's negative self-concept and fear of abandonment were often the focus of treatment. Much of the work addressed Joanna's profound feelings of shame and self-loathing. Like many people with a history of sexual abuse, Joanna felt disgusting and inherently damaged. She vacillated between intense anger and profound grief. She struggled to make sense of the expressions of tenderness that she had encountered in her relationships with members of the psychotherapy group. It was during this phase of treatment that the work began to assume a greater focus on couple's issues. The work revolved around two persistent themes: (1) "If I get close to someone I will be exploited," and (2) "I don't trust myself or others to maintain appropriate personal boundaries in relationships, so in any close relationship I will surely lose myself." Interventions focused on underscoring her ability to voice her needs in ways that would not compromise her boundaries. Joanna felt intense pain in response to her growing awareness of her emotional needs. Her husband, John, was invited to attend sessions.

The work was aimed at heightening the couple's awareness of their interactional and communication patterns. Specifically, Joanna either minimized her needs in a manner that left John feeling superfluous to her life or expressed an intensity of anger and frustration that rendered him helpless and ineffective. John exhibited features of a dismissive attachment style, a pattern of engagement that readily confirmed Joanna's view that others either abandon or ignore her. He appeared self-assured, confident, and emotionally self-sufficient. He was large and strong-looking.

Joanna's physical limitations and fear of emotional intimacy reinforced John's conviction that he should rely on no one. Couple therapy centered on challenging these beliefs and the manner in which they were manifested in the relationship. A number of tasks were critical to this phase of treatment. For example, John interpreted Joanna's anger as reflecting her criticism and disapproval of him. He responded either defensively or by counterattacking. The near-constant affective tone of hostility between the couple softened significantly when Joanna was able to say, "I'm angry about this pain and I'm angry with myself. I can't do the same things that I used to do for you and Jesse [the daughter] and I just feel useless to both of you. I'm afraid that at some point you'll just get tired of me and leave. I don't know why you've stayed even this long." John's eyes filled with tears when he became aware of Joanna's fear of abandonment. The therapist expended considerable energy helping John understand that Joanna's anger reflected her loneliness and the hurt that came from the belief that she was no longer valued. Joanna's longing for a deeper intimacy with John challenged his deep mistrust of others. At the outset of couple therapy John was reserved and emotionally constricted. Gradually, however, he began to express long-held resentment in response to Joanna's prepain competence and perfectionism. At one point he said, "For all these years you've always had your own life—working, cleaning, insisting that everything was perfect. Cleaning the toilet came before me. Even now with all this pain you complain of, I still come home and you're down on your knees scrubbing floors. I always felt that you had no room for me, so I relied on myself and be damned if I was going to ask for anything."

A great deal of repetition and "translation" by the therapist was needed before Joanna and John were able to hear each other differently. Interventions were aimed primarily at disarming the ways in which both partners defended themselves against their fear of abandonment. Gradually, they took greater risks in expressing their needs to each other. Joanna's need to justify her worth through tangible accomplishments lessened as John became more emotionally expressive. She became less driven by unrealistic expectations regarding housekeeping and employment. She told John about her history of sexual abuse. John became more tolerant of Joanna's need for a physical boundary and his sexual approaches became less aggressive. Joanna's pain and the limitations it imposed on the couple's life became less of a focus and the lifestyle adjustments that each had to make were made with less resentment and anger.

The termination phase of treatment evoked irritability and agitation in Joanna. She regressed to feeling useless and worthless and there was a brief reemergence of her perfectionism. Her affective response was interpreted as a reaction to separation and loss. This interpretation gave Joanna permission to voice feelings of grief, which she shared with John. At times Joanna had the impulse to run away rather than work through the termination. That was how she had dealt with previous departures. In closing, she noted that what had been most sacred to her in treatment was feeling cared about while discovering that there had been no ulterior motive.

CONCLUSIONS

Joanna is relatively representative of patients seen in rehabilitation facilities. She was recently contacted (i.e., 5 years posttreatment) in order to obtain consent to use this material. She was still married to John and feeling at peace in the relationship. Joanna reported that she was doing well despite the pain and that she was working several days a week as a volunteer in a local food bank. She noted that she and John have derived a deep sense of meaning from their role as grandparents.

Joanna was fortunate to be treated at a time when there was considerable latitude in how treatment was delivered. Her treatment extended on and off for a period of 4 years. Today's health care climate emphasizes short-term interventions. Most chronic pain patients are likely to be treated with a trial of physiotherapy and placed in an 8- to 12-week pain management group. A brief course of individual psychotherapy may be introduced if there is evidence of posttraumatic stress disorder. The patient is likely to be referred to a private practitioner if a history of abuse and/or significant marital issues are uncovered. Yet Joanna's case illustrates the importance of employing a coordinated multidisciplinary approach to treatment. In the early stages of treatment, it was essential that the psychologist work with other members of the team in addressing Joanna's fear of pain and touch. Similarly, the occupational therapist's efforts to teach Joanna various energy conservation and pacing strategies were instrumental in addressing Joanna's rigid perfectionism and her intense need for control. These were essential components of an integrated treatment plan. The responsiveness of group members when Joanna's mother was dying was critical. Joanna's core beliefs and expectations of relationships were challenged by their gestures of caring. But perhaps the key shift in treatment came when Joanna and John could hear each other's fear of abandonment and could come together in a corrective emotional experience to comfort and care for each other.

Joanna's experience is a reminder that the people we treat live in a complex interpersonal environment that is profoundly shaped by early and ongoing attachments. In order for interventions to be effective, an individual's relational context has to be honored and addressed. Joanna's ability to adapt to and manage her pain was enhanced as she became more securely attached to John. This secure attachment allowed her to ask that her emotional needs be met, thereby creating a secure base from which she could continue to adapt to a condition that was often unpredictable.

REFERENCES

Ahern, D. K., & Follick, M. J. (1985). Distress in spouses of chronic pain patients. *International Journal of Family Therapy, 7*, 247–257.

Ainsworth, M. S. (1979). Attachment as related to mother–child interaction. In J. S. Rosenblatt, R. A. Hinde, C. Beer, & M. Busnel (Eds.), *Advances in the study of behavior* (Vol. 9, pp. 1–51). San Diego: Academic Press.

Ainsworth, M. S., & Bowlby, J. (1991). An ethological approach to personality. *American Psychologist, 46*, 333–334.

Alden, L. E., Wiggins, J. S., & Pincus, A. L. (1990). Construction of circumplex scales for the Inventory of Interpersonal Problems. *Journal of Personality Assessment, 55*, 521–536.

Bartholomew, K., & Horowitz, L. M. (1991). Attachment styles among young adults: A test of a four-category model. *Journal of Personality and Social Psychology, 61*, 226–244.

Beecher, H. K. (1946). Pain in men wounded in battle. *Annals of Surgery, 123*, 96–105.

Block, A. R., & Boyer, S. L. (1984). The spouse's adjustment to chronic pain: Cognitive and emotional factors. *Social Science and Medicine, 19*(12), 1313–1317.

Bowlby, J. (1988). *A secure base: Parent–child attachment and healthy human development.* New York: Basic Books.

Collins, N. L., & Feeney, B. C. (2000). A safe haven: An attachment theory perspective on support seeking and caregiving in intimate relationships. *Journal of Personality and Social Psychology, 78*, 1053–1073.

Collins, N. L., & Reed, S. J. (1990). Adult attachment, working models, and relationship quality in dating couples. *Journal of Personality and Social Psychology, 58*, 644–663.

Cooper, M. L., Shaver, P. R., & Collins, N. L. (1998). Attachment style, emotional regulation, and adjustment in adolescence. *Journal of Personality and Social Psychology, 74*, 1380–1397.

Dura, J. R., & Beck, S. R. (1988). A comparison of family functioning when mothers have chronic pain. *Pain, 35*, 79–90.

Feeney, J. (1995). Adult attachment, coping style and health locus of control as predictors of health and behaviour. *Australian Journal of Psychology, 47*, 171–177.

Feeney, J., & Ryan, S. (1994). Attachment style and affect regulation: Relationships with health behaviour and family experiences of illness in a student sample. *Health Psychology, 13*, 334–345.

Flor, H., Turk, D. C., & Scholz, O. B. (1987). Impact of chronic pain on the spouse: Marital, emotional and physical consequences. *Journal of Psychosomatic Research, 31*, 63–71.

Fordyce, W. E. (1990). Learned pain: Pain as behavior. In J. J. Bonica (Ed.), *The management of pain* (2nd ed., Vol. 1, pp. 291–299). Philadelphia: Lea & Febiger.

Feuerstein, M., Sult, S., & Houle, M. (1985). Environmental stressors and chronic low back pain: Life events, family and work environment. *Pain, 22,* 296–307.

Gottman, J. M. (1994). An agenda for marital therapy. In S. M. Johnson & L. S. Greenberg (Eds.), *The heart of the matter: Perspectives on emotion in marital therapy* (pp. 256–293). New York: Brunner/Mazel.

Griffin, D. W., & Bartholomew, K. (1994). Models of the self and other: Fundamental dimensions underlying measures of adult attachment. *Journal of Personality and Social Psychology, 67,* 430–445.

Holzman, A. D., & Turk, D. C. (1986). *Pain management: A handbook of psychological treatment approaches.* New York: Pergamon Press.

Horowitz, L. M., Rosenberg, S. E., Baer, B. A., Ureno, G., & Villasenor, V. S. (1988). Inventory of interpersonal problems: Psychometric properties and clinical applications. *Journal of Consulting and Clinical Psychology, 56,* 885–892.

International Association for the Study of Pain, Subcommitte on Taxonomy. (1986). Classification of chronic pain: Descriptions of chronic pain syndromes and definitions of pain terms. *Pain,* (Suppl. 3), S1–S225.

Johnson, S. M., & Best, M. (2002). A systemic approach to restructuring adult attachment: The EFT model of couples therapy. In P. Erdman & T. Caffery (Eds.), *Attachment and family systems* (pp. 165–192). New York: Brunner/Routledge.

Johnson, S. M., & Whiffen, V. E. (1999). Made to measure: Adapting emotionally focused couples therapy to partners' attachment styles. *Clinical Psychology: Science and Practice, 64,* 366–381.

Kerns, R., & Turk, D. (1984). Depression and chronic pain: The mediating role of the spouse. *Journal of Marriage and the Family, 46,* 845–852.

Kiesler, D. J. (1996). *Contemporary interpersonal theory and research: Personality, psychopathology and psychotherapy.* New York: Wiley.

Maruta, T., Osborne, D., Swanson, D. W., & Halling, J. A. (1981). Chronic pain patients and spouses: Marital and sexual adjustment. *Mayo Clinic Proceedings, 56,* 307–310.

McWillians, L. A., Cox, B. J., & Enns, M. (2000). Impact of adult attachment styles on pain and disability associated with arthritis in a nationally representative sample. *Clinical Journal of Pain, 16,* 360–364.

Melzack, R., & Wall, P. (1965). Pain mechanisms: A new theory. *Science, 150,* 971–979.

Melzack, R., & Wall, P. (1982). *The challenge of pain.* New York: Penguin Books.

Mikail, S. F., & Frank, J. (1996). Communication with chronic pain patients: A perspective based on attachment and interpersonal theory. In *Communication with pain patients.* Symposium, presented to the Eighth World Congress on Pain, Vancouver, BC, Canada.

Mikail, S. F., Henderson, P. R., & Tasca, G. A. (1994). An interpersonally based model of chronic pain: An application of attachment theory. *Clinical Psychology Review, 14,* 1–16.

Mikail, S. F., & von Baeyer, C. L. (1990). The effects of parental chronic pain on children's adjustment. *Social Science and Medicine, 31,* 51–59.

Mohamad, S. N., Weisz, G. M., & Waring, E. M. (1978). The relationship of chronic pain to depression, marital adjustment and family dynamics. *Pain, 5,* 285–292.

Nicassio, P. M., & Radojevic, V. (1993). Models of family functioning and their contribution to patient outcomes in chronic pain. *Motivation and Emotion, 17,* 295–316.

Pianta, R. C., Egeland, B., & Adam, E. K. (1996). Adult attachment classification and self-reported psychiatric symptomatology as assessed by the Minnesota Multiphasic Personality Inventory–2. *Journal of Consulting and Clinical Psychology, 64,* 273–281.

Polatin, P. B., Kiney, R. K., Gatchel, R. J., Lillo, E., & Mayer, T. G. (1993). Psychiatric illness and chronic low back pain. *Spine, 18,* 66–71.

Robertson, J. (1952). *A two-year-old goes to hospital* [Film]. New York: New York University Film Library.

Romano, J. M., Turner, J. A., & Clancy, S. L. (1989). Gender differences in the relationship of pain patient dysfunction to spouse adjustment. *Pain, 39,* 289–295.

Romano, J. M., Turner, J. A., & Jensen, M. P. (1997). The family environment in chronic pain patients: Comparison to controls and relationship to patient functioning. *Journal of Clinical Psychology in Medical Settings, 4,* 383–395.

Schwartz, L., & Ehde, D. M. (2000). Couples and chronic pain. In K. B. Schmaling & T. G. Sher (Eds.), *The psychology of couples and illness: Theory, research and practice* (pp. 191–216). Washington, DC: American Psychological Association.

Simpson, J. A., Rholes, W. S., & Nelligan, J. A. (1992). Support seeking and support giving within couples in anxiety-provoking situations: The role of attachment styles. *Journal of Personality and Social Psychology, 62,* 434–446.

Sullivan, M. J. L., Reesor, K., Mikail, S., & Fisher, R. (1992). The treatment of depression in chronic low back pain: Review and recommendations. *Pain, 50,* 5–14.

Taylor, J., & Curran, N. (1985). *The Nurpirn pain report.* New York: Harris & Associates.

Turk, D. C., Meichenbaum, D., & Genest, M. (1983). *Pain and behavioral medicine: A cognitive-behavioral perspective.* New York: Guilford Press.

Turner, J. A., & Romano, J. M. (1984). Self-report screening measures for depression in chronic pain patients. *Journal of Clinical Psychology, 40,* 909–913.

PART V

CONCLUSION

19

What Attachment Theory
Can Offer Marital
and Family Therapists

VALERIE E. WHIFFEN

John Bowlby believed that attachment theory has the potential to make enormous contributions to the understanding and treatment of emotional distress. He was a man of vision and it has taken us a long time to fulfill his prediction. More than 30 years after the publication of his three volumes on attachment and after Mary Ainsworth's seminal work on mother–infant attachment, we are just beginning to apply attachment theory to the understanding and treatment of clinical problems. In this book, we have brought together the researchers and clinicians who are at the forefront of this development. They have described the application of attachment theory to family and couple systems, and to problems like conduct disorder and postpartum depression, which normally are considered manifestations of individual psychopathology. However, the field is nascent. There is little consensus on terminology; some topics have been extensively researched while others remain the domain of clinical practitioners. This concluding chapter has two basic goals. The first is to find the commonalities in the diversity of opinion represented, in order to answer basic questions of interest to clinicians. What causes insecure attachment? How do we change attachment insecurity? The second goal is to identify the missing links. What areas of clinical practice would benefit from further exploration from an attachment theory perspective? What unanswered questions do we need to keep in mind as this field develops?

WHAT CAUSES INSECURE ATTACHMENT?

The authors who contributed to this volume assume that many of the issues and symptoms that bring clients into our offices reflect the fundamental problem of attachment insecurity. Insecurity disrupts key relationships and creates emotional distress and psychopathology for the insecurely attached individual. If attachment insecurity is at the heart of the problems our clients bring to us, then to change it we first must understand how it develops.

There is convergence across several of the chapters in this volume that insecure attachment develops when an attachment figure repeatedly is emotionally unavailable. Attachment figures can be unavailable for a variety of reasons, each having different implications for change. First, attachment figures can be unavailable because they are insecurely attached themselves, specifically because they are avoidant of closeness in their relationships (*fearful* and *dismissing* strategies). Individuals who are avoidant of closeness feel uncomfortable being intimate with others and they are unsettled by vulnerable feelings, both their own and those of other people. Often these are people whose own attachment histories have been plagued by insecurity. As we know from Main's seminal work with mothers and infants (Main, Kaplan, & Cassidy, 1985), the failure to come to terms with one's own attachment history and to understand its impact on one's relationships interferes with the ability to become an effective attachment figure for one's spouse and children.

Susan M. Johnson, in Chapter 1, and Dory A. Schachner, Phillip R. Shaver, and Mario Mikulincer, in Chapter 2, point out that avoidant individuals tend to withdraw precisely when the people for whom they are attachment figures need them most. Thus, the avoidant parent is one who pushes away a distressed child, telling him to stop crying and control himself. Similarly, the avoidant spouse is one who looks away or seems bored when his wife cries in a therapy session. As Johnson observes, unavailability at critical moments has the potential to create an *attachment injury*. Guy S. Diamond and Richard S. Stern, in Chapter 10, identify a similar construct in the attachment histories of the depressed adolescents they treat, which they label a *family trauma*. Attachment injuries are powerful and enduring wounds that can profoundly influence the course of the relationship and interfere with the process of repair. They are concrete examples of the attachment figure's unavailability and are presumed to reflect his or her lack of care for the injured person. Unavailability at moments of intense need conveys the message that neediness and vulnerability are shameful and embarrassing emotions, which should not be articulated or acted upon, a message that also is likely to foster avoidance of closeness in its recipient.

In Chapter 6, Susan M. Johnson observes that feelings of anxiety and hopelessness typically underlie the unavailability of avoidant individuals. Unavailable attachment figures may feel anxious about their capacity to soothe and reassure, or they may have given up providing reassurance to a spouse or child who seems unable to benefit from their efforts. Reframing unavailability in terms of the unavailable person's anxiety can be a powerful intervention, both for the avoidant individual and for the one seeking comfort and reassurance. When one individual is unavailable, the other tends to believe that this unavailability reflects a fundamental lack of love and care. Reframing unavailability in terms of the attachment figure's *own* vulnerabilities enables the partner to avoid depression-inducing inferences about the causes of the unavailability, for instance, that she or he is unworthy of love and nurturance or that the attachment figure doesn't care.

Johnson goes on to state that longing underlies the interpersonal behavior of reassurance-seeking individuals. The authenticity and intensity of this longing can lead therapists to sympathize with reassurance-seeking individuals because we see them as being in touch with and articulate about their attachment needs. However, this perception can be misleading because, in distressed relationships, individuals who are seeking comfort and reassurance often do so in ways that exacerbate their attachment figures' unavailability. For instance, in working with maritally distressed couples, reassurance-seeker partners or pursuers in pursue–withdraw couples tend to be emotionally unavailable as attachment figures because they tend to express their longing for connection though blame, criticism, and invalidating the experience of their partners. When their partners make attempts to be emotionally available and responsive, initially reassurance-seeking partners mistrust and reject these efforts as inauthentic. Thus, while the unavailability of avoidant attached individuals may be easier to identify, it is important to recognize that anxiously attached individuals also tend to be emotionally unavailable, which makes them poor attachment figures in their relationships.

A tendency to be avoidant of closeness is only one reason that an attachment figure may be unavailable. As Roger Kobak and Toni Mandelbaum describe, in Chapter 8, unavailability also can occur when attachment figures are overwhelmed by negative emotions, such as feelings of anger, helplessness, and depression, or when they are preoccupied by their own difficult life situations. Negative affect and self-absorption interfere with the ability to be emotionally available, in part because these emotional states make it difficult to recognize and attune to the emotional needs of other people. Depressed attachment figures also may feel too helpless and inadequate to respond to others' needs even when such a need is recognized, and they may withdraw rather than risk failure.

All too often, depression and life stress are chronic or recurrent states (Coyne & Benazon, 2001). Individuals who are vulnerable to depression may spend as much as 15% of their adult lives in full-blown episodes of clinical depression (Judd et al., 1998). Similarly, the risk of depression increases exponentially with every episode suffered (Teasdale et al., 2002).

Thus, we can predict that chronic or recurrent depression will have a particularly deleterious impact on attachment relationships in families. Although little research has been done on this topic, we do know that chronic depression in married women is associated with attachment insecurity in their husbands, while delimited episodes of depression are not (Whiffen, Kallos-Lilly, & MacDonald, 2001). Clinicians who work with recurrently or chronically depressed individuals should expect to see high rates of attachment insecurity in their marriages and families.

In couples and families, attachment insecurity becomes part of a self-perpetuating cycle. Emotional unavailability promotes insecure attachment, and, in turn, insecure attachment promotes depression, anger, and emotional disengagement, all of which damage attachment relationships. Similarly, attachment security facilitates coping and reduces emotional distress, while attachment insecurity both creates emotional distress and impedes individuals' ability to use their relationships to cope. Thus, the emotional distress created by the attachment figure's unavailability is compounded by the absence of a relationship that can soothe, comfort, and reassure. Understanding that attachment insecurity is part of a reciprocal negative feedback loop makes sense of the clinical observation that the couples and families who come for treatment appear to be multiply stressed and distressed. Attachment theory gives us a way of understanding the coherence in the web of symptoms and interpersonal difficulties that our clients present, and to identify the most effective targets for change. Rather than intervening piecemeal with one person's depression, another's disengagement from the family, and the third's conduct disorder, an attachment perspective enables us to see how all parts of the system are linked to the fundamental problem of attachment insecurity. In this sense, attachment theory helps therapists who work with couples and families to truly think systemically about their difficulties.

I began this section by posing a question: What causes insecure attachment? The brief answer is "emotional unavailability." When attachment figures are emotionally unavailable, either because they have not known attachment security themselves or because they are overwhelmed by negative emotions and life stress, they can create attachment insecurity in their spouses and children. Furthermore, once attachment insecurity takes root in a system, it can become a self-perpetuating cycle in which the insecurity is both the problem and an impediment to the solution.

HOW DO WE CHANGE ATTACHMENT INSECURITY?

Most of the chapters in this book address the question of change, either directly or indirectly. Chapter 9, by Terry M. Levy and Michael Orlans, provides a description of the caregiving behaviors that are associated with secure attachment, which they summarize as "showing love and setting limits." However, as their case example compellingly demonstrates, the simple application of good caregiving practices may be insufficient when an individual has an insecure attachment history. In the case they present, the insecure attachment was to the biological parents, but the disruption of attachment security in that relationship also prevented the formation of a secure attachment to the adoptive parents. Their case shows that damage to an individual's ability to form secure attachments may have to be repaired *before* the individual can recognize and accept the efforts of other attachment figures to be available and responsive.

This observation leads to the question posed by both Elaine Scharfe in Chapter 4, and by Schachner, Shaver, and Mikulincer, in Chapter 2: Is some degree of attachment security needed for change to occur? The clinical cases presented by other authors in the book would seem to argue against the need for some measure of security. Reading the cases described by Diamond and Stern in Chapter 10; by J. Michael Bradley and Gail Palmer, in Chapter 14; by Valerie E. Whiffen, in Chapter 16; and elsewhere in this book would seem to suggest that attachment-based interventions are effective even in the treatment of intense attachment insecurity. However, attachment security is more than just the *absence of insecurity*; it is more than *not* being caught in the fear of rejection or abandonment. Attachment security involves a confident belief that attachment figures can and will be emotionally available and responsive. Perhaps change requires the individual to trust in the *possibility* of forming a secure attachment, even if the present attachment relationship is insecure. Belief in this possibility could be based on previously secure attachment relationships or on a previous time of security in the presently insecure relationship. It also could be based on specific perceptions of the attachment figure. For instance, one of the best predictors of outcome in EFT is the wife's belief in her husband's care for her (Johnson & Talitman, 1997). Believing that attachment figures are fundamentally caring may enable individuals to tolerate their unavailability.

Johnson, in Chapter 6; Kobak and Mandelbaum, in Chapter 8; and Diamond and Stern, in Chapter 10 provide the most explicit answer to the question of how we can create change. Whether working with couples, families, or depressed adolescents, these authors agree that individuals must be able to articulate their attachment concerns, and that the attachment figure must be helped by the therapist to respond appropriately. Diamond and Stern label this process a "conversation about attachment," and they observe that articulating these concerns can be a risky business. Individuals who are insecurely attached may feel that disclosure of their attachment concerns risks the attachment figure's criticism, rejection, or even abandonment. However, the perceived risks are minimized by an alliance with a therapist who is seen to be supportive, and by the appropriate response from the attachment figure. Diamond and Stern characterize the appropriate stance in terms of empathy and curiosity about the insecurely attached individual's experience of the relationship. Later in the process, attachment figures must take responsibility for their unavailability, that is, they must acknowledge their unavailability and do their best to give the insecurely attached person a coherent understanding of their unavailability, how it evolved, and why it occurred. Taking responsibility creates empathy for the unavailable individual. Rather than being demonized, the unavailable person can be understood and perhaps even forgiven and accepted.

What is the therapist's role in this process? Schachner, Shaver, and Mikulincer, in Chapter 2, review the empirical evidence showing that attachment operates like a schema. Schemas can be difficult to change because negative emotions and cognitions are triggered whenever the therapist approaches attachment issues. Schachner, Shaver, and Mikulincer point to research suggesting that individuals who can form a secure bond with the therapist may be able to use this bond to change existing attachment representations of their partners. Thus, the research suggests that the therapist needs to act as a temporary attachment figure for the insecurely attached individuals in a system to facilitate their conversations about attachment. This idea is reprised by Kobak and Mandelbaum, in Chapter 8, when the authors propose that the therapist become part of the "caregiving alliance" to enable parents to reflect upon their attachment experiences with their children.

There is some reason to believe that the therapist's role is more crucial in attachment-based interventions than is normally the case. For instance, Johnson and Talitman (1997) showed that the therapeutic alliance accounted for more of the variance in EFT outcome than is typically the case in therapy outcome studies. Therapists who work with attachment concerns need to be skilled at understanding and soothing the intense anxieties that are aroused by conversations about attachment. For insecurely attached individuals, attachment concerns have a life-or-death quality. For instance, one client in couple therapy told her unavailable partner that during a vulnerable period of her life she felt "like a cracked teacup on the verge of shattering." Such images reflect the intense emotion associated with attachment concerns. Unfortunately, these strong emotions can interfere with the insecurely attached person's ability to see that a previously unavailable attachment figure is trying to be available and responsive. Therapists using attachment-based interventions need to be able to empathize with and validate this intense emotion, but also to soothe and contain it, so that it does not derail the conversation about attachment.

The therapist's role may be especially important in working with couples. When a therapist is working with a parent–child attachment relationship, attachment is primarily the responsibility of the parent. However, with couples, attachment is a two-way street because ideally each person acts as an attachment figure for the other. This reciprocity can complicate the process of change considerably; it is difficult to be an effective attachment figure for one's spouse when one's own attachment needs are frustrated or when the spouse is the source of one's own attachment anxiety. Thus, when the spouse is the source of attachment insecurity, couples have a special need for the therapy session to be a safe haven and a secure base, which may create special challenges for the therapist.

Two of the couples chapters in this book make the case that therapists can integrate our knowledge about attachment relationships into existing behavioral interventions designed to prevent or repair distressed marriages. Rebecca J. Cobb and Thomas N. Bradbury, in Chapter 13, and Joanne Davila, in Chapter 7, argue that behavioral therapies traditionally have emphasized conflict resolution skills, but that attachment theory and research suggest that support-giving and support-receiving skills are more important determinants of attachment security. Cobb and Bradbury raise the interesting possibility that learning to enact such behaviors as giving and receiving support will facilitate change in attachment security. In essence, they are proposing that attachment insecurity arises in part because individuals simply do not know how to behave in a way that creates security with and for their attachment figures.

There is a long tradition in clinical psychology to argue the relative merits of skill-based, insight-based, and emotion-based approaches to change. I believe that much of the power of the interventions described in this book comes from the fact that they intervene directly at the level of changing the drama of problematic relationships, and therefore that they are inherently both behavioral and experiential. For instance, Nancy J. Cohen, Elisabeth Muir, and Mirek Lojkasek, in Chapter 11, show that helping the mother to become a more available caregiver to her infant not only changes the mother–infant relationship but also has an impact on the mother's insight into her own attachment history. It would be interesting to know if the other interventions described in this book similarly produce change at all three levels.

How does attachment insecurity change? Insecurely attached individuals need to have a conversation about attachment with the attachment figures to whom they are insecurely attached, and these attachment figures need to respond sensitively and empathically to the newly articulated attachment needs. This formulation changes the traditional role of the therapist, ironically making it both more and less central to the therapeutic process. The therapist who works with insecure attachment in families and couples is more a facilitator than a substitute attachment figure. The real-world attachment figure is in the room; the therapist's role is to provide a secure base in therapy sessions so that insecurely attached individuals can discuss their needs and previously unavailable attachment figures can be responsive. However, while the attachment therapist is not a player in the drama, his or her skill at creating a safe haven is critical to the success of the play. Without confidence in the therapist as an emotionally available and responsive director, the conversation about attachment may be too threatening, dangerous, and overwhelming for both insecurely attached persons and their attachment figures. Thus, such skills as creating a therapeutic alliance and conveying empathy, understanding, and compassion may be even more critical in attachment-based therapies than is normally the case.

MISSING LINKS

Any concluding chapter must include a discussion of the lacunae in our knowledge and a lament for the research that still needs to be done. Several of the chapters in this book demonstrate that there is much more to be known about the role of sexuality in adult attachment relationships (Cindy Hazan, Chapter 3), the use of attachment-based interventions with gay and lesbian couples (Gordon J. Josephson, Chapter 15), the link between attachment insecurity and adolescent violence (Marlene M. Moretti and Roy Holland, Chapter 12), and the impact of chronic illness on attachment security (Samuel F. Mikail, Chapter 18). In this section, I would like to focus on two issues that I think are particularly important.

First, I agree with Scharfe (Chapter 4) that we need to know much more about the impact of trauma on attachment security. Bowlby originally formulated attachment theory to explain what happens when children are separated for prolonged periods from their parents, an event that is inherently traumatic for a child. Returning to this conceptual tradition, Pamela C. Alexander, in Chapter 17, proposed that childhood sexual abuse has a negative impact on women's ability to form secure attachment relationships with adult attachment figures. In the decade since she first published this hypothesis, several empirical studies have shown that childhood sexual abuse survivors have attachment difficulties, both with romantic partners and with their children. Childhood sexual abuse survivors tend to be *fearful–avoidant* in their adult attachment relationships, particularly if their fathers or other family members sexually abused them. Similarly, childhood physical abuse is associated with the development of a *disorganized* attachment style in children, in which the child appears to lack a coherent strategy for maintaining proximity to the attachment figure and instead vacillates between approach and avoidance strategies (see review by Cassidy & Mohr, 2001).

In light of the research showing an impact of childhood trauma on attachment security, it is astonishing that there is *no* research on the impact of adult trauma on attachment security (see review by Whiffen & Oliver, in press). Clinicians who work with trauma survivors argue that trauma intensifies attachment needs for comfort and reassurance, while shattering trust in the benevolence of others (Cassidy & Mohr, 2001; Johnson, 2002). Thus, paradoxically, traumatized individuals seek out their attachment figures while simultaneously maintaining emotional distance from them. For example, a traumatized woman may pursue her partner for closeness, but reject him when he responds to her. These competing approach and avoidance behaviors are extremely difficult for attachment figures to understand and tolerate, and may be a significant factor in the perpetuation of marital distress, which is common among trauma survivors regardless of the type of trauma suffered. In light of the attention given by clinicians to the link between trauma and attachment, it seems imperative that more research be done on the impact of adult trauma on attachment security.

The second issue is the cultural construction of attachment relationships. Vivian J. Carlson and Robin L. Harwood remind us in Chapter 5 that most of the research on attachment has been done with participants from European-based cultures. In their case example, they show that caregiving behaviors that would be construed as "insensitive" in these cultures actually may promote attachment security in other cultures. Thus, they suggest that maternal sensitivity per se may be less important in the development of attachment security than is "mother–child harmony" in the service of producing culturally valued traits and behaviors in children.

Their chapter raises the interesting possibility that the role of attachment in marital and family relations varies across cultures. For instance, in European-based cultures, the current ideal for married couples combines sexual attraction with friendship. However, this definition of marriage is relatively recent, and may be the child of necessity because many married couples now live far away from their extended families and the social networks in which they grew up. Thus, the ideal couple may need to be best friends in North America and Europe because they are likely to be isolated from the other people who could have fulfilled this function in the past. It is important for clinicians to be sensitive to cultural variations in the nature of attachment relationships, and to recognize that the specific behaviors that promote attachment security may be different. This does not mean that the availability of the attachment figure would not be important in other cultures, but that availability may be expressed in ways that could be considered intrusive or neglectful in other cultural contexts.

WHAT CAN ATTACHMENT THEORY OFFER MARITAL AND FAMILY THERAPISTS?

Attachment theory offers clinicians a road map to the complex, mutually reinforcing systems that are couples and families. Attachment theory tells us that the fundamental problem in distressed couples and families is attachment insecurity. It tells us how this insecurity developed and shows us how it is manifested in the symptoms of emotional distress that some members of the system experience. It tells us how to change attachment insecurity by facilitating an authentic dialogue about attachment needs among the members of the system, and by encouraging the responsiveness of previously unavailable attachment figures. Finally, it specifies the role to be played by therapists in this process, as well as the skills they need to bring to the therapy room. Attachment theory offers clinicians guidelines for understanding and changing the relationships that are the source of so much pain for our clients, but which could be the source of so much joy.

REFERENCES

Cassidy, J., & Mohr, J. J. (2001). Unsolvable fear, trauma, and psychopathology: Theory, research, and clinical considerations related to disorganized attachment across the life span. *Clinical Psychology: Science and Practice, 8*, 275–298.

Coyne, J. C., & Benazon, N. R. (2001). Not agent blue: Effects of marital functioning on depression and implications for treatment. In S. Beach (Ed.), *Marital and family processes in depression* (pp. 25–43). Washington, DC: American Psychological Association.

Johnson, S. M. (2002). *Emotionally focused couple therapy with trauma survivors: Strengthening attachment bonds.* New York: Guilford Press.

Johnson, S. M., & Talitman, E. (1997). Predictors of success in emotionally focused marital therapy. *Journal of Marital and Family Therapy. 23*, 135–152.

Judd, L. L., Akiskal, H. S., Maser, J. D., Zeller, P. J., Endicott, J., Coryell, W., Paulus, M. P., Kunovac, J. L., Leon, A. C., Mueller, T. I., Rice, J. A., & Keller, M. B. (1998). A prospective 12–year study of subsyndromal and syndromal depressive symptoms in unipolar major depressive disorders. *Archives of General Psychiatry, 55*, 694–700.

Main, M., Kaplan, N., & Cassidy, J. (1985). Security in infancy, childhood and adulthood: A move to the level of representation. In I. Bretherton & E. Waters (Eds.), Growing points of attachment theory and research. *Monographs of the Society for Research in Child Development, 50*(1–2, Serial No. 209), 66–104.

Teasdale, J. D, Moore, R. G, Hayhurst, H., Pope, M., Williams, S., & Segal, Z. V. (2002). Metacognitive awareness and prevention of relapse in depression: Empirical evidence. *Journal of Consulting and Clinical Psychology, 70*, 275–287.

Whiffen, V. E., Kallos-Lilly, A. V., & MacDonald, B. J. (2001). Depression and attachment in couples. *Cognitive Therapy and Research, 25*, 577–590.

Whiffen, V. E., & Oliver, L. E. (in press). The relationship between traumatic stress and marital intimacy. In D. Catherall (Ed.), *Stress, trauma and the family.* Washington, DC: American Psychological Association Books.

Index

Sensitivity
  maternal. *See* Watch, Wait, and
    Wonder
  parental, and change of attachment,
    68–70
  to signals and cues, 168
Sensitivity hypothesis, 93–94
Separation
  issues of in older adults, 281–283
  unanticipated or unplanned, 151
Separation distress
  in couple relationships, 105–106
  response sequence, 6–7, 51
Sexual abuse history. *See* Childhood
  sexual abuse history
Sexuality
  adult attachment and, 108
  attachment and, 305–306
  attachment style and, 30–31
  as bond-promoting activity, 52–53
  See also Intimacy
Sexual strategies theory (SST)
  female preference and, 47–48
  fertility detection and, 47
  gender differences and, 48–49
  male preference and, 45–46
  mating as strategic process, 48, 56
  overview of, 43–45
  predictions of, 45
  short-term mating and, 46–47
Shared working model, 284–285
Sibling conflict, 179
Social expectations
  cultural assumptions and, 87
  within group vs. between groups, 88
Socialization goals, 89–92
Social-learning perspective on couple
  relationship, 125–126
Social psychology and attachment
  theory, 126
Social relations theory, 253–254
Social support behaviors, 132–133. *See
  also* Support
"Softenings," 36, 108, 289–290
Specificity theory, 367
Spouse as primary attachment figure,
  104–105, 327, 328, 330–331

Stability of attachment representations
  in adulthood, 72–77
  clinical significance of research on,
    78–80
  in infancy, 65–71
  from infancy to childhood, 71–72
  from infancy to young adulthood,
    77–78
  interview measures of, 76–77
Standards for self, personal vs.
  parental, in adolescence, 238,
  242–243
State of mind, 170
Strange Situation, 92–93, 344
Structure, clear and consistent, 169–
  170, 180
Support
  attachment security and, 260
  attachment style and, 28–29
  for caregiving, 155
  childbearing depression and, 325–326
  Compassionate and Accepting
    Relations through Empathy, 266–
    268
  seeking, skills for, 137–138
  sexual abuse survivors and, 350–351
  social support behaviors, 132–133
  targeting behaviors within marital
    context, 262–264
Systemic perspective of changes in
  attachment, 12
Systems theory and emotion, 106

T

Terminology, 10–11
Therapeutic contract, 183, 185
Therapeutic parenting, 174–176
Therapist
  reaction of to avoidant clients, 250
  role of, 179–181, 394–396
Threat
  activation of attachment system and,
    21–26
  attachment style and interpretation
    of, 29